SHELF-LIFE OBSTETRICS AND GYNECOLOGY

SHELF-LIFE OBSTETRICS AND GYNECOLOGY

Editors

Elizabeth Buys, MD
Assistant Clinical Professor
Department of Obstetrics and Gynecology
University of North Carolina School of Medicine
Mountain Area Health Education Center
Admitting Medical Staff Physician
Women's Services
Mission Hospital
Asheville, North Carolina

Kristina Tocce, MD, MPH
Assistant Professor
Medical Student Program Director
Assistant Director, Fellowship in Family Planning
Department of Obstetrics and Gynecology
University of Colorado, Anschutz Medical Campus
Denver, Colorado

Michele A. Manting, MD, MEd
Associate Professor and Director of
Interprofessional Education
Department of Obstetrics and Gynecology
Paul L. Foster School of Medicine
Texas Tech University Health Sciences Center
Director of Simulation
Department of Obstetrics and Gynecology
University Medical Center
El Paso, Texas

Series Editors

Veeral Sudhakar Sheth, MD, FACS
Director, Scientific Affairs
University Retina and Macula Associates
Clinical Assistant Professor
University of Illinois at Chicago
Chicago, Illinois

Stanley Zaslau, MD, MBA, FACS
Professor and Chief
Urology Residency Program Director
Department of Surgery/Division of Urology
West Virginia University
Morgantown, West Virginia

Robert Casanova, MD, FACOG
Assistant Dean of Clinical Sciences
Curriculum
Associate Professor Obstetrics and
Gynecology
Obstetrics and Gynecology Residency
Program Director
Texas Tech University Health Sciences
Center
Lubbock, Texas

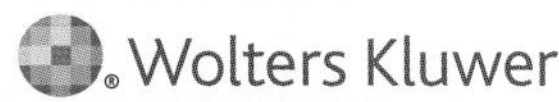

Health

Philadelphia • Baltimore • New York • London
Buenos Aires • Hong Kong • Sydney • Tokyo

Acquisitions Editor: Tari Broderick
Product Manager: Stacey Sebring
Marketing Manager: Joy Fisher-Williams
Production Project Manager: Alicia Jackson
Designer: Stephen Druding
Compositor: Integra Software Services Pvt. Ltd.

351 West Camden Street
Baltimore, MD 21201

Two Commerce Square
2001 Market Street
Philadelphia, PA 19103

Printed in China

9 8 7 6 5 4 3 2 1

Library of Congress Cataloging-in-Publication Data

Shelf-life obstetrics and gynecology / co-editors Elizabeth Buys, Kristina Tocce, Michele Manting.
p. ; cm.
Includes index.
ISBN 978-1-4511-9045-8
I. Buys, Elizabeth (Elizabeth A.) , editor of compilation. II. Tocce, Kristina, editor of compilation. III. Manting, Michele, editor of compilation. [DNLM: 1. Genital Diseases, Female—Problems and Exercises. 2. Obstetrics—methods—Problems and Exercises. 3. Gynecology—methods—Problems and Exercises. 4. Pregnancy Complications—Problems and Exercises. WQ 18.2]
RG111
618.10076--dc23

2013047865

To purchase additional copies of this book, call our customer service department at **(800) 638-3030** or fax orders to **(301) 223-2320**. International customers should call **(301) 223-2300.**

Visit Lippincott Williams & Wilkins on the Internet: http://www.lww.com. Lippincott Williams & Wilkins customer service representatives are available from 8:30 am to 6:00 pm, EST.

RRS1312

Contributors

Ashley S. Atkins, MSIV
Texas Tech University Health Sciences Center
Lubbock, Texas

Samuel Barker, MSIV
Texas Tech University Health Sciences Center
Lubbock, Texas

Jennifer Black, MSIII
University of Colorado Anschutz Medical Campus
Aurora, Colorado

Bennett Gardner, MD
Resident physician
Department of Obstetrics & Gynecology
Mountain Area Health Education Center
Asheville, North Carolina

Rachel Harper, MSIII
University of North Carolina School of Medicine
Chapel Hill, North Carolina

Sarah Jenkins, MSIII
University of Colorado Anschutz Medical Campus
Aurora, Colorado

Hollis Konitzer, MS III
University of North Carolina School of Medicine
Chapel Hill, North Carolina

Jon Larrabee, MD
Resident physician
Department of Obstetrics & Gynecology
Mountain Area Health Education Center
Asheville, North Carolina

Richard Loftis, MD
Resident physician
Department of Obstetrics & Gynecology
Mountain Area Health Education Center
Asheville, North Carolina

Melinda Ramage, FNP, RN
Mountain Area Health Education Center
Asheville, North Carolina

Amy Richards, MSIV
Texas Tech University Health Sciences Center
Lubbock, Texas

Amanda M. Roberts, MSIII
Texas Tech University Health Sciences Center
Lubbock, Texas

Sara Scannell, MSIII
University of Colorado Anschutz Medical Campus
Aurora, Colorado

Meghan Sheehan, MSIII
Texas Tech University Health Sciences Center
Lubbock, Texas

Susan Ulmer, MSIII
University of Colorado Anschutz Medical Campus
Aurora, Colorado

Anna van der Horst, MSIII
University of North Carolina School of Medicine
Chapel Hill, North Carolina

Introduction to the Shelf-Life Series

The Shelf-Life series is an entirely new concept. The books have been designed from the ground up with student input. With academic faculty helping guide the production of these books, the Shelf-Life series is meant to help supplement the student's educational experience while on clinical rotation as well as prepare the student for the end-of-rotation shelf-exam. We feel you will find these question books challenging but an irreplaceable part of the clinical rotation. With high-quality, up-to-date content, and hundreds of images and tables, this resource will be something you will continue to refer to even after you have completed your rotation.

The series editors would like to thank Susan Rhyner for supporting this concept from its inception. We would like to express our appreciation to Catherine Noonan, Laura Blyton, Amanda Ingold, Ashley Fischer, and Stacey Sebring, all of whom have been integral parts of the publishing team; their project management has been invaluable.

Veeral S. Sheth, MD, FACS
Stanley Zaslau, MD, MBA, FACS
Robert Casanova, MD, FACOG

Acknowledgments

It has been a pleasure to work with the staff at Lippincott Williams &Wilkins on the first edition of *Shelf Life Obstetrics and Gynecology*, especially with Laura Blyton, Catherine Noonan, and Stacey Sebring. Also, special thanks to Susan Rhyner who thought of me when developing this project.

I could not have done it without the help of my co-editors, Beth, Kristina, and Michele. My sincere thanks to you and to our student contributors who kept us focused.

I also want to thank the hundreds of medical students whom I have had the privilege to meet during my years as Clerkship Director. You have taught me more than you will ever know and it has been an honor to play even a small role in your medical education.

Finally, I want to thank our families who allowed us to spend endless hours developing and tweaking questions

Robert Casanova, MD, FACOG

Contents

CHAPTER

1

Preventive Care

1 A 32-year-old G4P2022 presents to your office for her annual examination. She has regular menses every 28 days, lasting 4 days each time. The patient reports 10 sexual partners in her lifetime, 3 in the past 6 months. She almost always uses condoms. The patient takes oral contraceptive pills but does not always remember to take them on a daily basis. She has never had an abnormal pap smear and the last one she had done was 3 years ago. The patient reports no significant past medical history and denies any health conditions in family members.

What testing and/or examinations should be done during today's visit?

(A) Pap smear
(B) Gonorrhea and chlamydia cultures
(C) Pap smear, gonorrhea, and chlamydia cultures
(D) Pregnancy test
(E) Mammogram

The answer is C: Pap smear, gonorrhea and chlamydia cultures. This patient is sexually active with multiple partners and does not always use condoms, so she needs to be screened for sexual transmitted diseases (STDs). Her last pap smear was 3 years ago, so even though she has never had an abnormal one she should receive one today. One would consider co-testing with human papillomavirus (HPV) and cytology every 5 years between the ages of 30 and 65. See Table 1-1. She is too young for a mammogram and a pregnancy test is not indicated.

2 A 19-year-old G0 presents to your office for her annual examination. Her last period was 3 weeks ago. She has regular menses every 28 days, lasting 4 days each time. She has had one lifetime partner for 3 years and uses condoms regularly. The patient does not take any medications and has no gynecologic concerns at this time.

What testing and/or examinations should be done during today's visit?

Table 1-1 Screening Method for Cervical Cancer

Age	Recommended Screening
<21 y	No screening
21–29 y	Cytology alone every 3 y
30–65 y	Human papillomavirus and cytology co-testing every 5 y Cytology alone (acceptable) every 3 y
>65	No screening necessary

(A) Pap smear
(B) Gonorrhea and chlamydia cultures
(C) Pap smear, gonorrhea, and chlamydia cultures
(D) Pregnancy test

The answer is B: Gonorrhea and chlamydia cultures. This is a sexually active woman in a high-risk age group for STDs (≤25 years old), so she should be tested for gonorrhea (GC) and chlamydia despite her safe sex practices. Pap smears should not be performed until the age of 21, regardless of how long the woman has been sexually active. The patient has not missed her period and has no concerns so a pregnancy test would not be a standard component of an annual examination.

3 Your next patient in the resident clinic is a 17-year-old G0 last menstrual period unsure who presents for "a prescription for pills." Menarche was at age 13 and she has regular, monthly periods lasting 4 to 5 days but does not keep track of them. She became sexually active about a year ago and has had six male partners. She has been with her current partner for the last 6 months. She wants pills to keep from getting pregnant. She smokes half a pack per day and drinks on weekends, but never more than a couple of beers. What are your recommendations for this patient?

(A) GC/chlamydia screening, pap, blood pressure (BP)
(B) GC/chlamydia screening, pap, tobacco and alcohol counseling, BP
(C) Seatbelt use, pap, tobacco and alcohol counseling, BP
(D) GC/chlamydia screening, seatbelt use, tobacco and alcohol counseling, BP

The answer is D: GC/chlamydia screening, seatbelt use, tobacco and alcohol counseling, BP. Pap is not indicated until age 21. GC/chlamydia screening should be performed in all sexually active women under 25. Motor vehicle accidents (MVAs) are the major cause of accidental death in the age group making screening for seatbelt use very important. BP screening should start at age 13 and repeated every 2 years in patients who are normotensive and yearly with higher levels. Alcohol and tobacco counseling should be part of every encounter with a patient who either abuses or is underage.

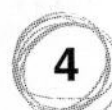

4 Your patient is a 20-year-old Asian woman G0 who recently transferred to a local university and wants to establish care. She has had no period on Depo-Provera for at least 2 years and is due for an injection this month. She is sexually active with the same partner for 6 months. She became sexually active at 17 and has had five lifetime male partners. She has no medical problems and has never had any surgery. She leads a relatively sedentary lifestyle now due to her college schedule although she used to engage in moderate aerobic exercise. She drinks moderately on weekends, but denies tobacco or drug use. On examination, she is in no acute distress (NAD). Her vital signs are stable and her BMI is 28. Her examination is unremarkable.

What are your recommendations for this patient?

(A) Stop Depo-Provera, get bone densitometry, pap, offer Gardasil
(B) Stop Depo-Provera, get STD testing, and offer Gardasil
(C) Continue Depo-Provera, get pap, and offer Gardasil
(D) Continue Depo-Provera, offer Gardasil, and get STD testing

The answer is D: Continue Depo-Provera, offer Gardasil, and get STD testing. Although there is evidence of bone loss with use of Depo-Provera over 2 years, it is not an indication for stopping it or for getting bone densitometry. STD testing is appropriate in sexually active women under 25. The American College of Obstetricians and Gynecologists (the College) currently recommends that all girls and women aged 9 to 26 years be immunized against human papillomavirus (HPV).

5 Your patient is a 35-year-old G2P2 last menstrual period 3 weeks ago who presents for contraceptive counseling. She got divorced about a year and a half ago and has had three male sexual partners since then. Since her husband had a vasectomy, she has tried to use condoms as much as possible but wants to review her options. She considers herself to be in good health with no medical problems and no previous surgeries. She denies smoking or drug use and only drinks moderately on weekends. Her last annual examination was 5 years ago after the birth of her last child. Her physical examination is unremarkable.

What are your recommendations for this patient?

(A) Pap, GC/Chlamydia, lipid profile, thyroid screening
(B) Pap, GC/Chlamydia, blood testing for STDs, thyroid screening
(C) Pap, GC/Chlamydia, blood testing for STDs, lipid profile
(D) Pap, GC/Chlamydia, blood testing for STDs

The answer is D: Pap, GC/Chlamydia, blood testing for STDs. Pap smears are performed every 3 years in this age group. She should have full sexual transmitted disease (STD) testing because of her recent sexual activities and poor use of condoms. Lipid profiles and thyroid screening begin at age 45.

---

6 Your patient is a 46-year-old G3P2012 status post tubal ligation who presents for her annual examination. Her past medical history is negative and her surgical history included an appendectomy as well as her tubal. Her periods are regular although getting lighter. She denies tobacco or drug use but admits to a glass of wine with dinner 4 to 5 times a week. Her family history is remarkable for hypertension and diabetes in both parents, and her brother had a heart attack at 45. She has always had normal paps and her last one was 2 years ago. On examination, she is in no acute distress (NAD). She is afebrile with normal vital signs. BMI is 30. Her physical examination is unremarkable.

What are your recommendations for this patient?

(A) Mammogram, colonoscopy, pap
(B) Mammogram, lipid profile, thyroid screening
(C) Mammogram, lipid profile, pap
(D) Lipid profile, colonoscopy, pap
(E) Thyroid screening, colonoscopy, pap

The answer is B: Mammogram, lipid profile, thyroid screening. Pap smears are recommended every 3 years in this age group and she had one 2 years ago. Yearly mammography starts at age 40. Colonoscopy screening begins at age 50 and continues every 5 years. Lipid profiles should start at age 45 plus she has a brother with premature cardiovascular disease (<50 years old in men or <60 years old in women). Women 45 and over should have thyroid screening every 5 years.

---

7 Your patient is a 70-year-old in good health who is new to an assisted living facility. Her husband recently died and her grown children live out of state. She is a G3P3 20 years postmenopause who has had no bleeding. She never had any abnormal paps in the past and she was religious about getting them along with mammograms, but because of her husband's protracted battle with cancer she has not seen a doctor in over 5 years. She denies hypertension or "sugar diabetes." She had her tonsils removed as a child and her appendix out at age 12. She takes no medications or supplements. She denies alcohol or tobacco use. On physical examination, she is a frail white woman with BP 128/84. She is 5′4″ and weighs 122 lb. Her physical examination is unremarkable except for atrophic vaginal changes.

What are your recommendations for this patient?

(A) Colonoscopy, pneumococcal vaccine, lipid screen, pap
(B) Mammogram, bone densitometry, pneumococcal vaccine, lipid screen, pap
(C) Mammogram, bone densitometry, colonoscopy, lipid screen, pap
(D) Mammogram, bone densitometry, colonoscopy, pneumococcal vaccine, pap
(E) Mammogram, bone densitometry, colonoscopy, pneumococcal vaccine, lipid screen

The answer is E: Mammogram, bone densitometry, colonoscopy, pneumococcal vaccine, lipid screen. A pap is not indicated for a woman over 65 years of age who has never had an abnormal pap and has had regular screening. Mammography starts at age 40. Colonoscopy screening begins at age 50 and continues every 5 years. Lipid profiles should start at age 45. Bone densitometry scanning for bone mineral density starts at 65. Pneumococcal vaccine is recommended at 65.

8 A 24-year-old white woman and her husband present for preconception counseling. She smokes 1 pack per day and is requesting a prescription to help her quit smoking. She has tried three times in the past to stop cold turkey. The last time was a year ago just before they were married. That time, her roommate continued to smoke and the temptation was too great for her, so after 10 days, she started again. She is planning to conceive this year and wants to try to quit before that time. Her husband is a smoker but in the interest of their future family, is willing to quit as well. Men and women may have different barrier to quit smoking.

Which of the following concerns are more likely to be an important barrier for her husband?

(A) Fear of weight gain
(B) Stress relief
(C) Depression
(D) Cravings

The answer is D: Cravings. Women are more likely to identify weight gain and stress relief as barriers to quit smoking. Men are more likely to identify cravings as a barrier.

9 You are seeing a distraught patient in your clinic. Her best friend has just been diagnosed with ovarian cancer at age 40 and she is concerned about her risk. She is a 38-year-old white woman G0 last menstrual period 2 weeks ago on birth control pills that she has used for about 20 years. She has no history of hypertension or diabetes. She had her tonsils and appendix removed while quite young. She is a lawyer and

lives with her boyfriend of 3 years. She became sexually active at age 17 and has had five lifetime partners. She has never had chlamydia or gonorrhea, but did have an abnormal pap in college that ultimately required a conization. Her paps have been normal ever since. Family history is remarkable for a paternal aunt with breast cancer around age 60. She is afebrile with normal vital signs and a BMI of 28. Her physical examination, including breast and pelvic, is unremarkable.

What is this patient's greatest risk for ovarian cancer?

(A) Long-term use of oral contraceptives
(B) Nulliparity
(C) Family history of breast cancer
(D) History of abnormal pap
(E) Obesity

The answer is B: Nulliparity. Nulliparity is associated with a greater risk of ovarian cancer. Long-term oral contraceptive use is actually protective against ovarian cancer (5 years of use confers approximately a 50% reduction in ovarian cancer). Second-degree relatives with breast cancer and cervical dysplasia do not change ovarian cancer risks. Although obesity does increase your risk of ovarian cancer, a BMI of 28 is not in the obesity range.

---

10 You are in clinic during Spring Break seeing a 17-year-old G0. She is starting college in the fall and her mother wants to make sure she is up on her vaccinations. She grew up in rural El Salvador up to age 8 and had chicken pox at age 6. She had regular immunizations through junior high but due to financial restraints has not had an annual examination since age 14.

What vaccinations would you recommend at this time?

(A) Gardasil
(B) Hepatitis A vaccine
(C) Varicella vaccine
(D) Flu vaccine

The answer is A: Gardasil. Gardasil is indicated in women ages 8 to 26. Hepatitis A is not routinely recommended. The patient had varicella at age 6 and therefore does not require vaccination. The flu vaccine would be recommended during flu season.

---

11 You are helping out in the OB clinic and are seeing a 30-year-old patient who has been pregnant five times, but only has two kids. She had an abortion at age 16 and an ectopic at age 17. She later had a baby at 32 weeks that died and twins at 36 weeks that are doing well.

What are her Gs and Ps?

(A) G5P0222
(B) G5P0322
(C) G6P0223
(D) G6P0322

The answer is A: G5P0222. Five pregnancies, no term deliveries, two preterm deliveries (twins does not increase this number), and two living children. G refers to the number of pregnancies regardless of multiples. P refers to the outcomes of the pregnancies and does not increase with multiples. The numbers refer to Term (> or = 37 weeks) Preterm (<37 weeks but >20 weeks), Abortions (<20 week abortion or ectopic), Living (number of children presently alive, not number of live births).

---

12 Your patient is a 29-year-old G0 referred by her family medicine doctor for evaluation of infertility.

Which menstrual history below would warrant further evaluation of her lipids and HgA1c?

(A) Menarche at age 8 with regular periods every 28 to 32 days lasting 5 days
(B) Menarche at age 14 with regular periods every 30 to 34 days lasting 7 days
(C) Menarche at age 16 with irregular periods every 40 to 60 days lasting 5 to 10 days
(D) Menarche at age 18 with regular periods every 28 to 32 days lasting 5 to 10 days

The answer is C: Menarche at age 16 with irregular periods every 40 to 60 days lasting 5 to 10 days. This menstrual history is suggestive of polycystic ovarian syndrome (PCOS) characterized by widely variable length between cycles. The patient is usually anovulatory. PCOS increases the patient's risk for metabolic syndrome. Her blood pressure, lipids, and HgA1c should be carefully monitored.

---

13 You are in the resident clinic seeing a 19-year-old white woman requesting an annual examination.

What information would best guide you in contraceptive counseling?

(A) Her obstetric history
(B) Her sexual history
(C) Her family history
(D) Her past medical history
(E) Her smoking history

The answer is B: Her sexual history. Although the other histories will help guide you, the sexual history is crucial for appropriate personalized patient centered contraceptive and safer sex counseling. The sexual history includes age of first intercourse, total lifetime partner, and number of partners in the last year or length of time with present partner. Often forgotten are questions about sexual practices and sexual preferences that may change risk factors as well as need or preference for various contraceptive methods.

---

14 Your patient is a 40-year-old white woman G2P2 status post total hysterectomy for fibroids at age 38 who presents for annual examination. She has a history of hypertension and diabetes but has not been taking her meds. She has had her tonsils and appendix removed in the past. Her family history is remarkable for hypertension and diabetes in both parents. Her father and brother both had heart attacks in their 40s. She has been married for 28 years and feels that she is in a stable relationship. She has a 30-pack-year history of tobacco use, but denies alcohol or drug use. On examination her vital signs are as follows: BP 150/94 P 90 T 97.8 BMI 35. Her examination is unremarkable except for moderate central obesity.

What are your recommendations for this patient?

(A) Pap, mammogram, lipid screening
(B) Pap, mammogram, thyroid testing
(C) Mammogram, lipid screening, smoking cessation
(D) Mammogram, lipid screening, thyroid screening

The answer is C: Mammogram, lipid screening, smoking cessation. Paps are not indicated in women who have undergone hysterectomy for benign conditions. Yearly mammography starts at age 40. This patient is at great risk for heart disease. Lipid profiles should start at age 45, but she has a brother and father with premature cardiovascular disease (<50 years old in men or <60 years old in women) along with hypertension and diabetes, thus warranting early screening. Smoking is a preventable risk factor for heart disease; the patient should be counseled on cessation. Thyroid screening is warranted in women over 45 every 5 years.

15 Your patient is a 63-year-old white woman G4P4 s/p hysterectomy in her 40s for fibroids who presents for her annual examination. She has a history of hypertension and diabetes both controlled with oral medication. She smoked half a pack per day until 3 years ago when she quit cold turkey. Her urine dip today is remarkable for 3+ blood. She denies dysuria, frequency, or urgency.

What is the next step?

(A) Cystoscopy
(B) MRI
(C) Renal US
(D) Culture and sensitivity for UTI

The answer is D: Culture and sensitivity. The most cost-effective course is culture and sensitivity. If this is negative, you may repeat the urinalysis and consider referral for cystoscopy.

CHAPTER 2

Ethics

1 A 13-year-old girl presents to a Title X clinic requesting birth control. While taking her history, it is discovered that she is sexually active with a partner who is 23 years of age. She states that they are in a monogamous relationship and that this is consensual. She is requesting a contraceptive implant to be inserted today.

What is the most appropriate next step in management?

(A) Contact law enforcement to report prohibited sexual activity
(B) Insert the implant, screen for sexually transmitted infections, and schedule a follow-up visit
(C) Contact the patient's parents to discuss the situation
(D) Encourage the patient to terminate her relationship with her boyfriend

The answer is A: Contact law enforcement to report prohibited sexual activity. Once this information is obtained on history, reporting to law enforcement is a mandatory requirement. Most states use designations of sexual assault and sexual abuse to identify prohibited sexual activity. These crimes are based on the premise that until a certain age, individuals are incapable of consenting to sexual intercourse. This makes it illegal for anyone to engage in sexual intercourse with an individual below a certain age or with a specified age difference. This age varies by state, with many setting it at age 16. Title X is a federal grant program established to provide comprehensive family planning to low-income or underserved populations.

2 A 32-year-old, G0, and her husband present for genetic counseling prior to conception. Although currently asymptomatic, her husband has Huntington disease. They are interested in understanding the risk of occurrence and the options for assisted reproductive technology, first-trimester genetic diagnosis, and pregnancy termination. The counselor has a conflict of conscience regarding pregnancy termination.

What is the counselor's obligation to the couple in this situation?

(A) Provide information on occurrence, assisted reproductive technology, and genetic diagnosis
(B) Provide all requested information in a nondirective way that will allow the couple to make informed decisions and act in accordance with their decisions
(C) Provide limited information that is consistent with his/her own personal moral commitments
(D) Utilize this opportunity to advocate his/her own moral position on various options in reproductive medicine

The answer is B: **Provide all requested information in a nondirective way that will allow the couple to make informed decisions and act in accordance with their decisions.** The counselor's function is not to dictate a particular course of action, but to provide information that will allow the couple to make informed decisions. Patients must be provided with accurate and unbiased information, so that they can make informed decisions about their health care. Health-care providers must disclose scientifically accurate and professionally accepted characterizations of reproductive health services. When conscience implores providers to deviate from standard practices (including abortion, sterilization, and provision of contraceptives), they must provide potential patients with accurate and prior notice of their personal moral commitments. Providers should not use their professional authority to advocate their own positions. At the very least, systems must be in place for counseling and referral for those services that may conflict with a provider's deeply held beliefs.

3 A 44-year-old, G2P2, has heavy menstrual bleeding secondary to a large fibroid uterus. She has failed medical management with hormonal contraceptives and is now interested in surgical treatment with hysterectomy. During the consent process, the risks, benefits, and alternatives are explained to the patient and she is given the opportunity to ask questions.

What is the primary purpose of the consent process?

(A) To disclose information relevant to the surgery
(B) To establish a satisfactory physician–patient relationship
(C) To uncover practitioners' biases
(D) To protect patient autonomy

The answer is D: **To protect patient autonomy.** The primary purpose of the consent process is to protect patient autonomy. The point is not to merely disclose information, but to ensure the patient's comprehension. Encouraging open communication while relaying relevant information enables the patient to exercise personal choice. This choice may include the refusal of recommended treatment. Such discussions are never completely free of the informant's biases and practitioners should seek to maintain objectivity while discussing options for treatment.

4 A 26-year-old, G0, with developmental delay is brought to the clinic by her older brother. He wishes to schedule a bilateral tubal ligation for his sister. Since their parents died, he has been caring for her. He is concerned that she will become pregnant while away at a vocational education program next month. The patient articulates that she does not want children at this time and is willing to sign the consent form; however, she repetitively asks when she can have her tubes "untied."

What is the most appropriate next step in obtaining informed consent?

(A) Advise the brother to legally establish guardianship, so he can sign the consent

(B) Disclose the relevant information regarding the procedure and allow the patient to sign the consent form

(C) Explore options for reversible contraception with the patient

(D) Make a report to child protective services

The answer is C: Explore options for reversible contraception with the patient. In order to give informed consent, the patient must understand her condition and the risks, benefits, and alternatives to the proposed treatment. This patient clearly does not understand the permanent nature of bilateral tubal ligation. A patient's capacity to understand depends on multiple factors and diminished capacity to understand is not always synonymous with incompetence. While recommending evaluation of capacity, reversible methods of contraception should be explored to prevent unintended pregnancy.

5 A 21-year-old, G3P2, has a positive urine toxicology screen for cocaine at 27 week's gestation. The patient also had a positive screen for cocaine at her first prenatal visit at 16 week's gestation. At that time, the patient was provided information regarding the consequences of drug use during pregnancy and referred to a treatment program.

What is the most appropriate next step in treating this patient?

(A) Notify the police and have her involuntarily committed to a treatment program

(B) Continue to provide accurate and clear information regarding the consequences of drug use and referrals to treatment facilities

(C) Notify child protective services and arrange for the infant to be taken away from the mother after delivery

(D) Involuntarily admit the patient to the psychiatry service

The answer is B: **Continue to provide accurate and clear information regarding the consequences of drug use and referrals to treatment facilities.** Medical ethicists have consistently maintained that the rights of the mother take precedence over those of the fetus. Obstetrician-gynecologists (OBGYNs) are obligated to respect the mother's autonomy, even if her choices and actions are harmful to herself and the fetus. In situations where the woman is engaging in harmful behaviors, the OBGYN should provide accurate and clear information regarding the consequences of such behavior. Referrals to appropriate treatment facilities are also appropriate.

6 A 29-year-old, G1P0, presents to labor and delivery at 38 week's gestation with ruptured membranes and contractions. Her membranes ruptured over 24 hours ago; however, she remained home until she felt regular contractions. On admission, her body temperature is 38.2°C (101.2°F), blood pressure is 110/60 mmHg, and pulse is 110 beats/min. Pelvic examination shows her cervix to be 3 cm dilated, 90% effaced, and –2 station. On external fetal monitoring, the fetal heart rate has a baseline of 165 beats/min, minimal variability, and repetitive late decelerations. Immediate Cesarean section is recommended by the obstetrician on call, but the patient wishes to continue labor. She will accept antibiotics for chorioamnionitis and oxytocin for augmentation of labor, but states that she will not consent to an operative delivery under any circumstances.

What is the physician's most appropriate course of action?

(A) Contact the legal department of the hospital and make arrangements to obtain a court order for Cesarean section
(B) Attempt to transfer the care of the patient to another provider who may be able to get her consent
(C) Convey clearly the reasons for the recommendations and examine her motives for refusing the recommended treatment
(D) Request a psychiatric evaluation to deem her incompetent to make decisions

The answer is C: **Convey clearly the reasons for the recommendations and examine her motives for refusing the recommended treatment.** The pregnant woman's autonomous decisions should be respected as long as she is competent to make informed medical decisions. This remains true even if the woman rejects medical interventions that may result in fetal complications or death. The obstetrician's response to the patient's unwillingness to consent for the recommended treatment should be to convey clearly the reasons for the recommendations. He/she should also explore the patient's reasons for refusal. While doing this, the obstetrician must continue to care for the patient, respect her autonomy, and not intervene against her wishes, regardless of the consequences.

7 A 19-year-old, G2P1, presents to her Obstetrician-gynecologist (OBGYN) 4 months after delivery with persistent nausea. She has a positive urine pregnancy test in the office and subsequent transvaginal ultrasound shows an intrauterine pregnancy at 6 week's gestation. The patient is distraught and requests an abortion. The OBGYN does not perform abortions as part of her practice.

Under what circumstance does this physician have a genuine claim of conscience?

(A) She finds abortion procedures unpleasant to perform
(B) She fears of criticism from family and/or society
(C) She wishes to utilize her professional authority and advocate her personal positions on abortion
(D) She feels performing abortions would risk her personal wholeness or identity

The answer is D: She feels performing abortions would risk her personal wholeness or identity. Conscience has been defined as the private, constant, ethically attuned part of the human character. Not to act in accordance with one's conscience is to risk personal wholeness or identity. Claims of consciences may not always be genuine. Providers who decide not to perform abortions because they find the procedure unpleasant or because they fear criticism do not have a genuine claim of consciousness.

8 An 18-year-old, G1P0, presents to labor and delivery at 20 weeks' hemorrhaging with a known placenta previa. On admission, her blood pressure is 80/40 mmHg and pulse is 130 beats/min. Hematocrit is 25%. On sterile speculum examination, there is brisk red bleeding and the cervix appears 3 cm dilated. In the few minutes that she is being examined, she loses approximately 500 cm^3 of blood. A blood transfusion is started and the patient is moved to the operating room. The obstetrician on call does not perform abortions, citing a conflict of conscience.

What is the most appropriate next step in management of this unstable patient?

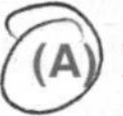

(A) Provide the medically indicated uterine evacuation regardless of personal moral objections
(B) Contact a provider that performs abortions and continue supportive care until his/her arrival
(C) Obtain consultation from the legal department
(D) Start labor augmentation

The answer is A: Provide the medically indicated uterine evacuation regardless of personal moral objections. The patient's well-being is paramount. A conscientious refusal that conflicts with a patient's well-being can only be accommodated if the primary duty to the patient can be fulfilled. In this emergent situation, a referral will compromise the patient's health and the on-call obstetrician is under an obligation to provide the medically indicated care regardless of their personal moral objections.

---

9 An Obstetrician-gynecologist (OBGYN) has been reporting to work late and has appeared disheveled. A practice partner observes her drinking alcohol alone in her office during lunch and realizes that she displays multiple signs of alcohol dependence. When he approaches her and suggests finding a treatment program, he is rebuffed and she emphatically denies alcohol use.

Which of the following ethical principles does she violate with her reaction?

(A) Autonomy
(B) Veracity
(C) Justice
(D) Paternalism

The answer is B: Veracity. The principle of veracity implies that physicians must deal honestly with patients and colleagues at all times. Misrepresentation of themselves through any communication is a violation of veracity. Behaviors such as substance abuse, which diminish a physician's capacity to practice, must be immediately addressed. This physician's reaction to her colleague's offer of assistance does not violate patient autonomy. Justice is the most complex ethical principle, dealing not only with physicians' obligation to render equal care but also with physicians' role in allocation of health resources. It is not directly violated by this physician's reaction to her colleague. Paternalism is not an ethical principle, but an attempt to override patient autonomy and to provide what the clinician sees as in the patient's best interest.

10 A 16-year-old girl is brought to the clinic by her mother because she believes that her daughter has become sexually active. She is very concerned that her daughter will experience an unintended pregnancy. During an interview alone, the daughter reports that she has become sexually active with her boyfriend over the past 6 months. Prior to becoming sexually active, she presented to a Title X clinic and received a contraceptive implant. At that time, both she and her boyfriend were tested for sexually transmitted infections and were found to be negative. The patient is not comfortable discussing this with her mother.

What is the next step?

(A) Inform the mother that her daughter is sexually active and using birth control
(B) Do not inform the mother that her daughter is sexually active or using birth control
(C) Tell the mother that her daughter is not at risk for pregnancy
(D) Question the mother as to why her daughter is not comfortable discussing these matters with her

The answer is B: Do not inform the mother that her daughter is sexually active or using birth control. Physicians and other health-care providers are charged with strict avoidance of discrimination on the basis of age, race, color, ethnicity, or any other factor. Discrimination jeopardizes the patient–physician relationship; personal information should not be disclosed to the parents of adolescents because of their minor status. No state or federal laws require minors to get parental consent for contraception. Title X is a federally funded program that provides funds to states for family planning services. Title X protects adolescents' privacy and prohibits parental consent requirements for teens seeking **contraception.**

---

11 A 29-year-old patient has delivered at 24 week's gestation, 12 days after premature rupture of the membranes. The estimated fetal weight is 400 g. The patient had discussed the fetal prognosis with her Obstetrician-gynecologist (OBGYN) and the neonatology team. She had all of her questions answered. She and her husband requested that no attempts at resuscitation should be made.

She precipitously delivered a small male infant before her OBGYN could arrive. At delivery, there were occasional gasping/breathing movements. The OBGYN arrived to discover that the pediatrician on call was demanding that intubation be done.

Who has the primary responsibility for the decision to intubate?

(A) Ethics committee
(B) Hospital attorney
(C) Mother
(D) Obstetrician
(E) Pediatrician

The answer is C: Mother. These situations are very difficult; however, it is important to remember that the child's mother has the primary responsibility for making care decisions in the delivery room. From an ethical standpoint, a plan was in place that was acceptable to the parents. Intact survival of a fetus less than 500 g is highly unlikely. Once the parents have made this decision, if health-care providers impose their personal preferences, it may cause the parents even more suffering than they are already experiencing. Issues of life and death at the extreme ends of the age's spectrum are fraught with complicated issues; however, it seems as if it is generally easier to let an elderly patient die than to let a baby of any gestational age die.

CHAPTER 3

Genetics

1 A 22-year-old G2P1001 comes to see you for a prenatal checkup. The patient's first child is male and the patient is excited because the 20-week anatomic screening ultrasound revealed that the current fetus is female. Both the patient and her husband are from Greece. The couple's first child was recently diagnosed with hemolytic anemia following consumption of fava beans, but neither parent suffers from hemolytic anemia. The patient is concerned that her second child could also develop this disease.

What is your next step?

(A) Advise the patient that her son likely has an autosomal dominant disease, and there is a significant chance that her daughter will also have hemolytic anemia
(B) Advise the patient that her son's disease is not a genetic disorder and there is almost no risk to her female fetus
(C) Advise the patient that the causes and inheritance of her son's disease is multifactorial and is not possible to assess the risk to the fetus
(D) Advise the patient that her son's disorder is X-linked recessive and her daughter has a 25% chance of being unaffected and a 25% chance of being a carrier
(E) Advise the patient that her son's disease is autosomal recessive and the risk to the female fetus is 25%

The answer is D: Advise the patient that her son's disorder is X-linked recessive and her daughter has a 25% chance of being unaffected and a 25% chance of being a carrier. Glucose-6-phosphate dehydrogenase (G6PD) deficiency is X-linked recessive (*Figure 3-1*). The disorder is identified at a higher frequency in men of Mediterranean and African descent. G6PD deficiency is known to cause a hemolytic anemia in response to a number of instigating factors including infection, medications, and various foods including fava beans. As this couple has one male child with the disorder, her

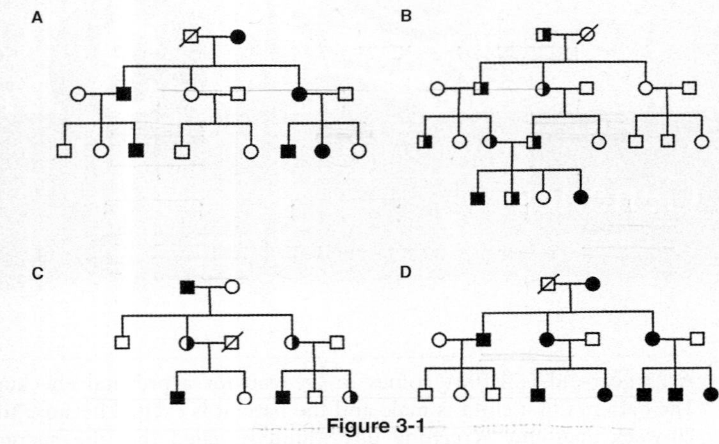

Figure 3-1

daughter has a 25% chance of being unaffected and a 25% chance of being a carrier. All other choices are incorrect as G6PD deficiency is inherited as an X-linked recessive disorder.

---

2 A 29-year-old G0 and her husband come to see you for preconception genetic counseling. The woman has numerous café-au-lait spots. The patient's father also has similar findings.

What is the inheritance pattern of this disorder?

(A) This is a result of mosaicism and therefore you are unable to accurately predict the inheritance pattern
(B) Autosomal dominant and therefore likely to recur in subsequent generations
(C) Autosomal recessive and therefore unlikely to affect her offspring
(D) X-linked and therefore likely to present more often in male offspring

The answer is B: Autosomal dominant and therefore likely to recur in subsequent generations. Neurofibromatosis is an autosomal dominant disorder; therefore, if one parent has neurofibromatosis, his or her children have a 50% chance of inheriting the disorder. Neurofibromatosis exhibits variable expressivity meaning that different individuals will be affected by the disease to different degrees.

---

3 A 34-year-old, G1P0, presents for genetic counseling at 12 week's gestation. The patient has two sisters and a brother; her father has hemophilia. Her siblings are not affected, but she has a nephew that is.

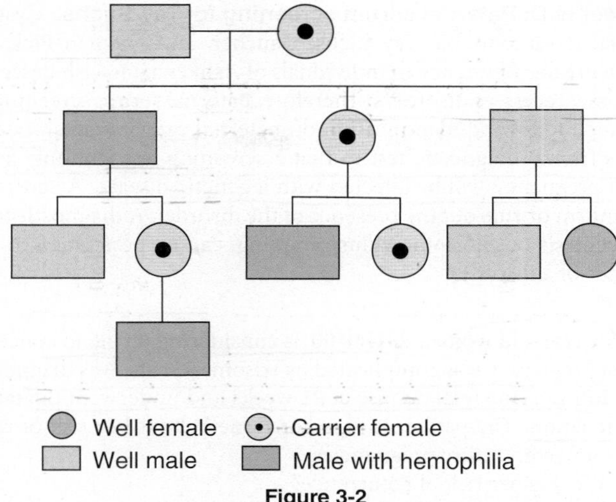

Figure 3-2

What is the inheritance pattern of this disorder?

(A) X-linked inheritance
(B) Autosomal recessive
(C) Mitochondrial inheritance
(D) Multifactorial inheritance

The answer is A: X-linked inheritance. Hemophilia is an X-linked recessive disease (see *Figure 3-2*). These diseases are more common in men than in women. An affected male will not pass the diseases to his sons, but all daughters will be carriers. X-linked recessive diseases are transmitted from carrier women to affected men.

4 While collecting a thorough family and personal history, a 24-year-old, G1P0, at 10 weeks is discovered to be of Ashkenazi Jewish descent. Her blood is sent for cystic fibrosis, familial dysautonomia, Tay-Sachs, Canavan, Gaucher, and Niemann-Pick disease screening. She is found to be a carrier for Tay-Sachs disease.

Which of the following is the most appropriate next step in determining the risk of fetal Tay-Sachs disease?

(A) Maternal first-trimester serum screening
(B) Amniocentesis in the second trimester
(C) Chorionic villus sampling in the first trimester
(D) Paternal serum screening for Tay-Sachs

The answer is D: Paternal serum screening for Tay-Sachs. Cystic fibrosis, familial dysautonomia, Tay-Sachs, Gaucher, and Niemen-Pick diseases occur with greater frequency in individuals of Ashkenazi Jewish descent. They are autosomal recessive disorders. Therefore, paternal serum screening should be performed following identification of maternal carrier status. A screening test differs from a diagnostic test in that a screening test will only assess the risk that a pregnancy will be affected with a genetic disease. A screening test cannot confirm or rule out the presence of the disorder. A diagnostic test, such as amniocentesis or chorionic villus sampling, can be performed to confirm the presence of a disorder.

5 A 36-year-old woman, G1P0100, is considering trying to conceive. Her first pregnancy was complicated by trisomy 18. She was diagnosed with an intrauterine fetal demise at 21 weeks and underwent dilatation and evacuation. The patient is now concerned about her risk of recurrent trisomy with future pregnancies.

What is her risk of recurrence?

(A) Not greater than her maternal age risk for chromosomal abnormalities
(B) Greater than 10 times her maternal age risk for chromosomal abnormalities
(C) 1.6 to 8.2 times her maternal age risk for chromosomal abnormalities
(D) Unknown

The answer is C: 1.6 to 8.2 times her maternal age risk for chromosomal abnormalities. Women with a previous pregnancy complicated by any trisomy, in which the fetus survived at least to the second trimester, are at risk for having a recurrence of the same or different trisomy. The risk of trisomy recurrence is 1.6 to 8.2 times the maternal age risk. This risk depends on several factors, including the maternal age during the index pregnancy, type of trisomy, and pregnancy outcome. Certain sex-chromosome abnormalities may also carry an increased risk of recurrence. Turner syndrome (XO) and XYY karyotypes carry a nominal recurrence risk; fetal XXX or XXY has an increased recurrence risk.

6 A 26-year-old, G3P2, presents for second-trimester ultrasound screening at 18 weeks. An intracardiac focus, echogenic bowel, and pyelectasis are diagnosed. The patient is counseled that the significance of these markers should be considered in the context of serum screening results.

What quadruple screen findings would further increase the probability of aneuploidy?

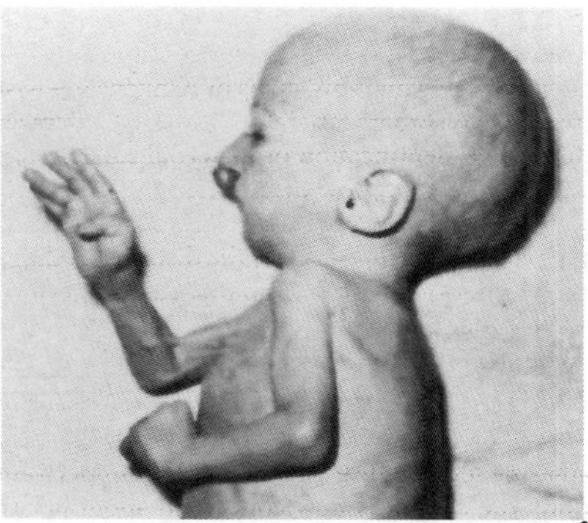

Figure 3-3

(A) Increased α-fetoprotein (AFP), decreased intact human chorionic gonadotropin (hCG), decreased estradiol, decreased inhibin A

(B) Increased AFP, normal intact hCG, normal estradiol, normal inhibin A

(C) Decreased AFP, decreased intact hCG, increased estradiol, normal inhibin A

(D) Decreased AFP, elevated intact β-hCG, decreased estradiol, increased inhibin A

The answer is D: Decreased AFP, elevated intact β-hCG, decreased estradiol, increased inhibin A. Ultrasonographic "soft markers" for trisomy 21 include intracardiac echogenic focus, echogenic bowel, pyelectasis, nuchal fold, mild ventriculomegaly, shortened femur or humerus, and absent nasal bone. The average maternal serum AFP level in trisomy 21 pregnancies is reduced to 0.74 multiple of the median (MoM). Intact β-hCG is increased in affected pregnancies (2.06 MoM) and estradiol is reduced (0.75 MoM). Adding inhibin A to the triple screen improves the detection rate for trisomy 21 to approximately 80%. Inhibin A is increased (1.77 MoM) in trisomy 21 pregnancies.

7 A 33-year-old, G4P2012, presents to a genetic counselor after receiving abnormal quadruple screen results. She has been told by her obstetrician that the pregnancy is at increased risk for trisomy 18.

What components of the quadruple screen were used to calculate this risk?

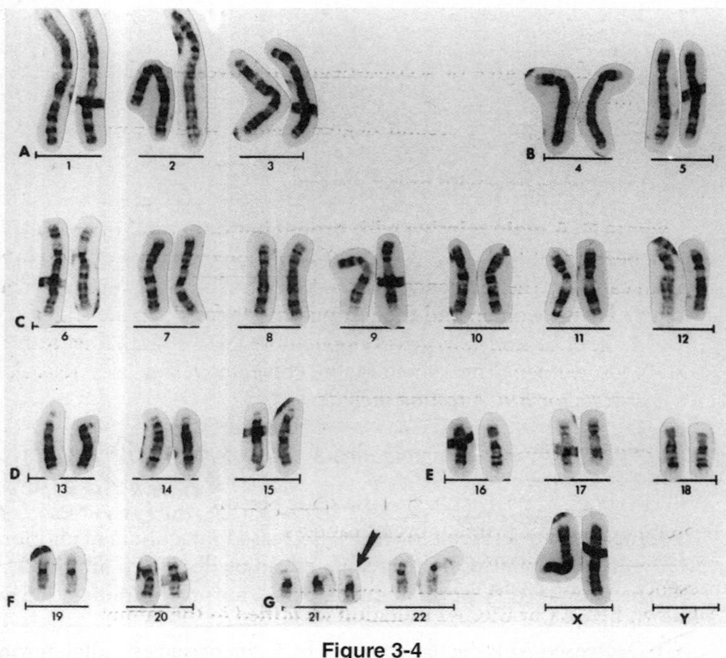

Figure 3-4

for trisomy 21, ↓ not 18

(A) α-fetoprotein (AFP), intact hCG, estradiol, inhibin A
(B) Intact hCG, estradiol, inhibin A
(C) AFP, estradiol, inhibin A
(D) AFP, intact hCG, inhibin A
(E) AFP, intact hCG, estradiol all ↓

The answer is E: AFP, intact hCG, estradiol. Inhibin A is not used in the calculation of risk for trisomy 18. Typically, the values of AFP, intact hCG, and estradiol are all reduced when the fetus is at increased risk for trisomy 18 (see *Figure 3-4*).

---

8 During a routine examination, a 28-year-old woman expresses concern about her risk for breast cancer because her mother recently died from the disease at 59 years of age. A thorough family history is taken. The patient is not of Ashkenazi Jewish descent. She has a maternal aunt with ovarian cancer and her paternal uncle was recently diagnosed with breast cancer.

What makes *BRCA* (breast cancer gene mutation) testing appropriate for this patient?

(A) One second-degree relative with breast cancer diagnosed at under age 50
(B) Two first-degree or second-degree relatives with breast cancer at any age
(C) A first-degree or second-degree relative with breast and ovarian cancers
(D) A male relative with breast cancer

The answer is D: A male relative with breast cancer. *BRCA 1* and *BRCA 2* genes have been identified as responsible for hereditary forms of both breast and ovarian cancers. The incidence of breast cancers linked to *BRCA* is higher in Ashkenazi Jewish women and the testing criteria for them are slightly different. In the general non-Jewish US population, *BRCA* mutations occur in 1 in 300 to 500 women. The United States Preventative Services Task Force (USPSTF) criteria for *BRCA* testing include:

- Breast cancer diagnosed before the age of 50
- Ovarian cancer diagnosed at any age
- Both breast and ovarian cancer in the same person
- Bilateral or multiple primary breast cancers
- Ashkenazi Jewish heritage with a history of breast and/or ovarian cancer
- Presence of male breast cancer in the family
- A known BRCA1 or BRCA2 mutation identified in the family

---

9 A 35-year-old woman presents with a chief complaint of abnormal uterine bleeding. Her cycles had been regular until approximately 6 months ago when they became closer together and heavier. There are no significant findings on pelvic examination and an endometrial biopsy was performed. When she returns to discuss her biopsy results, the patient reveals that she was recently diagnosed with Lynch II syndrome by genetic testing. In addition to uterine cancer, which gynecologic cancer is the patient at increased risk for developing?

(A) Cervical
(B) Fallopian tube
(C) Ovarian
(D) Vaginal

The answer is C: Ovarian. Lynch I syndrome (hereditary nonpolyposis colorectal cancer type A) increases the risk of developing colon, endometrial, ureteral, and renal cancers. Hereditary nonpolyposis colorectal cancer type B, or Lynch II syndrome, is an autosomal dominant inherited syndrome. There is an increased risk of developing all of the cancers in Lynch I syndrome as well as ovarian, gastric, and pancreatic cancers. Individuals with the presence of hereditary nonpolyposis colorectal cancer in two successive generations and the diagnosis of nonpolyposis colorectal cancer in at least three relatives can undergo genetic testing.

10 A couple in their 20s comes to see you for genetic counseling before deciding whether to have children. Several members of the husband's family have suffered progressive behavioral changes, uncontrollable movements, and dementia before age 50. All of his family members who develop these symptoms died within 15 years of onset. What advice would you provide for this couple?

(A) The disease is autosomal recessive and the husband is still within the at-risk age group and should be tested
(B) Genetic testing is unnecessary because a detailed family history will establish whether the father carries the gene
(C) The disease is likely due to environmental exposure to lead
(D) The disease is autosomal dominant and the husband should be tested to determine his status and the likelihood of passing on the gene
(E) The disease is autosomal dominant, and with a positive family history, the couple can forgo screening and use preimplantation genetic diagnosis with in vitro fertilization

The answer is D: The disease is autosomal dominant and the husband should be tested to determine his status and the likelihood of passing on the gene. Huntington disease is an autosomal dominant disease caused by a mutation in the Huntingtin gene. The disease causes progressive neurodegenerative changes leading to cognitive decline, loss of motor coordination, chorea, and psychiatric problems. Onset of symptoms typically occurs between 35 and 44 years of age with genetic anticipation leading to earlier development of the disease in subsequent generations. Since the couple in the question is in their 20s, the husband may elect genetic screening to determine both his own status and the risk of passing the gene onto his children. Choice E is incorrect as screening of the husband is recommended before any elective fertilization techniques are considered (see Figure 3-5).

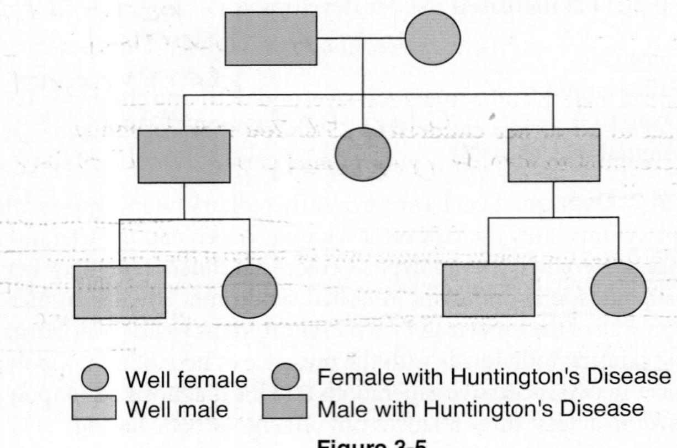

Figure 3-5

11 A 21-year-old G0 presents for preconception counseling. She has been told that she carries a balanced chromosome translocation and she is worried about the potential effects this could have on her future children.

Why are her future children at risk for chromosomal abnormalities?

(A) She has euploid and aneuploid gametes
(B) Balanced translocations are autosomal dominant
(C) Her chromosomes are more susceptible to breaks
(D) There is an increased risk of chromosomal nondisjunction

The answer is A: She has euploid and aneuploidy gametes. A balanced chromosome translocation is one in which there are chromosome structural abnormalities that do not change the total amount of genetic material. In an individual with a balanced translocation, meiosis gives rise to both aneuploid and euploid gametes. An aneuploid gamete will result in a fetus with an abnormal amount of genetic material which increases the risk of birth defects and mental retardation. Translocations are passed on through non-Mendelian inheritance patterns. Chromosome breaks result in rearrangement of the chromosome pieces, which gives rise to chromosome translocations. Chromosomal nondisjunction is an error resulting from chromosomes failing to separate at the centromere.

12 A 26-year-old G3P3003 comes to see you for her postpartum checkup and to discuss the results of the routine newborn screen. The testing showed a higher than normal level of immunoreactive trypsinogen, and you asked the patient to return when the baby was 1 month old for a confirmatory sweat test. The patient's two other children were born outside the United States, and they did not undergo such screening. The patient would like to know if screening the other children is indicated.

What is the next best step in managing the care of this patient?

(A) The disease is autosomal recessive, and with one child affected, the risk to all of her children is 25%. You may recommend genetic screening to identify asymptomatic carriers as well as those with the disease
(B) The infant's disease is likely due to drug-eluting stent exposure in utero and the siblings should only be tested if they were also exposed
(C) The infant's disease can occur as a result of over 1,000 mutations, and therefore a negative screen cannot rule out disease, and you do not recommend screening of asymptomatic siblings
(D) The infant's disease is X-linked recessive, and the mother is an asymptomatic carrier; therefore, you recommend screening of all the male children

The answer is A: The disease is autosomal recessive, and with one child affected, the risk to all of her children is 25%. You may recommend genetic screening to identify asymptomatic carriers as well as those with the disease. Cystic fibrosis is an autosomal recessive disease resulting from an abnormality in the cystic fibrosis transmembrane conductance regulator (*CFTR*) gene for chloride channels. If one child is affected, then both parents must be carriers of the gene and therefore the risk to all children of being affected by the disease is 25% and genetic screening may be recommended. Choice C is true in that the disease can occur as a result of over 1,000 mutations but screening is still recommended even though there remains a small chance that a child with a negative screen could still have the disease.

CHAPTER 4

Obstetrics

1 A 19-year-old G2P0101 presented at term in the active phase of labor with spontaneous rupture of membranes. This is her second delivery and her baby is estimated to be 3,600 g. Her first delivery was preterm and her baby weighed only 2,500 g. She has been dilated 6 cm for the last 2 hours. She has an epidural and is comfortable.

What is the next step in her management?

(A) Perform a Cesarean section due to arrest of dilation
(B) Place an intrauterine pressure catheter (IUPC) to measure Montevideo units (MVUs)
(C) Start a fluid bolus to ensure adequate hydration
(D) Place a fetal scalp lead to monitor the baby for distress

The answer is B: Place an intrauterine pressure catheter (IUPC) to measure Montevideo units (MVUs). MVUs (the area under the uterine contraction curve) should be monitored in a patient whose labor is not progressing. This is done with a pressure catheter inside the uterine cavity. MVUs should be ≥200 U/10 minutes to qualify as adequate.

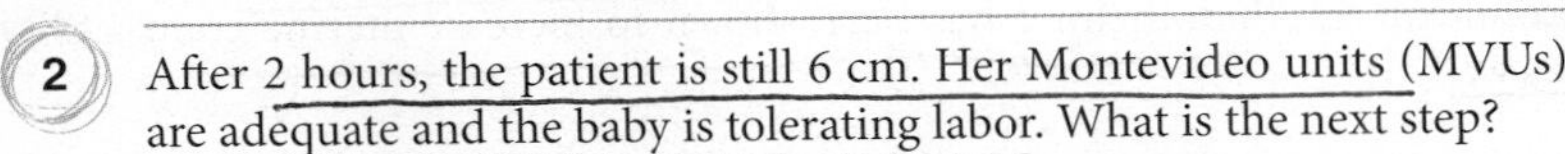

2 After 2 hours, the patient is still 6 cm. Her Montevideo units (MVUs) are adequate and the baby is tolerating labor. What is the next step?

(A) Proceed with Cesarean section; the pelvis is too small
(B) Increase Pitocin to strengthen the contractions
(C) Apply oxygen to help the baby with the stress of labor
(D) Start antibiotics to help decrease infection with increased risk of a long labor
(E) Reexamine the patient in 2 hours

The answer is E: Reexamine the patient in 2 hours. Two hours of adequate contractions is not enough to diagnose cephalopelvic disproportion or arrest of labor. The parameters to determine if labor is progressing satisfactorily may need to be expanded. With the availability of technology to assess maternal and fetal well-being, labor should be allowed to progress past the rigid 2-hour time limit for the second stage of labor artificially imposed on women in some childbirth settings. Adequate MVUs obviate the need for increasing Pitocin. Antibiotics and oxygen are not used for treatment of the course of labor.

---

3 A 23-year-old G1P0 at 38/3 weeks arrives at outpatient labor and delivery (L&D) with periodic contractions that have increased in frequency over the last 4 hours. The patient has blood pressure (BP) 124/79 mmHg, heart rate (HR) 85 beats/min, and category 1 fetal tracing, denies vaginal bleeding or loss of fluid, and feels the baby moves frequently. Cervical examination is dilation 1 cm, effacement 25%, and fetal station –4.

Which of the following factors is not involved in preparing the uterus for labor (activation phase)?

(A) Endothelin 1
(B) Decreased connexin-43
(C) Increase in size and number of gap junctions
(D) Increase in myometrial receptors for oxytocin and prostaglandins (PGs)
(E) Estrogen

The answer is B: Decreased connexin-43. Connexin-43 is also known as gap junction α-1 protein and will be increased in relation to the increasing gap junctions necessary for uterine contractility during labor. The four phases of labor are quiescence, activation, stimulation, and involution. Quiescence involves the suppression of uterine contractility by the action of progesterone, prostacyclin, relaxin, nitric oxide, parathyroid hormone–related peptide, and possibly other hormones. During the activation phase, estrogen begins to facilitate the expression of myometrial receptors for PGs and oxytocin, which results in ion channel activation and increased gap junctions, thus connexin-43. Endothelin-1 has been shown to increase uterine contractility as well.

---

4 A 26-year-old G2P1001 arrives in your office for routine prenatal visit. She has a history of a prior Cesarean section at term. She remembers that her doctor told her the baby "wasn't going to fit" after she had labored for several hours. You perform pelvimetry and recognize the rationale for that doctor's statement.

What type of pelvis is she most likely to have (*Figure 4-1*)?

(A) Gynecoid
(B) Anthropoid
(C) Android
(D) Platypelloid

The answer is C: Android. The gynecoid pelvis is the classic female shape. The anthropoid pelvis with its exaggerated oval shape of the inlet, largest anterioposterior diameter, and limited anterior capacity is more often associated with delivery in the occiput posterior position. The android pelvis is male in pattern and theoretically has an increased risk of cephalopelvic disproportion, and the platypelloid pelvis with its broad, flat pelvis theoretically predisposes to a transverse arrest.

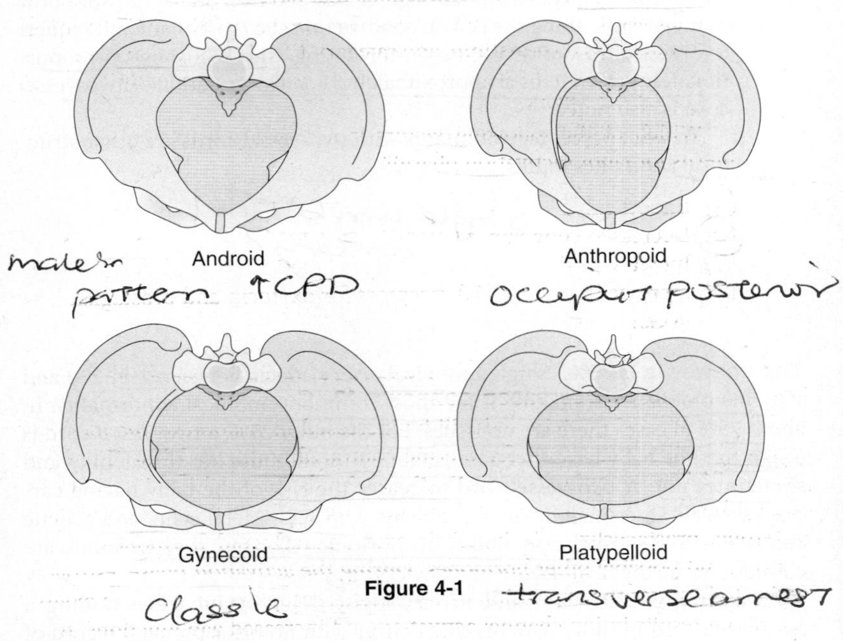

Figure 4-1

5 A 21-year-old G1P0 at 39/6 weeks arrives at the hospital painfully contracting. Cervical check is 6 cm. She is admitted and requests an epidural for pain management. She progresses to complete and begins pushing. After 3.5 hours, the baby is at +1 station.

Which of the following conditions is associated with a prolonged second stage of labor?

(A) Decreased bonding
(B) Postpartum depression
(C) Worsened neonatal outcome
(D) Uterine atony

The answer is D: Uterine atony. Neonatal outcomes have not shown to be decreased with longer second stages. Uterine atony increases with prolonged labor. Though nulliparous women may have increased complications, 3 hours should be used as a threshold and each woman should be evaluated independently for factors influencing the increased duration, including fetal position, adequate contractions, and pushing effort.

6 A 32-year-old G3P2002 presents for initial prenatal visit. She states she has not a period for several months though did not take a pregnancy test until recently. Two weeks ago, it was positive. She is not sure how many months along she is. You confirm that she is pregnant and request a formal ultrasound (U/S) scan for dating. The U/S shows a proportionately grown fetus at approximately 31 week's gestation. A two-vessel cord is also noted.

In what percentage of infants with two-vessel cords are other structural anomalies found?

(A) 1%
(B) 5%
(C) 15%
(D) 25%
(E) 50%

The answer is B: 5%. Single umbilical artery affects between 1 in 100 and 1 in 500 pregnancies, making it the most common umbilical abnormality. In about 75% of cases there are no issues. For the other 25%, a two-vessel cord is a sign that the baby has other abnormalities—sometimes life-threatening and sometimes not. A two-vessel cord increases the risk of the baby having cardiac, skeletal, intestinal, or renal problems. U/S scans, fetal echo, and genetic counseling to discuss the possibility of chorionic villus sampling or amnio are common to further evaluate.

Alerting pediatricians and neonatologist is important when finding a two-vessel cord in those patients that deliver with no prior prenatal record of the abnormality.

7 A 23-year-old G2P1001 is seen at 18-week gestational age (GA) for her first prenatal visit. The patient has no complaints and no significant medical or surgical history. The patient delivered her first child at term via an uncomplicated vaginal delivery. You last saw the patient 5 months ago for her annual examination. At that time, the Pap smear was normal, and gonorrhea and chlamydia assays were negative. During the appointment, the patient informs you that she is planning to travel to Haiti with a humanitarian aid group. As part of her travel requirements, multiple vaccinations are recommended, and the patient would like to know your recommendations regarding the safety of her fetus. In addition to the patient's up-to-date hepatitis B virus, MMR

(measles, mumps, and rubella), and DPT vaccination status, you recommend the patient receive the following:

(A) Administer hepatitis A, typhoid, rabies, and cholera vaccinations with addition of small pox and yellow fever vaccinations if endemic in that country
(B) Administer typhoid and cholera vaccinations, but hepatitis A, rabies, smallpox, and yellow fever vaccinations are contraindicated in pregnancy
(C) Administer hepatitis A and typhoid vaccinations with addition of cholera, rabies, and yellow fever vaccinations if endemic in that country
(D) Administer cholera, rabies, and yellow fever vaccinations, but avoid hepatitis A and typhoid vaccinations during pregnancy

The answer is C: Administer hepatitis A and typhoid vaccinations with addition of cholera, rabies, and yellow fever vaccinations if endemic in that country. Hepatitis A, typhoid, cholera, rabies, and yellow fever vaccinations are recommended during pregnancy before traveling to a high-risk country. Choice A is incorrect as smallpox has been eradicated and therefore no routine immunization is required. Choices B and D are incorrect as the hepatitis A, typhoid, rabies, and yellow fever vaccinations are all safe in pregnancy. Remember that pregnant patients do not receive the MMR vaccine until postpartum if needed.

---

8 A 27-year-old G1 comes to you for her first prenatal visit. The patient follows a strict vegetarian diet and wants to know if her dietary choices are optimal for her baby's development. The patient voices her willingness to change her diet if it will benefit the baby.

Compared with the less stringent lacto ovo vegetarian diet, this patient's diet is more likely to be deficient in which of the following?

(A) Vitamin A
(B) Vitamin B_{12}
(C) Vitamin C
(D) Folic acid
(E) Calcium

The answer is B: Vitamin B_{12}. Vitamin B_{12} is found solely in animal-derived foods, including eggs and milk. Therefore, in comparing a strict vegetarian diet to a lacto ovo vegetarian diet, the lacto ovo vegetarian is less likely to be deficient in vitamin B_{12}. Vitamin A, C, folic acid, and calcium should be adequate in both diets.

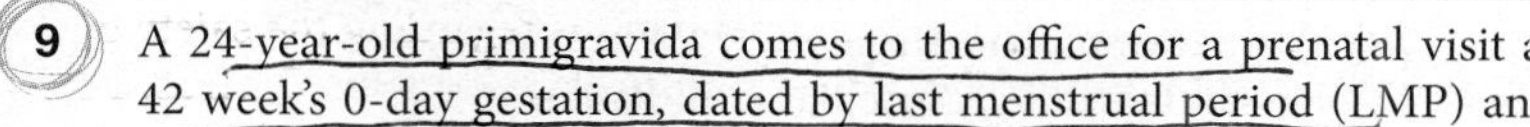

9 A 24-year-old primigravida comes to the office for a prenatal visit at 42 week's 0-day gestation, dated by last menstrual period (LMP) and

8-week fetal ultrasound (U/S). She has had an uncomplicated pregnancy, and her only complaint is mild discomfort due to her gravid uterus. Fetal movement is reassuring, and the patient denies regular contractions, vaginal bleeding, or loss of fluid. Bedside U/S reveals a cephalic infant and an amniotic fluid index of 3 cm (normal = 5 to 15 cm). A fetal nonstress test is reactive. Sterile vaginal examination is notable for a posterior cervix of medium consistency, 1-cm cervical dilation, 70% cervical effacement, and fetal station of −2.

Which of the following is the best course of management for this patient?

(A) Have the patient return to the clinic in 1 week to check the nonstress test and amniotic fluid index
(B) Have the patient return to the clinic in 3 days to check the nonstress test and amniotic fluid index
(C) Admit the patient to the hospital now and induce labor
(D) Admit the patient to the hospital now and perform Cesarean section
(E) Expectant management

The answer is C: Admit the patient to the hospital now and induce labor. Indications for immediate delivery of a postterm infant include oligohydramnios (as in this patient) or any evidence of fetal compromise. Although this patient has an unfavorable cervix (Bishop score of 6), it is reasonable to allow her a trial of labor via medical induction before proceeding to Cesarean section.

Induction of labor at 41 weeks results in statistically lower perinatal fetal mortality and no difference in rate of Cesarean section compared with expectant management. However, the mortality benefit is modest, and in patients without indications for immediate delivery, expectant management may be a reasonable option for patients if they choose to do so after a thorough discussion of the risks and benefits.

---

10 A 29-year-old, G4P3, at 42-week 3-day gestation by last menstrual period (LMP) and 10-week ultrasound (U/S) presents to her obstetrician (OB) for a prenatal visit. The patient denies regular contractions, vaginal bleeding, or loss of fluid. Fetal movement is reassuring and a nonstress test is reactive.

Which of the following complications is this patient at greatest risk for?

(A) Fetal meconium aspiration
(B) Polyhydramnios
(C) Eclampsia
(D) Postpartum hemorrhage
(E) Disseminated intravascular coagulation

The answer is A: Fetal meconium aspiration. Postterm pregnancy is a pregnancy that is ≥42-week 0-day gestation. The risk of antenatal fetal and early perinatal demise increases with increasing gestational age (GA) after 40 week's gestation. Mechanisms for this increased risk include intrauterine infection, placental insufficiency, oligohydramnios, cord compression, and meconium aspiration. Passing of meconium can be an indication of fetal distress and/or fetal maturity, and risk of fetal meconium aspiration increases with increasing GA after its nadir at 31 weeks.

---

11 An 18-year-old primigravida who did not receive any prenatal care presents in labor to the emergency department at 42+ weeks by last menstrual period (LMP). Labor is complicated by meconium-stained fluid and shoulder dystocia, but the fetus is successfully delivered with the McRoberts maneuver and does not appear to aspirate upon delivery. On the pediatrician's examination, the infant is unusually long and lean, with a large amount of hair, no laguna, long fingernails, thin wrinkled skin, and a "wide-eyed" look.

What is the most likely diagnosis?

(A) Fetal dysmaturity syndrome
(B) Potter syndrome
(C) Trisomy 18
(D) Prune belly disease
(E) Prader-Willi syndrome

The answer is A: Fetal dysmaturity syndrome. This infant's examination is most consistent with fetal dysmaturity syndrome from postterm pregnancy. Pregnancies greater than 40 weeks are at increased risk for meconium aspiration, shoulder dystocia, fetal macrosomia, and fetal dysmaturity syndrome. Besides the physical findings on examination, these infants do not appear to have long-term consequences that are different from term infants. Potter syndrome is a term used to describe the triad of lung hypoplasia, limb deformities, and flattened facies seen in severe cases of oligohydramnios, typically in the setting of fetal renal disease. The appearance of infants with trisomy 18 is characterized by small size, micrognathia, prominent occiput, and overlapping fingers. Prune belly syndrome describes the triad of abdominal muscle deficiency, urinary tract abnormalities, and bilateral cryptorchidism in men. Neonatal hypotonia, poor feeding, and genital hypoplasia are features of Prader-Willi syndrome.

---

12 A 37-year-old G2P1001 at 39-week 1-day gestational age (GA) presents to labor and delivery (L&D) with severe pain with contractions. Her previous pregnancy resulted in a Cesarean section via a low transverse uterine incision secondary to arrest of cervical dilation after premature rupture of membranes (PROMs) at 37-week 2-day GA. This pregnancy has been complicated by gestational diabetes. External monitoring shows the fetal heart rate (HR) to be 60 beats/min.

Which of the following is an indication for Cesarean delivery in this patient?

(A) Nonreassuring fetal HR
(B) Advanced maternal age
(C) History of arrest of cervical dilation
(D) Previous Cesarean section
(E) History of PROMs

The answer is A: Nonreassuring fetal HR. Indications for Cesarean delivery include nonreassuring fetal HR, placental abruption, hemorrhage from placenta previa, prolapse of umbilical cord, and uterine rupture. If a patient has had a "classical" (vertical) or T-shaped incision with previous pregnancies, they are recommended to have a Cesarean with subsequent pregnancies due to the risk of uterine rupture. However, in patients who have only had one previous Cesarean delivery via a low, transverse incision they are candidates for vaginal delivery with subsequent pregnancies. Advanced maternal age, history of cervical dilation arrest, and previous premature rupture of membrane (PROM) are not independent indications for Cesarean delivery.

---

13 A 28-year-old G1P0 at 35-week 2-day gestational age (GA) presents for a return obstetrician (OB) visit and wants to discuss her birth plan with her physician. Her pregnancy has been uncomplicated thus far and she has no underlying comorbidities. She has decided that she would like to undergo an elective Cesarean section, as she does not wish to deliver vaginally. If lung maturity in the fetus has not yet been documented and there are no medical indications for Cesarean section, at what GA can an elective Cesarean section be performed?

(A) 36 weeks
(B) 37 weeks
(C) 38 weeks
(D) 39 weeks
(E) 40 weeks

The answer is D: 39 weeks. Cesarean section by maternal request is very controversial, but should not be performed before 39-week GA unless lung maturity can be documented. In general, elective Cesarean section by maternal request is not recommended for women who desire several children, as Cesarean section increases the risk of placenta previa, placenta accreta, and gravid hysterectomy with each Cesarean delivery.

14 A 19-year-old woman G1P0 at 27-week 5-day gestational age (GA) presents to her obstetrician (OB) for a routine return obstetrician (OB) visit. She has no complaints today, her vitals are stable, and physical examination is benign. On routine urinalysis, she is found to have pyuria and bacteriuria. She is subsequently diagnosed with a urinary tract infection (UTI). She denies dysuria, frequent urination, or urgency.

What is the next step in the management of this patient?

(A) Doxycycline pending culture
(B) Nitrofurantoin pending culture
(C) Confirmatory urine culture before starting treatment

The answer is B: Nitrofurantoin pending culture. All UTIs, whether symptomatic or not, should be treated in pregnancy. Of the choices given, only nitrofurantoin is safe to give in pregnancy. Doxycycline should be avoided in pregnancy, as it can cause skeletal malformation as well as teeth discoloration in the fetus. A urine culture should be sent, but the confirmatory results are not necessary prior to initiating treatment in pregnant patients who present with asymptomatic bacteriuria.

15 A 34-year-old G1P0 presents in labor and is completely dilated. She has an epidural, has had no complications with her pregnancy, and has no medical problems. Her BMI is 33 and at 35 week's gestation, she was found to be group B strep negative. She begins pushing and has pushed for 2 hours. You are asked to assess her labor progression.

Which component of your examination will give you the most pertinent information regarding her labor progression?

(A) The fetal sutures
(B) The maternal position for pushing
(C) The amount of lower extremity edema present
(D) The fundal height of the patient's uterus

The answer is A: The fetal sutures. The fetal sutures are used to determine the position of the fetal head and possibility of the baby being asynclitic, occiput posterior, or have a compound presentation, all important aspects that can alter the progression of labor during the second stage. Maternal position and lower extremity edema are not focal aspects of the examination needed to assess labor progression. The fundal height is not accurate once the fetal head has begun its descent into the birth canal.

16 A 23-year-old G1P0 at 20-week gestational age (GA) presents to your office complaining of difficulty finishing her regular aerobic exercise class. She has always been athletic and in good physical condition, but lately she is more aware of her breathing and has shortness of breath during her workouts. In addition, she sometimes feels her heart beating. On physical examination, her HR is 85 beats/min, BP is 100/70 mmHg, and lungs are clear to auscultation with nonlabored symmetric breathing. Which of the following is the most likely etiology of this patient's current symptoms?

(A) Increase in the tidal volume
(B) Increase in the total lung capacity
(C) Increase in the respiratory rate
(D) Increase in the $PaCO_2$ level

The answer is A: Increase in the tidal volume. The tidal volume increases during pregnancy and the total lung capacity decreases due to the elevation in the diaphragm. The respiratory rate remains constant. The increased tidal volume and increased minute ventilation often cause pregnant patients to experience dyspnea and feel that they are hyperventilating. The $PaCO_2$ decreases which causes an increased CO_2 gradient between the mother and the fetus which facilitates oxygen delivery to the fetus.

---

17 A 26-year-old G0 at 30-week gestational age (GA) comes to see you for a regularly scheduled prenatal appointment. The patient reports increased fatigue and weakness over the past few weeks. In addition, the patient tells you that she now quickly becomes short of breath with normal activities such as cleaning. The patient is worried that the baby is pressing on her lungs and that she might need bed rest. On physical examination, the patient's heart rate (HR) is rapid, her skin is cool and pale, and there is marked pallor of the patient's conjunctiva. You reassure the patient that she will not require bed rest. What is the most likely cause of the patient's presentation?

(A) A benign physiologic decrease in hematopoiesis that occurs in pregnancy due to the transfer of metabolic energy to the growing fetus
(B) A normal change in the hematologic system seen in pregnancy due to the dilutional effect of increased plasma volume
(C) A dilution of red blood cells (RBCs) in the maternal circulating blood by sequestration into the fetal circulation
(D) Decreased oxygenation of the blood due to increased HR which does not require bed rest

The answer is B: A normal change in the hematologic system seen in pregnancy due to the dilutional effect of increased plasma volume. There is a normal dilutional anemia seen in pregnancy due to the increase in the plasma volume. Despite pregnancy being a hypercoagulable state there is no increase in the clotting and bleeding time.

---

18 A 29-year-old G2P1 at 30-week gestational age (GA) comes to see you with new-onset gastric reflux not responsive to antacids. The patient reports that she did not experience these symptoms during her first pregnancy at age 20. What physiologic changes of pregnancy explain these symptoms?

(A) Increased gastric emptying times
(B) Increased large bowel motility
(C) Decreased water absorption in the small bowel
(D) Decreased gastroesophageal sphincter tone

The answer is D: Decreased gastroesophageal sphincter tone. Progesterone causes decreased gastroesophageal sphincter tone and prolonged gastric emptying times. These changes lead to increased gastroesophageal reflux.

---

19 A 22-year-old G1 at 32-week gestational age (GA) comes to see you for a routine prenatal visit. The patient reports that she is doing well and has no current health concerns. The patient's only medication is her prenatal vitamin. On examination, the patient appears healthy, fundal height is consistent with GA, and fetal heart tones (FHTs) are in the 140s. She is concerned because she received lab work from an insurance physical that shows decreased blood urea nitrogen, decreased creatinine, and trace glucose in her urine. You reassure the patient that these changes are normal due to:

(A) An increase of 50% in the glomerular filtration rate that occurs in the first trimester and is maintained until delivery
(B) The mass effect of the uterus on the bladder leading to compression and temporary physiologic changes
(C) The direct effects of progesterone on the bladder during pregnancy
(D) Mild gestational diabetes that can be managed by dietary changes

The answer is A: An increase of 50% in the glomerular filtration rate that occurs in the first trimester and is maintained until delivery. The glomerular filtration rate increases early and significantly in pregnancy. The progesterone effect on the rest of the system causes dilation of the ureters and the uterus itself often causes hydronephrosis (more on the right than the left). The flexibility of the bladder is not affected, but the size of the bladder is often decreased as the uterus grows in size.

---

20 A 24-year-old G2P1 presents at 4 cm with 50% effacement c/o spontaneous rupture of membranes 3 hours ago. Reevaluation 4 hours after arrival confirms an examination of 4 cm with 50% effacement. The patient is concerned because a friend of hers underwent a Cesarean section when she "got stuck" at 4 cm for 3 hours. Of the following, which best outlines the evidence with regard to the course of labor:

(A) A prolonged latent phase is considered a risk factor for Cesarean section
(B) Modern labor patterns confirm the findings of Friedman in the 1950s
(C) Multiparous women begin active labor at lesser dilation than primiparous women
(D) Ninety percent of women will be in active labor at 5-cm dilation
(E) Perceived pain level has been demonstrated to be reliable at differentiating latent from active phase of labor

The answer is D: Ninety percent of women will be in active labor at 5-cm dilation. Only 60% of labors will be in active phase by 4 cm, but 90% of women will be in active labor by 5 cm. All other alternatives are false.

---

21 A 23-year-old G1P0 at 36 weeks presents for a routine prenatal visit. Her pregnancy has been complicated by an anxiety disorder exacerbated by the fact that her husband was deployed to Afghanistan. Attempts at other nonpharmacologic methods to reduce stress and improve sleep patterns have met with little success and the patient is currently taking lorazepam. What is the main reason for tapering to the lowest dose of lorazepam?

(A) Crying
(B) Transient tachypnea
(C) Hypothermia
(D) Hypotonia
(E) Aggressive sucking response

The answer is C: Hypothermia. Lorazepam is the optimal choice among benzodiazepine when a patient is refractory to nonpharmacologic measures. One of the neonatal symptoms of withdrawal is hypothermia.

---

22 A 32-year-old G3P2 presents at term with a cervical examination of 6/90/high. Fetal head is palpated but not yet engaged. Two hours later, the examination has not changed. A decision is made to artificially rupture membranes and place an intrauterine pressure catheter (IUPC) in anticipation of augmenting labor. When artificial rupture of membrane was performed and the IUPC placed, the initial fetal heart tracing remained category 1.

However, after 10 minutes, severe variables were noted that progressed to persistent bradycardia in the 60s. What is the next appropriate step?

(A) Administer terbutaline subcutaneously
(B) Digital examination
(C) Positional changes
(D) STAT Cesarean section
(E) Turn off Pitocin

cord prolapse?

The answer is B: Digital examination. Given the timing, patient risk profile, and tracing changes, this patient is at high risk to have cord prolapse that can be detected on digital examination. It is not recommended that a prolapsed cord be replaced and labor allowed to continue. Preparation for immediate delivery via Cesarean section should begin if vaginal delivery is not imminent. Avoid handling loops of cord outside the vagina because this can cause vasospasm. Having an assistant elevate the head to prevent compression has only anecdotal support in the literature, whereas placing the mother in knee–chest position has been shown to prevent further cord compression. Tocolysis should only be considered if the delivery will need to be delayed.

---

23 A 29-year-old G2P2 woman reports that her last menstrual period (LMP) was 3 weeks ago, and she is in the emergency room complaining of excruciating right-sided pain that began 2 hours ago. She rates the pain as 8 on a 10-point scale. Her vital signs are BP 104/56, P 92, T 37°C, R = 22. She gives a history of regular menstrual cycles that occur every 28 days and last for 4 days. She has a negative history for sexually transmitted diseases, is currently married, and is mutually monogamous with the father of her children. Her past medical history is significant for asthma that is well controlled and irritable bowel syndrome that has responded to diet change. Her past surgical history is significant for a bilateral tubal ligation 7 years ago. She is currently taking no medications. She is visibly uncomfortable. Her physical examination is significant for rebound and guarding in the right lower quadrant. In addition, pelvic examination reveals a mass approximately 5 cm in diameter in the right adnexal area. What is the next step in management?

(A) Hemoglobin and hematocrit
(B) Kidneys, ureters, and bladder x-ray of the abdomen
(C) Surgery consultation
(D) Transvaginal ultrasound (U/S)
**(E)** Urine pregnancy test

The answer is E: Urine pregnancy test. Although the patient will certainly require a pelvic sonogram, the best answer for this question initially is to perform a simple pregnancy test. In the outpatient setting, the pregnancy test of choice is urine due to false positives that can occur with serum testing. If the pregnancy test is positive, a quantitative beta human chorionic gonadotropin (β-hCG) should be performed. In the emergency room, they typically perform serum testing with a reflex quantitative titer. If the pregnancy test is positive, this patient is at over 30% risk for an ectopic pregnancy given that she previously had a bilateral tubal ligation.

---

24 A 31-year-old G2P0010 at 5 week's gestation presents for her first prenatal visit complaining of vague abdominal cramping and bleeding that is slightly less than her normal menstrual period. The most appropriate steps you take to evaluate this patient are:

(A) β-hCG and progesterone
(B) Qualitative beta human chorionic gonadotropin (hCG) and complete blood count (CBC)
(C) Serial quantitative β-hCG
(D) ultrasound (U/S) and CBC
(E) Quantitative β-hCG, then U/S

The answer is E: Quantitative beta human chorionic gonadotropin (β-hCG), then U/S. This patient has first-trimester bleeding. The differential diagnosis for this presentation is ectopic pregnancy, threatened abortion, and molar pregnancy. Ectopic pregnancies occur about 20/1,000 pregnancies. Ectopic pregnancy is the leading cause of maternal mortality in the first trimester. The studies that will most appropriately differentiate among these conditions are the quantitative β-hCG and transvaginal U/S. If the quantitative level is above 1,500 mIU/L, a gestational sac on transvaginal U/S should be visible. If no gestational sac is visible, an ectopic pregnancy must be ruled out.

---

25 A healthy 23-year-old woman presents to the emergency room after passing out at work. Her medical and surgical history is remarkable: chlamydia treatment 6 months ago and an appendectomy at the age of 6. She describes a menstrual period 4 weeks earlier followed by 2-week history of intermittent vaginal spotting. Her menstrual cycles are typically every 23 days. The most appropriate initial step to evaluate this patient is:

(A) Serial quantitative beta human chorionic gonadotropin (β-hCG)
(B) CBC c. serum progesterone
(C) Transvaginal ultrasound (U/S)
(D) Qualitative β-hCG

The correct answer is D: Qualitative β-hCG. In women of reproductive age presenting with abnormal bleeding, ruling out pregnancy should be the first consideration. If this patient is pregnant, she is at risk for ectopic, molar pregnancy, or a threatened abortion in which case additional studies are performed that typically include a quantitative β-hCG and transvaginal U/S. This patient is at an increased risk for ectopic pregnancy due to her history of chlamydia and an appendectomy.

---

26 A 31-year-old G1P0 at 40 weeks presents with premature rupture of membranes (PROM). Her cervix is cl/th/high. She progressed to 4 cm after a single dose of misoprostol, but over the past 3 hours, she has not changed her cervix. An intrauterine pressure catheter (IUPC) is placed and the Montevideo units (MVUs) per 10 minutes equal 40. The source of the failure to dilate at this point is most likely:

(A) Fetal presentation
(B) Infant size
(C) Shape of the pelvis
(D) Arrest of labor
(E) Uterine contractility

The correct answer is E: Uterine contractility. An arrest disorder of labor cannot be diagnosed until the patient is in the active phase and the contraction pattern exceeds 200 MVUs for 2 or more hours with no cervical change. Extending the minimum period of oxytocin augmentation for active-phase arrest from 2 to 4 hours may be considered as long as fetal reassurance is noted with fetal heart rate (HR) monitoring.

---

27 A 34-year-old G2P1 is traveling with her family for a vacation when she notes a gush of fluid vaginally and reports to the nearest labor and delivery (L&D) for evaluation. She does not have her prenatal records with her, but states that she is 39 week's pregnant. An ultrasound (U/S) that is performed in triage places her at 42 week's gestation. A biophysical profile (BPP) score of 10/10 and evaluation of the vaginal secretions yields no pooling or ferning. Cervix is 2/50/–2. When she receives the U/S report, she asks if she should be induced because her dates have now changed. Why is induction of labor not indicated?

(A) She has a normal fetal evaluation
(B) No prenatal labs are available
(C) Her cervix is not favorable
(D) Third-trimester U/S confirms her estimated gestational age (EGA)
(E) She does not have placental sulfatase deficiency

The answer is D: Third-trimester U/S confirms her estimated gestational age (EGA). The accuracy of U/Ss in pregnancy varies with gestational age (GA). In the first trimester, it is accurate within 1 week, in the second trimester it is accurate within 2 weeks, and in the third trimester it is accurate within 3 weeks. This means if the last menstrual period (LMP) is within that limit of accuracy, the LMP is confirmed. If it is outside the zone, the EGA is changed to the sonographic dating. In this case, the patient has a cervix favorable for induction, but given that her membranes are intact and she has a reassuring fetal status due to the 10/10 BPP, induction of labor is not indicated. Placental sulfatase deficiency is associated with failure to initiate labor spontaneously. The absence of prenatal labs is not a reason to delay an indicated induction of labor.

---

28 A 26-year-old woman, G1P0, presents to labor and delivery (L&D) at 34-week gestation complaining of visual changes and right upper quadrant pain. BP on arrival is 165/105. Urine protein is 3+ on dipstick.

She is painfully contracting regularly every 3 minutes. The fetal heart tracing is category I and her cervical examination is initially 5 cm but changes within 1 hour to 6 cm. After admission, magnesium sulfate is administered in order to:

(A) Accelerate fetal lung maturity
(B) Decrease BP
(C) Prevent seizures
(D) Provide maternal relaxation
(E) Stop uterine contractions

The correct answer is C: Prevent seizures. This patient most likely has severe preeclampsia, and although she is currently in preterm labor, she is currently in active labor. Magnesium sulfate is indicated in this case to prevent maternal seizure activity not to stop uterine activity. Antihypertensives such as labetalol are used to lower BP. There is insufficient time to administer steroids to accelerate fetal lung maturity.

---

29 A 22-year-old G2P2 with late prenatal care presented to labor and delivery (L&D) at 33-week's gestation with 7 cm of dilation. She delivers a male infant with Apgar score of 5/6. The infant does not look completely normal, appearing symmetrically small for dates with some hypotonia, a cleft palate, and polydactyly. What is the most likely chromosomal diagnosis?

(A) Trisomy 21
(B) Trisomy 18
(C) Trisomy 13
(D) Turner syndrome (monosomy X)
(E) Cri du chat (del 5p) syndrome

The answer is C: Trisomy 13. Trisomy 13 occurs in about 1 in 16,000 newborns. Sometimes called Patau syndrome, it is a chromosomal condition associated with severe intellectual disability and physical abnormalities in many parts of the body. Individuals with trisomy 13 often have heart defects, brain or spinal cord abnormalities, microphthalmia, polydactyly, cleft lip, and hypotonia. The prognosis is poor; only 5% to 10% of children with this condition live past their first year, while most die within the first few days to weeks of life. The quad screen does not determine the risk status for this chromosomal abnormality. It is typically diagnosed when ultrasound (U/S) findings reveal typical anomalies, and an amniocentesis is performed. A chorionic villus sampling can also diagnose this condition antenatally.

---

30 A 45-year-old G2P1 is currently 13 week's pregnant. Her blood type is O negative. She is planning on an amniocentesis in 2 weeks and is reluctant to accept the recommended Rhogam after the procedure. She asks if there is a way she might be able to avoid the injection. Paternal testing is offered and the father of the baby is found to be homozygous RHD. What is the probability that their child will have an Rh-positive blood type?

(A) 0%
(B) 25%
(C) 50%
(D) 75%
(E) 100%

The answer is E: 100%. The RHD gene is dominant so a person is considered to be Rh (D)-positive whenever this gene is present, even though the gene may have been inherited from only one parent. Conversely, a person will be Rh (D)-negative if no RHD gene is inherited from either parent. If the partner were heterozygous for the RHD gene, there would be 50% chance that the baby will inherit the dominant gene. The only way the patient can assure that the baby will not be Rh positive is if the partner was homozygous RHD negative.

---

31 A 25-year-old G4P3 presents to the emergency room 2 hours after Thanksgiving dinner with her family. She is at 10-week gestation and just noted scant vaginal bleeding. Uterine size on pelvic examination was 6 to 8 weeks. An ultrasound (U/S) reveals an intrauterine pregnancy consistent with 6-week gestation with absent fetal heart motion. Which of the following is an inappropriate management plan for this patient?

(A) Expectant management
(B) Immediate dilation and curettage (D&C)
(C) Misoprostol
(D) Office aspiration
(E) Suction curettage in ambulatory surgical center.

The answer is B: Immediate dilation and curettage (D&C). It is inappropriate to perform an immediate D&C in this stable patient with a full stomach. All of the other options are reasonable depending on the patient's wishes.

---

32 A 28-year-old G3P0020 has been trying to conceive for the past 3 years. After her second spontaneous abortion at 6 week's gestation, she has now maintained a pregnancy to 18 weeks. She and her husband are very concerned about her risk of miscarrying again. A routine anatomy ultrasound (U/S) is normal and confirms a viable male infant with normal anatomy. You reassure the patient and inform her that approximately 80% of spontaneous abortions occur by what gestational age (GA)?

(A) 6 weeks
(B) 8 weeks
(C) 10 weeks
(D) 12 weeks
(E) 14 weeks

The answer is D: 12 weeks. There is a dramatic decrease in pregnancy loss after 12 weeks.

---

33 A patient presents at 8 week's pregnant or at 8 week's gestation for her prenatal visit. Her main complaint is nausea and occasional vomiting. Her weight is the same as her prepregnancy weight. What do you tell her?

(A) She has hyperemesis gravidarum
(B) She has delayed gastric emptying due to progesterone effect
(C) She could have appendicitis and needs a computed tomography (CT) scan
(D) She has anorexia due to her lack of weight gain

The answer is B: She has delayed gastric emptying due to progesterone effect. Patients will have nausea and vomiting commonly in pregnancy. Hyperemesis gravidarum can only be diagnosed if a patient has lost 5% of her body weight and had ketosis. Progesterone effect along with beta human chorionic gonadotropin (hCG) cause nausea in pregnancy.

---

34 A 31-year-old G3P2002 woman presents to obstetrician (OB) clinic at 39 weeks 3 days complaining of contractions that occur two to three times per hour and last about 20 seconds. The patient has received prenatal care throughout her pregnancy and has had no complications. Her chart indicates that she has a hemoglobin of 8.0 g/dL measured at 36 weeks and a history of anemia. Her other labs show type O+ blood, rubella immune, HIV negative, and group B strep (GBS) positive. Her BP today is 133/77 with a pulse of 88. Fetal heart tones are in the 150s. Physical examination shows a gravid uterus with a fundal height of 36 cm. The baby is found to be vertex by Leopold maneuvers. Speculum examination shows an anterior, soft, thinning cervix with some serous discharge. Microscopic examination of the vaginal discharge shows few bacteria, 0 to 5 white blood cells (WBCs)/hpf (high power field), 0 to 5 RBCs/hpf. No ferning was noted. Manual cervical examination indicates that she is dilated 3 cm, 75% effaced, and at 0 station.

What is the next step in the management of this patient?

(A) Schedule patient for a Cesarean section at 40 weeks
(B) Expectant management
(C) Admit the patient to the labor and delivery (L&D) and admit the patient to L&D and start antibiotics
(D) Order an ultrasound (U/S) to verify the baby's status, station, and orientation
(E) Schedule a biophysical profile (BPP) for the following day

Table 4-1 The Bishop Score 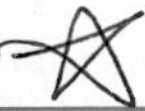

Score	Cervical Dilation	Cervical Effacement	Station of Baby	Cervical Position	Cervical Consistency
0	Closed	0–30%	–3	Posterior	Firm
1	1–2 cm	40–50%	–2	Mid-line	Moderately firm
2	3–4 cm	60–70%	–1, 0	Anterior	Soft (ripe)
3	5+ cm	80%+	+1, +2		

Add 1 point to overall score for preeclampsia and for each prior vaginal delivery.

Subtract 1 point off overall score to postdate pregnancy, no prior births, and premature or prolonged rupture of membranes. A score below 5 is considered unfavorable, while a score of 6 or above is favorable. A score of 9 or higher indicates a very high likelihood of a successful induction of labor with a subsequent vaginal delivery.

The answer is B: Expectant management. The Bishop score is an algorithm that was developed to determine the likelihood of successful spontaneous induction of labor in an obstetrical patient. The basic components of the score are cervical dilation, cervical position, cervical consistency, cervical effacement, and fetal station. Occasionally, the following modifiers are added: number of previous vaginal deliveries, presence of preterm premature rupture of membranes (PROM), being postdates, and preeclampsia status. This patient scores points for multiparity, favorable cervical position, consistency, and effacement. Also the station is favorable for spontaneous labor. In a patient where spontaneous labor is anticipated, expectant management is appropriate (Table 4-1). A score below 5 is considered unfavorable, while a score of 6 or above is favorable. A score of 9 or higher indicates a very high likelihood of a successful induction of labor with a subsequent vaginal delivery. This patient is not a candidate for a medically indicated Cesarean section at this time. U/S and a BPP are unnecessary as the position is known and no other comorbidities are present.

35 A 19-year-old G0 presents to the clinic as a new patient complaining of nausea, vomiting, and malaise. She states that her last period was 11/20/2012. She is sexually active with multiple partners and uses condoms for contraception intermittently. Her last sexual encounter was on 12/25/12, but she states that she had more than 15 partners in the past 2 months. An office pregnancy test confirms that she is pregnant.

Assuming regular periods, what is her most likely due date?

(A) Cannot be determined without ultrasound (U/S)
(B) 8/20/2013
(C) 8/27/2013
(D) 9/17/2013
(E) 9/27/2013

The answer is C: 8/27/2013. Naegele rule states that the estimated date of delivery can be accurately estimated by subtracting 3 months from the date of the last menstrual period (LMP) and adding 1 week.

---

36 A 31-year-old G1P0 at 40 5/7 weeks is currently admitted to labor and delivery (L&D). The patient has been laboring for 16 hours with intact membranes. Fetal heart tracing is category 1 with moderate variability. Her cervix is 6 cm dilated, 80% effaced, and −2 station. The decision to perform amniotomy is made. The fluid is turbid, greenish black, and contains a large quantity of tar-like substance.

What is the next step in the management of this patient?

(A) Expectant management
(B) Amnioinfusion
(C) Urgent Cesarean section
(D) Intravenous antibiotics
(E) Transabdominal ultrasound (U/S)

The answer is B: Amnioinfusion. The amniotic fluid is stained with thick meconium. In the absence of fetal distress signs on the fetal heart tracing, continued nonsurgical management is appropriate. To that end, amnioinfusion of saline is beneficial to thin the meconium and may prevent meconium aspiration syndrome in the neonate.

37 A 32-year-old G4P2011 at 40 1/7 weeks is laboring in labor and delivery (L&D). On admission, her vital signs were as follows: BP 133/68 mmHg, HR 84 beats/min, temperature 98.8°F, fetal heart tones (FHTs) 145 and reactive, fundal height 33 cm. During her sixth hour of labor, her membranes spontaneously rupture, and the fluid is noted to be dark with thick meconium present. FHT continues to be reactive with periodic variable decelerations. The patient's cervical examination shows 7 cm, 80% effaced, and 0 station.

What is the next step in the management of this patient?

(A) Urgent Cesarean section
(B) Forceps-assisted vaginal delivery
(C) Amnioinfusion
(D) Expectant management
(E) Call anesthesia to place an epidural

The answer is C: Amnioinfusion. Amniotic fluid stained with thick meconium is an important indication for amnioinfusion. Amnioinfusion decreases the risk of meconium aspiration syndrome by diluting and thinning the meconium making it easier for the baby to clear her lungs. Deep variable decelerations on the fetal heart tracing can be an indication of early fetal distress. Meconium aspiration syndrome is a cause of significant morbidity to the neonate that would necessitate a neonatal intensive care unit admission. It would be inappropriate to place an epidural at this time as this would not address the meconium stained fluid. The baby has not demonstrated the arrest of descent or other complications of delivery that would require immediate procedural intervention. In the presence of thick meconium, expectant management would not be appropriate due to the risk to the baby.

---

38 A 16-year-old G2P1001 at 39 1/7 weeks by dates has been laboring in labor and delivery (L&D) for 18 hours. She was admitted for active labor, and she has had no prior prenatal care. On admission her fundal height was 32 cm. estimated gestational age (EGA) was appropriate on ultrasound (U/S) but she was noted to have low fluid. The fetal heart tracing was reactive with HRs hovering around the 140s, and she was contracting every 4 to 5 minutes. Her cervical examination showed a 5-cm dilated cervix, 80% effacement, and –2 station. The nurse reports that the patient felt a gush of fluid and requests your verification. On examination, a small amount of pooling is seen in the vaginal vault, and ferning is present when the fluid is analyzed microscopically. She completed her previous dose of Penicillin G 3 hours ago. Her cervical examination is now 8/100/–1. As you are talking with the patient, you notice a change in the fetal heart tracing. Variable decelerations are noted. The decision is made to place an intrauterine pressure catheter (IUPC) and a scalp electrode. Her contractions are about 3 minutes apart and measure 260 Montevideo units (MVUs) per 10 minutes.

What is the next step in the management of this patient?

(A) Order a third dose of Penicillin G
(B) Amnioinfusion
(C) Expectant management
(D) Perform an operative vaginal delivery
(E) Perform an emergent Cesarean section.

The answer is B: Amnioinfusion. In the situation of a mother who has oligohydramnios who is experiencing repetitive variable decelerations, amnioinfusion is indicated to facilitate a vaginal delivery as long as there are no contraindications or urgent concerns for the safety of mother or baby. The patient's contractions are adequate as determined by the measurement being greater than 200 MVUs. In a GBS-positive or unknown patient, Penicillin G therapy prior to delivery is indicated to prevent neonatal Guillain-Barre syndrome (GBS) infection. An initial dose of 5 million IUs is given followed by 2.5 million units every 4 hours thereafter until the baby is delivered. Ideally, the patient should receive at least two doses before delivery. Expectant management could be considered in the absence of the combination of oligohydramnios and variable decelerations. There is no evidence of arrest of descent or other indication for operative vaginal delivery. There are also no medical indications for a Cesarean section at this time.

39 A 28-year-old G1P0 presents to the clinic for her 42-week appointment. She states that she is tired all the time, and her feet swell when she stands for too long. When her cervix is checked by the physician, it is noted that it is posterior, closed, thick, and very firm. As discussion begins regarding the possibility of induction, the patient asks what can be done to improve her chances of having her baby vaginally.

What do you tell her as her care provider?

(A) Cesarean section is the best option for the baby at this point
(B) The cervix must ripen on its own
(C) Induction with artificial ripening agents is an option
(D) Sexual intercourse always ripens the cervix
(E) A transvaginal ultrasound (U/S) will tell us if your cervix is ready to deliver

The answer is C: Induction with artificial ripening agents is an option. Current guidelines indicate that it is acceptable to allow a pregnancy to continue up to 42 weeks of gestational age (GA) without any intervention. Once the 42-week threshold is reached, prompt delivery by Cesarean section or induction is indicated. Cesarean section is not mandated. The earliest GA that an elective induction can be considered is 39 weeks. Artificial induction of labor is generally accomplished by three ways: intravenous Pitocin, intravaginal misoprostol, and bulb dilation of the cervix. Cervical ripening agents such as dinoprostone can also be utilized to soften the cervix. Anecdotally, sexual intercourse softens the cervix and can induce labor, but it is not 100% successful. The semen contains prostaglandins (PGs) that promote ripening of the cervix. A transvaginal U/S will not add any new or useful information at this stage and is indicated. The Bishop score of this patient is −2. See *Table 4-1* that outlines the Bishop score. A score of 6 or higher indicates high likelihood of a successful induction.

40 A 27-year-old G2P1011 presents to your clinic for preconception counseling. Two years ago she had a second-trimester miscarriage and postmortem examination of the fetus detected spina bifida. She desires another child and wants to know how to prevent a recurrence.

Which of the following recommendations can decrease the risk of another fetus being affected with spina bifida?

(A) 100 μg/d folic acid
(B) 200 μg/d folic acid
(C) 400 μg/d folic acid
(D) 2 mg/d folic acid
(E) 4 mg/d folic acid

The answer is E: 4 mg/d folic acid. Women with a history of pregnancies affected by neural tube defects (NTDs) are encouraged to take

4 mg/d of folic acid to decrease the chance for a recurrence. About 400 μg/d is the current daily folic acid recommendation for pregnant women with no history of a pregnancy affected by an NTD. About 50 to 100 μg/d is the current daily folic acid intake recommendation for nonpregnant women.

---

41 A 23-year-old G2P1001 at 10 week's gestation presents to the emergency room with acute right-sided abdominal pain of 2-hour duration. She is diaphoretic and restless. Her vitals are as follows: HR 110, RR 22, BP 90/65, temperature 98.7. Abdominal ultrasound (U/S) reveals fluid in the right lower quadrant. She has no significant past medical history and her last pregnancy was a spontaneous vaginal delivery with no complications. At her first prenatal visit, 2 weeks ago, an intrauterine pregnancy was seen on U/S.

What is the most appropriate course of action, following fluid resuscitation, in caring for this patient?

(A) Observation
(B) CT scan
(C) Transvaginal U/S
(D) Surgical exploration
(E) Surgical exploration followed by weekly progesterone injections

The answer is D: Surgical exploration. This patient likely has a hemoperitoneum secondary to a ruptured corpus luteum cyst. She is unstable on presentation and therefore the first steps in management should address her hemodynamic status. After the patient is stable, surgical exploration is necessary to ensure bleeding has stopped from the ruptured corpus luteum. At 10 week's gestation, the placenta is providing sufficient progesterone to maintain the pregnancy so progesterone injections following surgery to remove the ruptured corpus luteum are not necessary. Transvaginal U/S would be necessary to evaluate a possible ectopic pregnancy, but this patient had a documented intrauterine pregnancy at her previous prenatal visit. CT scan is not indicated as this patient is hemodynamically unstable and the findings are not likely to change the treatment plan.

42 A 23-year-old G1P0 presents for prenatal care during her first trimester. Despite an up-to-date vaccination record, the initial labs reveal that she is not immune to rubella. She has heard about the "blueberry muffin" babies and wants to prevent any chance of this happening to her child.

What is the most appropriate step to address this young mother's concerns?

(A) Administer MMR immunoglobulin at this visit
(B) Administer the MMR vaccination postpartum
(C) Administer the MMR vaccine after the first trimester
(D) Administer the MMR vaccination when the infant stops breast-feeding
(E) Recommend routine prenatal care as the mother is not at risk for rubella

The answer is B: Administer the MMR vaccination postpartum. The MMR vaccine is a live attenuated vaccination and is contraindicated during pregnancy due to a risk of teratogenicity. Women are regularly tested for immunity to rubella during prenatal lab workup due to the risk for congenital rubella syndrome. The appropriate management of a rubella nonimmune patient is to administer the vaccine postpartum. This is not a contraindication for breastfeeding.

---

43 An 18-year-old G2P1001 at 10 week's gestation presents for initiation of prenatal care. Her previous pregnancy was uncomplicated and she has no relevant past medical history. As part of her initial prenatal evaluation she tests positive for gonorrhea. What is the appropriate management at this time?

(A) Ceftriaxone 125 mg IM
(B) Azithromycin 1,000 mg PO
(C) Metronidazole 2 g PO
(D) Ceftriaxone 125 mg IM + azithromycin 1,000 mg PO
(E) Ceftriaxone 125 mg IM + azithromycin 1,000 mg PO + metronidazole 2 g PO

The answer is D: Ceftriaxone 125 mg IM + azithromycin 1,000 mg PO. Up to 40% of women with gonorrhea also have concomitant chlamydia infection. It is necessary to treat both infections so this patient must receive ceftriaxone and azithromycin. A test of cure is only necessary if symptoms fail to resolve with treatment. Repeating the gonococcus (GC) test during the third trimester is recommended because reinfection is common.

44 A 27-year-old G2P1001 at 37 week's presents to your clinic for a routine prenatal care visit. She complains of mild discomfort while urinating so you decide to perform a urinalysis. The urinalysis shows large leukocytes, positive nitrites, negative protein, and trace blood. What is the most appropriate next step in managing this patient?

(A) Treat with a 7- to 10-day course of amoxicillin
(B) Treat with a 7- to 10- day course of cephalexin
(C) Treat with a 7- to 10-day course of nitrofurantoin
(D) Perform a urine culture prior to initiating any form of treatment
(E) Treat with nitrofurantoin daily for the remainder of the pregnancy

The answer is B: Treat with a 7- to 10-day course of cephalexin. This patient has a symptomatic urinary tract infection (UTI) which much be treated to prevent progression to pyelonephritis. Performing a urine culture prior to treating the UTI can be useful for determining specific bacteria sensitivities; however, it is not necessary to initiate treatment as the urinalysis is diagnostic for a UTI. Nitrofurantoin is commonly used to treat UTIs in pregnant women; however, it is contraindicated at full term because of the risk of hemolytic anemia. Amoxicillin is another commonly used drug to treat UTIs; however, cephalexin has better coverage for *Escherichia coli*, the most common cause of UTIs.

---

45 A 25-year-old G1P0 presents for her routine obstetrician (OB) visit. On her previous visit, she has 3+ leukocytes and positive nitrites on urinalysis so you sent the specimen for culture. The results today show she has an *E. coli* urinary tract infection (UTI). This is the second occurrence of a UTI in her pregnancy. She asks you why she has another infection when she had never had a problem before becoming pregnant. Which of the following statements is most accurate regarding UTI incidence in pregnancy?

(A) Bacteria are present in higher quantities during pregnancy, making the need for good hygiene of increased importance
(B) There is no known reason for increased incidence; the patient should be reassured
(C) During pregnancy, there is decreased bladder tone and ureteral dilation which increases the risk of UTI
(D) All kinds of infection, including UTI, are increased during pregnancy due to hormonal changes

The answer is C: During pregnancy, there is decreased bladder tone and ureteral dilation which increases the risk of UTI. Progesterone causes smooth muscle relaxation which decreases bladder tone and causes dilation of the ureter. There is also mechanical obstruction on the ureters caused by the enlarged uterus which adds to the urine stasis and increases UTI risk as well as pyelonephritis risk.

---

46 A G2P1 presents to your office complaining of dysuria at 28 week's gestation. Her urinalysis shows many WBCs and positive nitrites, as well as trace blood. She has not had any complications throughout this pregnancy and has no past medical conditions. You diagnose her with a urinary tract infection (UTI). Which of the following statements is most accurate regarding the treatment of her infection?

(A) The antibiotic of choice should cover gram-negative rods
(B) She should have a 3-day course of antibiotics
(C) She does not require a test of cure after completion of antibiotics
(D) The treatment is based on urinalysis alone, making a culture unnecessary.

The answer is A: The antibiotic of choice should cover gram-negative rods. Most UTIs (70%) are caused by *E. coli*, so the first-line antibiotic choice should cover this bacteria (most frequently used are bactrim and nitrofurantoin). Although you can treat based on a urinalysis, a urine culture should always be sent to ensure you have chosen the correct antibiotic with appropriate sensitivities. A 5- to 7-day course of antibiotics is preferred during pregnancy. A repeat urinalysis should be done at each visit to monitor for repeat infection.

---

47 A 24-year-old G1P0 at 8 weeks by last menstrual period (LMP) comes to clinic to establish new obstetrician (OB) care. She has no history of hypertension, diabetes, or other medical condition and takes no medications other than PNVs. She denies any spotting or discharge. She has not had any surgeries. She has had regular Pap smears since the age of 21 with no abnormal results. She reports working as a waitress. She reports eating a healthy diet and exercising at least 30 minutes daily up to 6 days a week for the past 3 years. Her exercise regimen includes moderate aerobics and yoga. She expresses fear of gaining too much weight during the pregnancy and wants to know how much she can exercise. What advice do you give?

(A) She should switch to light exercise not to exceed 30 minutes daily

(B) She can continue a moderate-intensity exercise regimen

(C) She should switch to exercise that does not elevate the HR above 55% of the maximum HR for her age

(D) She should switch to weight training but avoid exercise in the supine position

(E) She should not exercise while pregnant

The answer is B: She can continue a moderate-intensity exercise regimen. Recommendations in pregnancy for exercise in patients with no other medical conditions or obstetric complications include 30 minutes of moderate exercise on most days. Pregnant patients are actually encouraged to engage in moderate physical activity to obtain the same benefits prior to pregnancy. Some physical activities that could potentially lead to abdominal trauma by contact or with a high risk of falling should be discouraged. Warning signs that exercise may need to be terminated include vaginal bleeding, chest pain, headache, dyspnea prior to exertion, decreased fetal movement, or amniotic fluid leak. Previously inactive pregnant women should be evaluated before exercise recommendations can be made. Since this woman was previously and consistently active, she can continue a regimen with modifications that include safe physical activity and avoiding a supine position after the first trimester as well as understanding warning signs that would indicate a need to see her physician and discontinue exercise.

 A 17-year-old girl presents to the emergency room with acute onset of constant sharp right lower quadrant pain. She reports having a positive pregnancy test 1 week ago in clinic. Her last menstrual period (LMP) was about 2 months ago. The patient denies any vaginal bleeding or fever. On physical examination, you find the patient to be tachycardic with BP 90/50. Physical examination reveals some abdominal distention with right lower quadrant abdominal tenderness and guarding but no rebound. Lab values show a hemoglobin of 8 and hematocrit of 24 with a normal WBC count and a beta human chorionic gonadotropin (β-hCG) of 2,200. You perform a vaginal ultrasound (U/S) and find an empty uterus and fluid in the cul-de-sac. Based on this presentation what is the next step?

(A) Consult general surgery
(B) Order a CT scan
(C) Proceed to the operating room
(D) Admit for transfusion

The answer is C: Proceed to the operating room. The presentation is consistent with ectopic and the patient is anemic and unstable.

 A 25-year-old G3P2002 at 36 week's gestation comes for her routine prenatal visit. Her first pregnancy resulted in a term vaginal delivery without complication. Her last pregnancy was complicated by footling breech presentation and she underwent a Cesarean section. She asks you if she will have to have another Cesarean section this pregnancy. Which of the following is the most appropriate counseling regarding her situation and past obstetrical history?

(A) Trial of labor after Cesarean section (TOLAC), if unsuccessful, has more complications than a repeat Cesarean section
(B) The most serious complication for a TOLAC is arrest of descent
(C) Her age makes her less likely to have a successful TOLAC
(D) Her previous vaginal delivery does not favor a successful TOLAC because it was before her Cesarean
(E) Less than half of women who attempt TOLAC after one Cesarean are successful

The correct answer is A: Trial of labor after Cesarean section (TOLAC), if unsuccessful, has more complications than a repeat Cesarean section. If a TOLAC is successful, it has fewer complications than a Cesarean section. However, if it is unsuccessful, then the complications exceed that of a Cesarean section. The most serious complication of a vaginal birth after Cesarean section (VBAC) is uterine rupture, which is considered a medical emergency that can lead to hemorrhage, maternal death, or fetal demise. Favorable factors for a successful TOLAC include previous vaginal delivery, including previous VBAC, favorable cervix, spontaneous labor, and breech as indication for previous Cesarean. Negative factors include increased number of prior Cesarean deliveries, gestational age (GA) over 40 weeks, and birth weight over 4,000 g. Classical or unknown Cesarean scar is a contraindication.

---

50 A 21-year-old G2P0010 presents to your clinic to establish prenatal care. She has a history of chlamydia and an ectopic pregnancy which was treated with methotrexate. She has asthma that is well controlled and has no surgical history. Her last menstrual period (LMP) was 9 weeks ago and she is concerned that this pregnancy is also ectopic because of her history.

What evaluation would best determine that the current pregnancy is normal?

- **(A)** No intervention needed
- **(B)** Perform a pelvic examination as well as a transvaginal ultrasound (U/S)
- **(C)** Abdominal CT to rule out ectopic pregnancy
- **(D)** Perform bimanual examination to assure uterine size correlates with gestational age (GA)

The answer is B: Perform a pelvic examination as well as a transvaginal ultrasound (U/S). A full physical examination including a pelvic should be done to rule out any abnormalities of the uterus that could affect implantation. A beta human chorionic gonadotropin (β-hCG) level will help to rule out any pathologies such as a molar pregnancy. At nine weeks, the U/S should confirm that the pregnancy is intrauterine.

---

51 A 28-year-old G1P0 at 30 week's gestation comes to your office because of increased swelling in her ankles. The patient works as a nurse and reports increased swelling in her ankles over the past 2 weeks, especially by the end of the work day. She denies any headache, changes in vision, or abdominal pain. Physical examination shows vitals within normal limits and 1+ pitting edema to the level of her mid-calf. She has had good prenatal care with no complications during the pregnancy.

What other information would you initially need to make a diagnosis of physiologic edema of pregnancy?

- **(A)** Serial BPs over a 6-hour period
- **(B)** Urine dipstick to test for protein
- **(C)** 24-Hour urine protein collection
- **(D)** Electrocardiogram
- **(E)** Admission to hospital for 24-hour observation

The answer is B: Urine dipstick to test for protein. While other tests may be needed for further evaluation if the patient has additional symptoms in the future, you can effectively rule out preeclampsia as a cause for the edema with a negative urine dip for protein. The other choices listed would be more important in a patient with a positive past medical history for a heart condition, hypertension, or preeclamptic disease.

---

52 A 32-year-old G6P3105 at 37 3/7 week's gestation presents to the hospital in active labor. Upon performing a vaginal examination, you find the patient to be dilated to 3 cm and 90% effaced and are able to palpate a foot. The patient wants to know if she will be able to have a vaginal delivery.

Which of the following counseling statements is most accurate?

(A) This is a footling breech, which is a contraindication to vaginal delivery incomplete
(B) This is a complete breech, which can be delivered vaginally depending on the skill of the physician
(C) This is a frank breech, which can be delivered vaginally depending on the skill of the physician
(D) No breech should ever be delivered vaginally

The answer is A: This is a footling breech, which is a contraindication to vaginal delivery. The palpation of a foot at the cervix is indicative of a footling breech presentation which is a contraindication to vaginal delivery. This patient should be taken for a Cesarean section. The figure below illustrates the different breech presentations (see *Figure 4-2*).

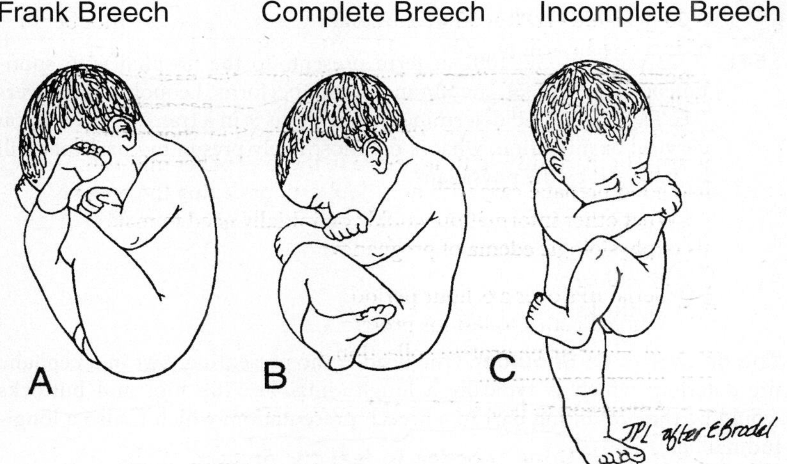

Figure 4-2

Frank or complete breech presentations may be delivered vaginally, but the decision is dependent on the availability of an experienced health-care provider.

---

53 A 27-year-old woman presents to your clinic after having a positive pregnancy test. She reports menarche at age 13, and irregular menses occurring every 1 to 3 months. She is unsure of her last menstrual period (LMP) but believes that it was around 6 weeks ago. Her past medical history includes type 2 diabetes which is well controlled with metformin. What is true about the dating of her pregnancy?

(A) Her LMP would be the most reliable dating method
(B) Perform an U/S; if she is in the first trimester, the accuracy is within 1 week of GA
(C) Perform an U/S; if she is in the second trimester, the accuracy is within 1 week of GA
(D) Due to her irregular menses, you will not be able to reliably date her pregnancy

The answer is B: **Perform an U/S; if she is in the first trimester, the accuracy is within 1 week of GA.** When dating a pregnancy you can use the LMP if it is a sure date or the pregnancy was achieved via in vitro fertilization or intrauterine insemination. If the LMP is unknown or the first-trimester ultrasound (U/S) gives a due date more than 8 days off from the LMP, the dates will be changed/set at the due date determined by U/S. U/Ss in the first trimester are most accurate, within 3 to 5 days of the actual gestational age (GA).

---

54 A 22-year-old G2P1001 at term presents to the hospital with spontaneous rupture of membranes. You perform Leopold maneuvers (see *Figure 4-3*) and determine that the fetus is in a transverse lie. Upon cervical examination, what is the most likely presenting part that will be palpated by the physician?

(A) Head
(B) Foot
(C) Shoulder
(D) Buttocks

The answer is C: **Shoulder.** The head is the presenting part in a cephalic presentation, which is typically a longitudinal lie. The foot and buttocks would be the presenting part in a breech presentation, which is also a longitudinal lie.

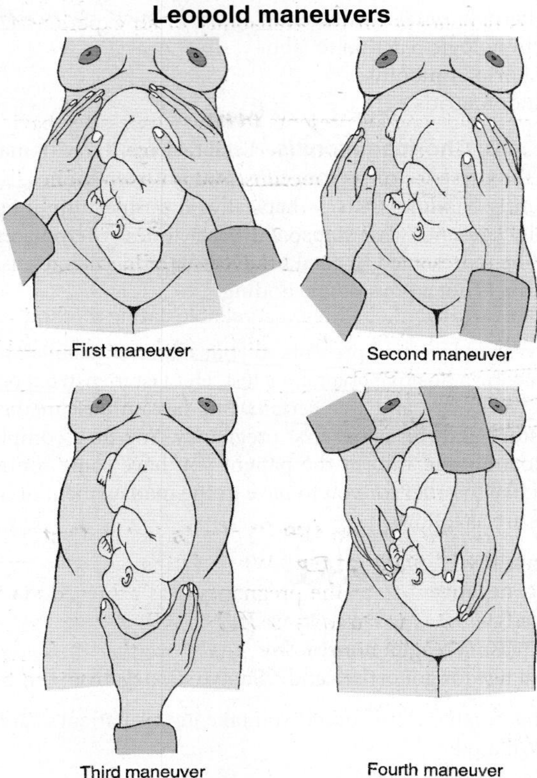

Figure 4-3

55 A 27-year-old G4P2103 at 37 week's gestation presents to labor and delivery (L&D) triage with contractions every 5 minutes. She feels like she has been leaking fluid for the past 2 days but thought that it was part of her normal vaginal discharge. On speculum examination, she is found to have a positive pooling test and you are able to identify ferning under the microscope. The Doppler shows fetal heart tones (FHTs) consistently over 180 beats/min. There are no decelerations. Vital signs of the patient include a temperature of 102.0°F and an HR of 107. All other vital signs are stable and there are no other significant findings on physical examination.

Based on these findings, what is the most likely etiology of the fetal tachycardia?

(A) Fetal anemia
(B) Uteroplacental insufficiency
(C) Physiologic reaction to labor
(D) Chorioamnionitis
(E) Endometritis

The answer is D: Chorioamnionitis. Fetal tachycardia with maternal fever, especially in the presence of prolonged rupture of membranes, is most likely chorioamnionitis. Endometritis is typically a postpartum infection. Fetal anemia usually presents with sinusoidal heart tones. Uteroplacental insufficiency would be represented by fetal bradycardia or decelerations. Consistent fetal tachycardia is not a physiologic finding.

---

56 A 22-year-old woman presents to your clinic to establish prenatal care after having a positive pregnancy test. Her last menstrual period (LMP) was 5 weeks ago and was certain. She has no past medical or surgical history and this is her first pregnancy. You do a complete physical examination and inform the patient you have some routine labs you would like to order for you to have in the management of her care. The results are as follows:

HIV: negative
HbsAg: negative
Rubella IgG: 10
Rapid plasma reagin: nonreactive
GCC (a test for gonorrhea and chlamydia): negative

What further steps should you take in this patient's care from these results, if any?

(A) Repeat GCC during the second trimester
(B) Get a full hepatitis panel and viral load
(C) Immunize the patient for hepatitis B
(D) Immunize the patient with MMR postpartum
(E) Order a treponemal antibody test

The answer is D: Immunize the patient with MMR postpartum. A patient is considered to be rubella immune when they have a titer >20. Due to the theoretical capability of the MMR vaccine to infect the fetus because it is a live vaccine, it cannot be administered until the postpartum period.

CHAPTER

5

Obstetrics Screening and Surveillance

1 A 19-year-old G1P0 is laboring at 38 weeks. Her pregnancy is complicated by minimal prenatal care. On the fetal monitor, you notice a baseline fetal heart rate (FHR) 140 with absent variability and recurrent late decelerations (see *Figure 5-1*). The maternal vital signs are as follows: heart rate (HR) 88, blood pressure (BP) 120/76, T 98.2. Based on the patient's fetal monitor, what would be the best course of management?

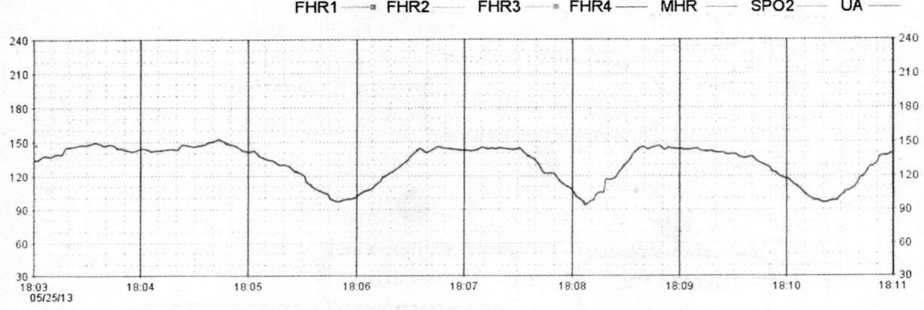

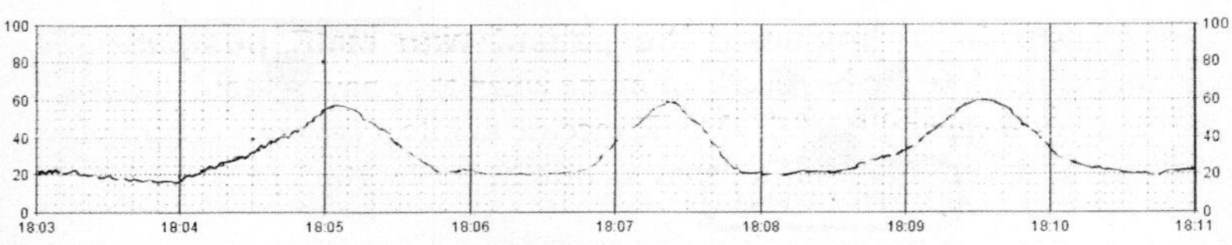

Figure 5-1

(A) Delivery by Cesarean section
(B) Expectant management of vaginal delivery
(C) Send the patient home with directions of when to follow up in the office
(D) Schedule an induction of labor for the next day

The answer is A: Delivery by Cesarean section. This patient has a category 3 FHR tracing which is associated with increased risk of fetal hypoxic acidemia. Category 3 strips are defined as FHR tracings with absent baseline FHR variability and recurrent late decelerations, recurrent variable decelerations, or bradycardia. Patients with these tracings should be prepared for delivery. Category 3 tracings are linked neonatal hypoxic-ischemic encephalopathy. Scalp stimulation can be attempted to provoke FHR acceleration, but delivery should be accomplished expeditiously if no improvements are seen (see *Figures 5-2 to 5-5*).

The Basics

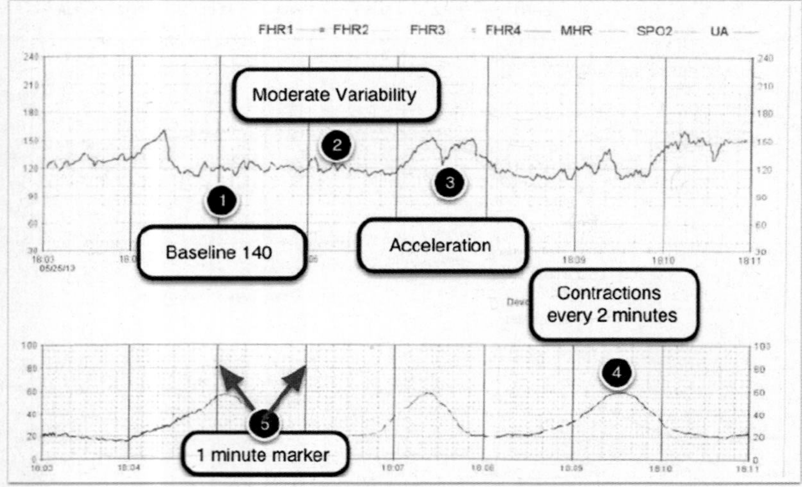

Figure 5-2

Variable Decelerations

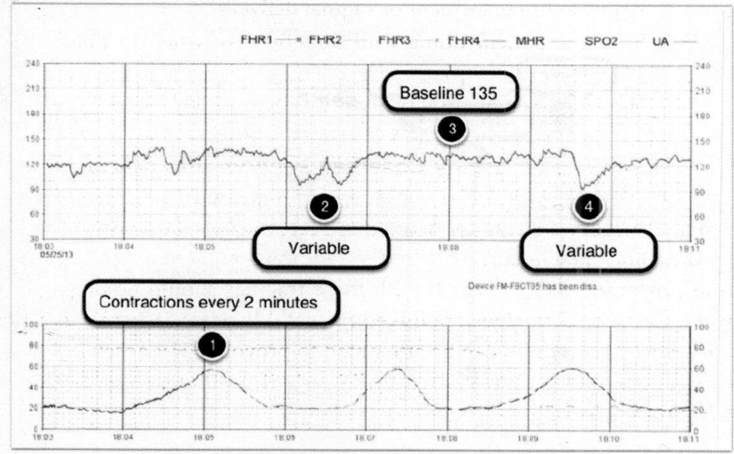

Figure 5-3

Early Decelerations

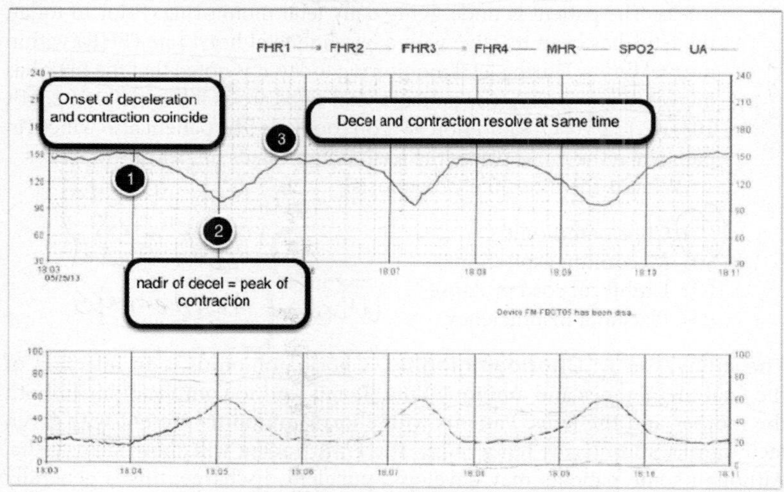

Figure 5-4

Late decerations

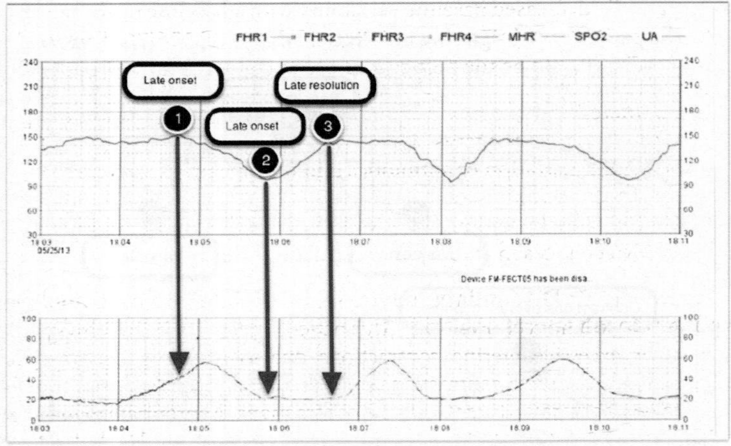

Figure 5-5

---

2 A 31-year-old patient has been on the maternal fetal medicine floor for 2 weeks due to preterm premature rupture of membranes (PPROM) at 28 weeks. The patient is undergoing daily fetal monitoring. Prior to today, the fetus has been reactive with a baseline fetal heart rate (FHR) within normal limits. During fetal monitoring today, it is noted that the FHR has increased and is 180. The patient's vital signs are as follows: T 101.2, HR 103, BP 122/76, O_2 saturation 98% on room air. The patient also winces in pain when the nurse places the fetal monitor pads on her gravid uterus.

What is the most likely diagnosis?

(A) Chorioamnionitis
(B) Meconium aspiration
(C) Umbilical cord prolapse
(D) Placental insufficiency

The answer is A: **Chorioamnionitis.** Chorioamnionitis is an infection of the fetal membranes and amniotic fluid. It can lead to complications in both the mother and the fetus. Patients with chorioamnionitis present with fever, tachycardia, and uterine tenderness. The FHR tracing will show tachycardia. Although some patients may develop a purulent discharge, this is generally considered a late presentation of uterine infection. Patients with PPROM are at increased risk for developing chorioamnionitis.

---

3 A 28-year-old G2P1 at 42 weeks is undergoing induction of labor. She was started on oxytocin a few hours ago and is currently receiving 10 mU/min. She has complained of seven very painful contractions

over the past 10 minutes. You notice that the fetal strip is showing dramatically decreased baseline variability with a baseline heart rate of 170. The patient's vital signs are as follows: HR 90, BP 126/76, T 98.9.

What would be the best course of management for this patient?

(A) Increase oxytocin to 12 mU/mL and continue monitoring the patient and the fetus
(B) Administration of antibiotics and immediate Cesarean section
(C) Discontinue oxytocin, administer oxygen, and place the patient in left lateral position
(D) No changes in care need to be made at this time

The answer is C: **Discontinue oxytocin, administer oxygen, and place the patient in left lateral position.** This patient appears to be in tachysystole—abnormal or excessive uterine contractions due to oxytocin. Tachysystole is defined as more than five contractions in 10 minutes. In this scenario, the fetus appears to be poorly tolerating the strong contractions. Appropriate management should focus on resorting uterine adequate uterine perfusion and includes discontinuing oxytocin, administering oxygen, and placing the patient in lateral position. Aggressive IV fluid administration may also be beneficial. After tachysystole and fetal heart rate (FHR) changes have been resolved, oxytocin can be resumed.

---

4 A 26-year-old laboring patient at 40 weeks presents to labor and delivery (L&D) with spontaneous rupture of membranes (ROMs). Prior to today, her pregnancy has been uncomplicated. On fetal monitoring, fetal heart rate (FHR) appears to be 140 with good variability. There are also three deep V-shaped decelerations which last 20 seconds with quick recovery to baseline.

What is the most probable cause of the decelerations?

(A) Decreased uterine perfusion
(B) Chorioamnionitis
(C) Fetal head pressure against the birth canal
(D) Umbilical cord compression

The answer is D: **Umbilical cord compression.** The question describes variable FHR decelerations that are abrupt decreases in FHR below the baseline FHR. The decrease in FHR is 15 beats/min or more, with duration of 15 seconds or more. They should not last more than 2 minutes. Variable decelerations can occur before, during, or after a contraction. These are usually associated with umbilical cord compression due to oligohydramnios. Most of the time, these decelerations can be resolved by repositioning the patient.

---

5 A 32-year-old G2P1 is laboring while you are on service. Past medical history for this patient is significant for prior Cesarean section with her first delivery. She desires a trial of labor after Cesarean section (TOLAC).

When you last checked the patient, she was 6 cm dilated and 1+ station. Her fetal strip has been category 1 throughout the morning. Over the past few minutes, you have observed a few variable and late decelerations on the fetal strip. The maternal vital signs are as follows: HR 105, BP 90/52, T 98.9. When you check on the patient, she appears to be dizzy and confused. She is complaining of severe abdominal pain. Bimanual examination shows that the cervix is 6 cm dilated and the fetus is −1 station.

What is the most likely diagnosis?

(A) Chorioamnionitis
(B) Placental abruption
(C) Natural progression of labor
(D) Uterine rupture

The answer is D: Uterine rupture. This patient is at increased risk for uterine rupture due to history of Cesarean section. Uterine rupture is a rare but severe complication during labor. Signs of uterine rupture include nonreassuring fetal heart rate (FHR) changes, regression of fetal station, maternal abdominal tenderness, maternal tachycardia, and hypotension. Fetal strip may show variable and late decelerations. It may also show fetal bradycardia. A high index of suspicion is needed for this diagnosis as it can lead to multiple adverse outcomes, including severe hemorrhage, hysterectomy, and infant morbidity or death.

---

6 A 24 year old G_1P_0 at 39 week's presents to triage and believes she may be in labor. Fetal monitoring shows a baseline of 149bpm with moderate variability and some visually apparent increases in FHR from 140 to 160 that last 30 seconds. One deceleration is present that seems to mirror the patient's uterine contraction. On bimanual exam she is 5cm dilated. Patient's contractions appear to be regular and every 3 minutes. Patient is unable to speak through contractions due to pain.

Which of the following would be the best strategy in management for this patient?

(A) Immediate Cesarean section
(B) Send the patient home due to false labor
(C) Admission and expectant management on L&D
(D) Repeat the cervical examination in 2 hours to evaluate for active labor

The answer is C: Admission and expectant management on L&D. This patient appears to be in labor. She is having regular contractions and is dilated to 5 cm. Her fetal strip is category 1 and reassuring due to moderate variability, accelerations, and only an early deceleration. She should be admitted to labor and delivery (L&D) for expectant management.

7 A 25-year-old woman G2P0101 presents to the hospital in active labor. She has received no prenatal care. She is 5 cm dilated and states she had a gush of fluid more than 24 hours prior to her presentation to the hospital. You obtain an ultrasound that shows she is 41 week's pregnant, and she has a negative urine drug screen. Her labor is progressing normally and the fetal heart rate (FHR) tracing is category 1. She should be treated for:

(A) Gestational diabetes
(B) Group B strep
(C) Preeclampsia
(D) Preterm labor given no prenatal care

The answer is B: Group B strep. Patients without screening for group B strep should be treated based on risk factors. Risk factors are rupture of membranes (ROMs) greater than 18 hours, fever during labor, labor before 37 weeks, urinary tract infection (UTI) during pregnancy with GBS, or prior infant infected with GBS. There is no evidence in this patient for diabetes, preeclampsia. An ultrasound showing 41 week's gestation should exclude preterm labor.

---

8 A 34-year-old primigravida presents in active labor at 36 + 6 weeks. Her pregnancy has been complicated by gestational diabetes as well as having a body mass index of 33. At 35 weeks, she tested positive for group B strep. She is having contractions every 4 minutes and is 5 cm dilated. She has no allergies to any medications.

Which antibiotic should she receive upon hospital admission?

(A) Ciprofloxacin 400 mg IV
(B) Vancomycin 1 g IV
(C) Penicillin G 5 M units IV
(D) Clindamycin 900 mg IV

The answer is C: Penicillin G 5 M units IV. The first-line antibiotic for group B strep is penicillin G. Many hospitals do not have access to Penicillin G and the substitution to ampicillin is used. Clindamycin is the antibiotic of choice for patients with a significant penicillin allergy. Vancomycin is used if the patient has penicillin allergy and the sensitivities to clindamycin are unknown. Ciprofloxacin is not used to treat Guillain-Barré syndrome (GBS) or used in pregnancy.

---

9 A G2P1 presents for her routine prenatal care visit at 36 weeks 2 days by sure last menstrual period and consistent with a second-trimester ultrasound. She has chronic hypertension but her BPs have been stable on nifedipine. She has no other complications with her pregnancy. She plans to use the intrauterine device for postpartum birth control.

What test is indicated at this visit?

(A) Rectovaginal culture for group B strep
(B) Quad screen
(C) Transvaginal ultrasound for cervical length
(D) Hemoglobin A1c

The answer is A: Rectovaginal culture for group B strep. Screening for group B strep is performed between 35 and 37 weeks for all patients unless they have had a urinary tract infection (UTI) with group B strep during their current pregnancy. The asymptomatic colonization is 10% to 35%. None of the other tests listed are indicated at this gestational age.

---

10 A G2P1001 comes to your office concerned about the health of her child. Her first child is now 8 years old and displays behavioral problems and poor performance in school. The patient had read that exposure to or ingestion of certain substances during pregnancy can lead to her child's current difficulties.

Which of the following substances is associated with poor school performance and behavioral difficulties?

(A) Cocaine
(B) Caffeine
(C) Peyote
(D) Marijuana
(E) Tobacco

The answer is E: Tobacco. Of the listed substances, tobacco use during pregnancy has been most definitively shown to be associated with poor school performance and behavioral difficulties. Tobacco use during pregnancy has also been associated with premature birth, miscarriage, placental abruption, placenta previa, preterm labor, low birth weights, cleft lip and palate, and sudden infant death syndrome.

---

11 A 36-year-old, G2P1, decides to undergo first-trimester genetic screening. At 11 weeks, her blood is drawn and an ultrasound performed. The results are positive for a risk of trisomy 21 above her age-related risk. She is offered chorionic villus sampling (CVS) as a diagnostic test.

Which of the following findings was most likely seen on her first-trimester screening?

(A) Decreased level of human chorionic gonadotropin (hCG)
(B) Decreased level of pregnancy-associated plasma protein A (PAPP-A)
(C) Decrease in size of the nuchal transparency (NT)
(D) Decrease level of α-fetoprotein (AFP)

The answer is B: Decreased level of pregnancy-associated plasma protein A (PAPP-A). First-trimester screening consists of two biochemical markers: free or total hCG and PAPP-A. An elevated level of hCG (1.98 of the median observed in euploid pregnancies [MoM]) and a decreased level of PAPP-A (0.43 MoM) have been associated with Down syndrome. The size of the NT is an ultrasonographic marker for Down syndrome; an increase in the size of the NT between 10 4/7 and 13 6/7 weeks is recognized as an early presenting feature of a variety of chromosomal, genetic, and structural abnormalities. Second-trimester screening utilizes AFP; low maternal serum AFP is associated with Down syndrome.

---

12 A 28-year-old, G1P0, was referred to a genetic counselor to discuss chorionic villus sampling (CVS) in the first trimester. Her first-trimester screening results indicated an increased risk of trisomy 21: ultrasound revealed a significantly increased size of the nuchal translucency and maternal serum screening for two biochemical markers were abnormal.

Which of the findings most likely reflect the patient's serum test results?

(A) Decreased levels of hCG and pregnancy-associated plasma protein A (PAPP-A)
(B) Elevated level of hCG and decreased level of PAPP-A
(C) Decreased level of hCG and increased level of PAPP-A
(D) Elevated levels of hCG and PAPP-A

The answer is B: Elevated level of hCG and decreased level of PAPP-A. First-trimester screening assesses the risk of trisomies 13, 18, and 21. This is performed between 10 and 14 weeks' gestation. Screening consists of two biochemical markers and an ultrasonographic marker. Free or total hCG and PAPP-A are measured in the maternal serum. An elevated level of hCG (1.98 MoM) and a decreased level of PAPP-A (0.43 MoM) have been associated with trisomy 21. Nuchal translucency is measured on ultrasound between 10 and 14 week's gestation. Increased size is recognized as an early presenting feature for a variety of chromosomal, genetic, and structural abnormalities. Combining the nuchal translucency measurement with the maternal serum biochemical markers yields an 82% to 87% detection rate of trisomy 21 with false-positive rate of 5%. Women found to have increased risk after first-trimester testing should be offered genetic counseling and diagnostic testing for definitive diagnosis. CVS can be performed in the first trimester. Amniocentesis is performed in the second trimester.

---

13 A 38-year-old, G1P0, presents for her first obstetric (OB) visit at 16 weeks. She is concerned about her fetus' risk of chromosomal abnormalities, especially since she is of advanced maternal age (AMA). After counseling, she decides to pursue noninvasive genetic screening.

Which of the following describes the advantages of the quadruple screen over the triple screen?

(A) Adding inhibin to the triple screen improves the detection rate of trisomy 21 to approximately 80%
(B) Adding hCG to the triple screen improves the detection rate of trisomy 21 to approximately 80%
(C) Adding inhibin to the triple screen improves the detection rate of trisomy 18 to approximately 80%
(D) Adding hCG to the triple screen improves the detection rate of trisomy 18 to approximately 80%

The answer is A: **Adding inhibin to the triple screen improves the detection rate of trisomy 21 to approximately 80%.** With the triple screen, the levels of α-fetoprotein (αFP), intact hCG, and estradiol are used to modify the maternal age-related trisomy 21 risk. The detection rate is 70% and approximately 5% of all pregnancies will have a false-positive result. Adding inhibin A to the triple screen (quadruple screen) improves the detection rate for trisomy 21 to 80%. Inhibin A is not used in the calculation of risk for trisomy 18.

---

14 A 33-year-old, G4P3, had normal first-trimester genetic screening at 12 weeks. Her pregnancy has been uncomplicated and she presents for a routine obstetric (OB) visit at 18 weeks.

Which second-trimester screening test is the most appropriate to further screen her pregnancy for aneuploidy?

(A) Independent second-trimester serum screening with the quadruple screen
(B) Ultrasound screening once at 26 week's gestation
(C) Serum screening if being performed as a component of integrated or sequential screening
(D) Amniocentesis

The answer is C: **Serum screening if being performed as a component of integrated or sequential screening.** Women who have had first-trimester screening for aneuploidy should not undergo subsequent independent second-trimester screening. The false-positive rates are additive and will lead to unnecessary invasive procedures. The results of both first- and second-trimester screening and ultrasound can be combined to increase the detection of aneuploidy. There are several ways to do this: integrated (nuchal transparency [NT], pregnancy-associated plasma protein A [PAPP-A], and hCG in the first trimester followed by quadruple screen in the second trimester; results are reported after both first- and second-trimester screening are complete), serum integrated (PAPP-A in the first trimester followed by quadruple screen in the second trimester; results are available after both first and second-trimester screening are complete), stepwise sequential (NT, PAPP-A, and hCG in the first trimester followed by quadruple screen in the second trimester; first report is available after first-trimester screening is completed; final report follows second-trimester screening), and contingent sequential screening (following first-trimester screening, those at very low and very high risk receive results; those at moderate risk proceed to second-trimester screening and obtain a final report). Integrated screening provides the highest sensitivity with the lowest false-positive rate; however, having to wait 3 to 4 weeks between initiation and completion of integrated screening can create a lost opportunity to consider chorionic villus sampling (CVS) if the first-trimester portion indicates a high risk of aneuploidy. CVS in the first trimester and amniocentesis in the second trimester are diagnostic tests.

---

15 A 38-year-old G0 and her 39-year-old husband have been trying to conceive for the last 8 months without success. Neither the patient nor the husband has any medical problems. In addition, there are no known genetic diseases in either family. The patient's periods occur at regular intervals and an at-home kit indicates ovulatory cycles. The patient has had regular Pap smears since age 21 with no abnormalities. The patient was diagnosed with bacterial vaginosis 6 months ago, and was treated with metronidazole 500 mg orally two times a day for 7 days with a normal test of cure. Today the patient appears in good health with HR 70, BP 110/72, RR 18, T 98.6, H 63, W 125. Neither the patient nor her husband smoke, drink, or use illicit drugs.

What is the next best step in management of this couple's infertility?

(A) Inform the patient that it is likely due to advanced maternal age (AMA) and immediately begin an infertility workup with a semen analysis to rule out the male factor

(B) Counsel the couple on good conception practices and if still unsuccessful at 12 months tell the couple to return for infertility assessment

(C) Perform a hysterosalpingogram to evaluate possible tubal infertility secondary to scaring from the patient's bacterial vaginosis infection

(D) Refer the couple for genetic counseling, as the infertility may be associated with maternal and/or paternal genetic abnormalities

(E) Due to AMA, schedule an appointment in 1 month to harvest eggs and plan for in vitro fertilization at 12 months if the couple has not conceived naturally

The answer is A: Inform the patient that it is likely due to advanced maternal age (AMA) and immediately begin an infertility workup with a semen analysis to rule out the male factor. The patient in the question is older than 35 and therefore is considered to be of AMA. In AMA, infertility assessment starts after 6 months of failure to conceive, whereas in younger patients 12 months are allowed before starting the workup. Semen analysis is typically the first step in any infertility workup so that the male factor can be ruled in or out. Hysterosalpingogram is not indicated at this time. The other choices may need to be explored in the future but are not part of the initial workup for infertility.

---

16 A 32-year-old G0 and her husband come to see you for preconception counseling. Both the patient and her husband are of Ashkenazi Jewish descent and are concerned about the risk of having a child with a genetic disorder. The husband informs you that he had one sister who died at 4 years of age after suffering progressive developmental delay and seizures. In addition, the patient's sister had genetic screening performed, which showed that she is a carrier for a genetic disorder, but neither she, nor her two daughters are affected.

What is the next best step in counseling this couple?

(A) Advise the couple to pursue alternative parenting options such as adoption, as their genetic offspring will likely inherit a severe genetic disorder

(B) Since the patient's nieces are not affected, the couple is only at risk for having a child who may be an unaffected carrier and they should continue to pursue pregnancy

(C) The patient and her husband should be screened for Tay-Sachs disease. Depending on the test results, the couple should be informed that invasive in vitro testing may be warranted

(D) The patient and her husband should be screened for Tay-Sachs disease and, if positive, the couple should be informed that they have a 50% chance of having an affected child

(E) The patient and her husband should undergo genetic screening for Tay-Sachs disease, β-thalassemia, and α-thalassemia before further recommendations can be made

The answer is C: **The patient and her husband should be screened for Tay-Sachs disease. Depending on the test results, the couple should be informed that invasive in vitro testing may be warranted.** Tay-Sachs is an autosomal recessive disease that is noted to have an increased prevalence in the European Ashkenazi Jewish population. The genetic background of the couple and their family history place them at high risk for having a child inherit this disease and therefore screening is appropriate. Based on the results of the screen, fetal diagnosis can be performed if both the mother and the father are found to be carriers of the genetic disorder. Choices A, B, and D are incorrect because, until screening of the parents is complete, the risk to a potential fetus cannot be assessed. Choice E is incorrect, as this couple currently needs to be screened for Tay-Sachs disease.

17 A 17-year-old woman, G2P0010, presents for a second prenatal appointment. Estimated gestational age is currently 10 weeks. A urine culture performed at her first prenatal visit was positive for *Escherichia coli*. To her knowledge, she has never had a urinary tract infection (UTI) and she denies any urinary symptoms whatsoever. The appropriate management for this asymptomatic pregnant patient in the first trimester of pregnancy is:

(A) Alkalization of the urine with cranberry juice
(B) Alterations in sugar and carbohydrate intake
(C) Treatment with antibiotics
(D) Changes of sexual behavior
(E) No treatment

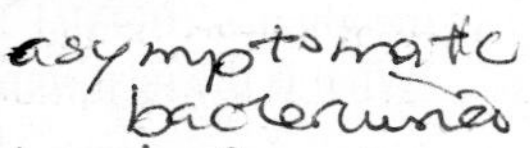

The answer is C: Treatment with antibiotics. Although there is no evidence to support treating asymptomatic bacteriuria (ASB) in the non-pregnant state, the correct answer for this pregnant patient is C, treat with antibiotics. ASB confers significant risk of pyelonephritis as well as preterm birth, low birth weight, and perinatal mortality. Studies have proven that treating this asymptomatic condition provides significant benefit and the routine screening for ASB now is considered a standard of care in early pregnancy. Choices A, B, and D are strategies that have been suggested to help reduce the risk of recurrent UTIs.

18 A 22-year-old G2P1 at 13 weeks presents for routine prenatal care. In review of her routine prenatal labs, a positive urine culture *Staphylococcus saprophyticus* is noted. A urinalysis today reveals negative nitrites. Upon review of systems, she denies any urinary frequency, urgency, or other symptoms.

What is your rationale for antibiotic treatment?

(A) Prevent kidney stones
(B) Prevent preterm labor
(C) Prevent development of antibiotic resistance
(D) Decrease the risk of chorioamnionitis
(E) Prevent second-trimester bleeding

The answer is B: Prevent preterm labor. Up to 10% of pregnancies are complicated by asymptomatic bacteriuria (ASB). Of these, about 30% will develop pyelonephritis if left untreated. Pregnancies complicated by pyelonephritis have been associated with low-birth-weight infants and prematurity. Thus, pregnant women should be screened for bacteriuria by urine culture at 12 to 16 week's gestation. The presence of 100,000 colony-forming units of bacteria per milliliter of urine is considered significant. The common urine dipstick may register negative for nitrites because *S. saprophyticus* does not reduce them metabolically. *S. saprophyticus* is the second most common causative agent for urinary tract infections (UTIs) in women. Although less common than *E. coli*, it is more aggressive. Patients infected with *S. saprophyticus* are more likely, even in non-pregnant patients to develop pyelonephritis and recurrent infection. Multiparous patients are more likely to present with ASB.

---

19 A 30-year-old G2P1 with an uncomplicated prenatal course now at 41 weeks presents in active labor. The fetal heart tracing is category 1. Not long after an examination, reveals she is 5/90/0. She has spontaneous rupture of membranes (ROMs). Light meconium-stained amniotic fluid is noted.

What is the next step?

(A) Amnioinfusion
(B) Close electronic monitoring of fetal status
(C) Fetal scalp blood sampling
(D) Immediate Cesarean section
(E) Periumbilical blood gas measurement

The answer is B: Close electronic monitoring of fetal status. Meconium is present in up to 25% of pregnancies. Pregnancies approaching 42 weeks are associated with more meconium than earlier in gestation. Typically, thick meconium and abnormalities in the fetal heart tracing are associated with meconium aspiration syndrome. However, this fetus is exhibiting a reassuring status and there is no reason to intervene.

---

20 A 29-year-old G3P2 at 40 weeks presents in active labor. She has had an uncomplicated pregnancy. As you are examining her cervix, it changes rapidly from 4 to 8 cm. Shortly thereafter, membranes rupture and meconium-stained amniotic fluid is discovered. Reexamination of the cervix reveals that she is currently 9 cm and feeling the urge to push. Fetal heart tones (FHTs) are in the 120s with occasional variable decelerations into the 90s that first occurred after rupture of membranes (ROM). The tracing also has accelerations and no evidence of late decelerations.

What is the next step?

(A) Amnioinfusion
(B) Close electronic monitoring of fetal status
(C) Epidural placement
(D) Immediate Cesarean section
(E) Vacuum extraction

The answer is B: Close electronic monitoring of fetal status *(see Figure 5-6)*. In light of this patient's history and rapid progress through labor, she will likely deliver soon. Accelerations are reassuring, and since the

FHT does not have repetitive late decelerations or severe variable decelerations, there is no reason currently to expedite the delivery of this fetus with a Cesarean section or a vacuum-assisted delivery. There is no evidence that supports an amnioinfusion given this patient's current status. While placement of an epidural is a consideration, this multiparous patient is likely to deliver before it can be placed. The overall best answer to this question is B.

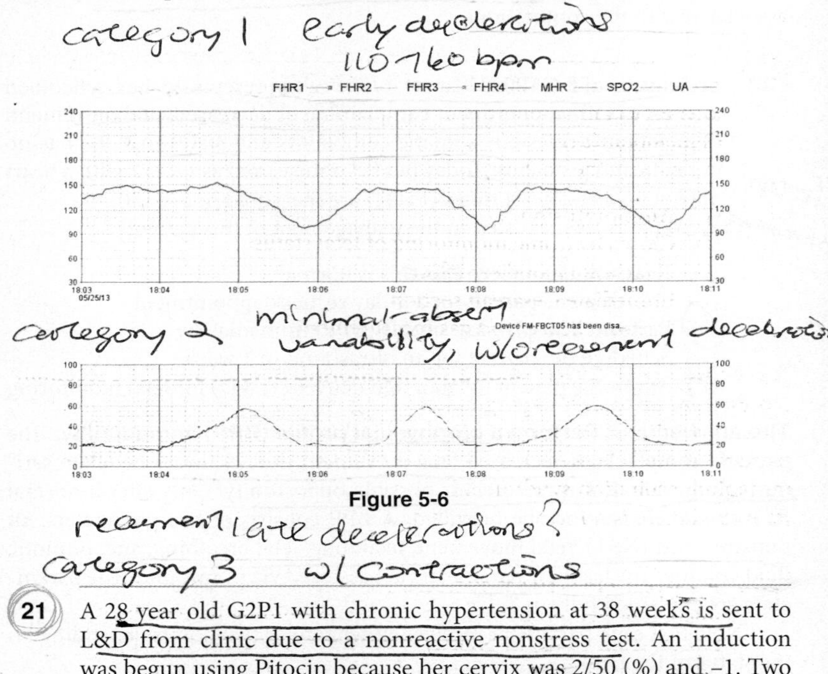

Figure 5-6

21 A 28 year old G2P1 with chronic hypertension at 38 weeks is sent to L&D from clinic due to a nonreactive nonstress test. An induction was begun using Pitocin because her cervix was 2/50 (%) and −1. Two hours into the induction, you are called to review the tracing above. The patient is currently 4 cm dilated. This tracing is particularly worrisome because it is associated with:

(A) Variable decelerations
(B) Early decelerations
(C) Tachysystole
(D) Decreased fetal heart rate (FHR) variability
(E) Tachycardia

The answer is D: Decreased fetal heart rate (FHR variability). FHR variability is categorized as absent, minimal (<5 BPM), moderate (6 to 25 beats/min), and marked (>25 beats/min). Persistently minimal or absent FHR variability is considered the most significant sign of fetal compromise. Periods of fetal sleep or administration of certain medication can alter the FHR patterns.

A category 1 tracing has a baseline between 110 and 160 beats/min and may have early decelerations. No late or variable decelerations are present.

A category 2 tracing may have minimal to absent variability without recurrent decelerations. It is not predictive of abnormal fetal acid–base status but requires continued surveillance and periodic reevaluation.

This tracing would be category 3 if it also had recurrent late decelerations associated with the contractions.

---

22 A 36-year-old G5P0222 at 31 6/7 weeks presents to her scheduled obstetric (OB) appointment complaining of decreased fetal movement. The patient denies any somatic complaints and states that she has no other health problems. Today her BP is measured as 125/77 with a heart rate of 66. Fetal heart tones (FHTs) are measured in the 130s.

What is the next step in the management of this patient?

- **(A)** Reassure the patient that this is normal
- **(B)** Schedule the patient for a 3-day recheck appointment
- **(C)** Perform a biophysical profile (BPP) immediately.
- **(D)** Schedule the patient for an ultrasound in 1 week
- **(E)** Admit the patient to labor and delivery (L&D) for fetal monitoring

The answer is C: Perform a biophysical profile (BPP) immediately. The patient's complaint of decreased fetal movement should always be taken seriously and evaluated at the earliest possible opportunity. Only after a normal BPP should reassurance be provided. A BPP consists of five parameters: an nonstress test (NST), fetal movement, fetal tone, fetal breathing, and amniotic fluid volume. The last four parameters are assessed via ultrasound. The parameters are explained fully in *Table 5-1*.

Note that each parameter receives either zero or two points depending on the status of the fetus.

The totals are significant as noted in *Table 5-2*.

A total BPP score that is 8 or greater is considered reassuring. A BPP is indicated when an NST is nonreactive, oligohydramnios is present, or the fetus is at an increased risk for stillbirth from other risk factors.

---

23 A 16-year-old G4P0131 at 30 3/7 weeks presents to your clinic complaining of occasional contractions. The patient states that they occur sporadically a few times per hour and last for less than 30 seconds. She states that she has not felt well and has not been eating. Records show that she has gained 15 lb during the course of this pregnancy and has not gained any weight in the past 4 weeks. Her BP is 122/65 with a heart rate of 77. Fetal heart tones (FHTs) are measured in the 120s. Fundal height is 26 cm.

Table 5-1 Criteria for Coding Fetal Biophysical Variables as Normal or Abnormal

Biophysical Variable	Normal (Score = 2)	Abnormal (Score = 0)
Fetal breathing movements	One or more episodes of ≥20 s within 30 min	Absent or no episode of ≥20 s within 30 min
Gross body movements	Two or more discrete body/limb movements within 30 min (episodes of active continuous movement considered as a single movement)	<2 episodes of body/limb movements within 30 min
Fetal tone	One or more episodes of active extension with return to flexion of fetal limb(s) or trunk (opening and closing of hand considered normal tone)	Slow extension with return to partial flexion, movement of limb in full extension, absent fetal movement, or partially open fetal hand
Reactive fetal heart rate	Two or more episodes of acceleration of =15 beats/min and of >15 s associated with fetal movement within 20 min	One or more episodes of acceleration of fetal heart rate or acceleration of <15 beats/min within 20 min
Qualitative Amniotic fluid volume	One or more pockets of fluid measuring ≥2 cm in the vertical axis	Either no pockets or largest pocket <2 cm in the vertical axis

From Anbazkagan A. Obstetric ultrasound and biophysical scoring. *Obs Gynae & Midwifery News*. Harrogate, North Yorkshire: Barker Brooks Communications Ltd., 2012.

Table 5-2 Implications of Biophysical Profile Score

Score	Implication
8–10	No cause for concern
6	Ambiguous, repeat test in 24 h and decide management plan depending on clinical picture
2–4	Concerning for hypoxia and acidosis, immediate delivery
0	Immediate delivery

From Anbazkagan A. Obstetric ultrasound and biophysical scoring. *Obs Gynae & Midwifery News*. Harrogate, North Yorkshire: Barker Brooks Communications Ltd., 2012.

What is the next step in the management of this patient?

(A) Reassure the patient that this is normal
(B) Schedule the patient for a 2-week recheck appointment
(C) Send the patient to the perinatal center for a biophysical profile (BPP)
(D) Schedule the patient for an ultrasound in 2 weeks
(E) Admit the patient to labor and delivery (L&D) for fetal monitoring

The answer is C: Send the patient to the perinatal center for a biophysical profile (BPP). This patient should be scheduled for a BPP to evaluate possible oligohydramnios and ensure that the fetus is stable in light of mother's poor weight gain.

---

24 A 25-year-old G3P2002 presents for her 32-week prenatal visit and states that she is not feeling the baby move as much as she did in her previous pregnancies. The patient's BP is 114/76 with a pulse of 66. Fetal heart rate (FHR) is in the 120s by Doppler. Fundal height is measured to be 33 cm.

What is the next step in the management of this patient?

(A) Reassure the patient that all babies are different
(B) Send the patient for an nonstress test (NST)
(C) Order a complete blood count, complete metabolic panel, and fetal ultrasound
(D) Admit her for 24-hour observation
(E) Urgent Cesarean section

The answer is B: Send the patient for an nonstress test (NST). Decreased fetal movement is a frequent and serious concern of a pregnant mother. If you see and examine the patient, you have a high index of suspicion that the fetus has decreased movement, an NST would provide an objective measure of the baby's status.

---

25 A 26-year-old G2P1001 presents to clinic for her 20-week prenatal visit. She excitedly reports that she no longer feels sick all the time and also denies any complaints. Her BP is 118/64 with a pulse of 76. The uterus is midway between the pubis and the umbilicus. Fetal heart tones (FHTs) are in the 150s.

What is the next step in the management of this patient?

(A) Perform amniocentesis
(B) Perform chorionic villus sampling (CVS)
(C) Reassurance
(D) Perform obstetric (OB) ultrasound
(E) Perform Leopold maneuvers

The answer is D: Perform obstetric (OB) ultrasound. The patient is 20 weeks by dates and only 16 weeks by size (see *Figure 5-7*).

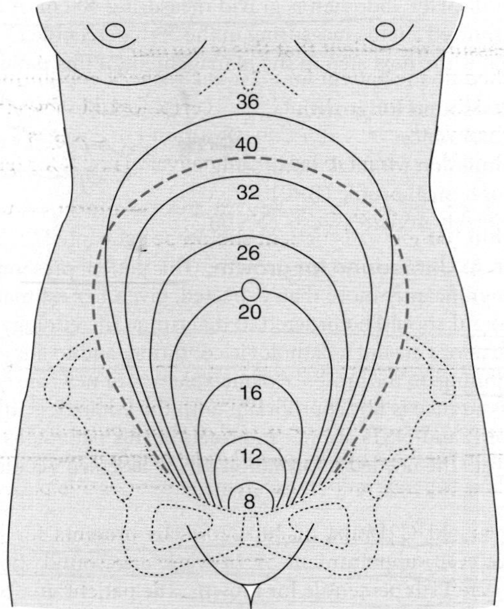

Figure 5-7

With a fundal height that is 4 weeks less than expected, reassurance is not an appropriate course of action. The best answer is to ultrasound the patient and verify dates as well as the amniotic fluid levels and ascertain if there are any gross fetal anomalies that would make the fetus small for dates at this early stage. Amniocentesis is appropriately performed between 15 and 17 weeks; however, noninvasive testing should be performed and results analyzed prior to any invasive testing. CVS is normally performed after the 10th week. This patient should receive noninvasive testing prior to any invasive testing. Leopold maneuvers would not provide any useful information at this stage of pregnancy.

---

26 A 35-year-old G3P1102 at 35 2/7 weeks presents for her scheduled obstetric (OB) visit. The patient denies any complaints today and states that she feels the baby move "some." Her pregnancy course was complicated by bleeding early in the pregnancy that subsided by week 10. She has had no complications since then. The patient denies recent vaginal discharge or bleeding. She states that she is experiencing occasional Braxton-Hicks contractions but denies other signs of labor. Fetal heart tones (FHTs) are in the 130s. Her abdomen is gravid measuring 40 cm. A 20-week ultrasound showed a fetus measuring in the 55th percentile.

What is the next step in the management of this patient?

(A) Ultrasound for growth
(B) Reassurance
(C) Admission for fetal monitoring
(D) Biophysical profile (BPP)
(E) Biweekly nonstress tests (NSTs)

The answer is A: Ultrasound for growth. This patient presents with a fundal height that is significantly more than expected, given her estimated gestational age. An ultrasound should be ordered to determine the etiology of the discordance, to confirm or rule out a pathologic condition, and to allow for appropriate delivery planning. In the presence of unexplained or new-onset fundal height anomalies, reassurance is not appropriate until the etiology is understood. The admission, a BPP, and NSTs are not indicated in this patient, as monitoring is not necessary yet. The needed information can be assessed via ultrasound.

---

27 A 22-year-old G2P0101 at 30 4/7 weeks presents for her scheduled obstetric (OB) appointment. A 24-week ultrasound showed the fetus to be in the 11th percentile for growth. The patient missed the previous three appointments but came today and denies any complaints today. The patient's previous pregnancy was complicated by preterm labor with delivery at 34 weeks. The patient denies vaginal discharge, bleeding, or abdominal cramping. Abdominal examination today shows a gravid uterus measuring 25 cm. Fetal heart tones (FHTs) are in the 140s.

What is the next step in the management of this patient?

(A) Schedule an appointment in 4 weeks
(B) Schedule a growth ultrasound
(C) Schedule biweekly nonstress tests (NSTs)
(D) Admit to hospital for fetal monitoring
(E) Schedule a biophysical profile (BPP)

The answer is B: Schedule a growth ultrasound. This patient presents with a gestation that is small for gestational age that should be evaluated promptly. This patient should be followed with serial ultrasounds to monitor the growth of the baby and allow for appropriate delivery planning. Fetal monitoring would be indicated if the baby's heart tachycardic or bradycardic or if the mother or physician was concerned about decreased fetal movement.

---

28 A 37-year-old G6P3205 at 34 4/7 with gestational diabetes moderately controlled with insulin presents for her scheduled obstetric (OB) appointment. During the course of the visit, the patient notes that the fetus is moving, but "sleeps a lot." Her previous pregnancy was also complicated by gestational diabetes and fetal macrosomia. Her BP is 138/85. Fetal heart tones (FHTs) are in the 130s. Fundal height measures 36 cm. Her last ultrasound was at 28 weeks and showed a fetus in the 93rd percentile.

What is the next step in the management of this patient for this visit?

(A) Schedule biweekly nonstress tests (NSTs)
(B) Schedule a growth ultrasound
(C) Draw preeclampsia labs and send her to triage for evaluation
(D) Reassure her and return to clinic in 2 weeks
(E) Refer to a maternal–fetal specialist for further management

The answer is A: Schedule biweekly nonstress tests (NSTs). Gestational diabetes is an important indication for scheduled NSTs. Fetal monitoring is imperative in a mother with significant comorbidities such as diabetes. Her BP is borderline, but she does not meet the criteria for preeclampsia.

---

29 A 28-year-old G2P1001 at 34 weeks presents to the clinic for her regular obstetric (OB) visit. Her pregnancy has been complicated by gestational diabetes initially managed by diet. She missed her last appointment. The patient's blood glucose log indicates postprandial glucose measurements now ranging from 180 to 360. She has an ultrasound scheduled in 2 weeks. In addition to starting the patient on insulin therapy, what would be the next step in the care of this patient?

(A) Refer the patient to a maternal fetal medicine specialist
(B) Schedule biweekly nonstress tests (NSTs)
(C) Schedule an ultrasound (U/S) for growth tomorrow
(D) Schedule a follow-up appointment to repeat the A1C in 8 weeks
(E) Counsel the patient about the importance of maintaining a hemoglobin A1C below 6.5 to prevent birth complications

The answer is B: Schedule biweekly nonstress tests (NSTs). Gestational diabetes is an important indication for scheduled NST monitoring. Scheduling additional ultrasounds is not indicated at this point. Counseling of patients is very important and should be done, but scheduling NSTs is the next step. Gestational diabetes is a risk factor for fetal macrosomia, organodysgenesis, and postpartum fetal hypoglycemia.

---

30 The patient is a 36-year-old G1P0 chronic hypertensive at 29 5/7 weeks. She denies somatic complaints today. She has been on methyldopa during this pregnancy with good results. Her BP today is 139/88 and the patient comments that that is "good for her." Her urine is negative for protein. On her 20-week ultrasound, it was noted that the fetus was in the 25th percentile. She denies vaginal bleeding, discharge, and abdominal cramping.

What is the next step in the management of this patient?

(A) Begin hydralazine therapy
(B) Schedule biweekly nonstress tests (NSTs)
(C) Schedule a growth ultrasound
(D) Schedule patient for follow-up in 2 weeks

The answer is B: **Schedule biweekly nonstress tests (NSTs).** This mother has a history of chronic hypertension and demonstrates poor fetal growth. NSTs should be scheduled to monitor the status of the baby to prevent adverse outcomes. Hydralazine therapy is not indicated at this time. Hydralazine therapy is generally reserved for inpatient use.

31 A 37-year-old G8P6107 has been laboring on labor and delivery (L&D) for 14 hours. She has a history of diabetes mellitus, hypertension, and Marfan syndrome, all diagnosed prior to pregnancy. Her membranes are still intact, and she is contracting regularly. She states that "she feels it coming" and adamantly wants to continue walking as she labors. As her physician, you convince her to go back to her room for a few minutes so that you can perform intermittent monitoring (see *Figure 5-8*). On examination, the cervix is dilated 6 cm, 95% effaced, and at +1 station. The strip below is recorded.

What is the likely etiology of the recorded tracing?

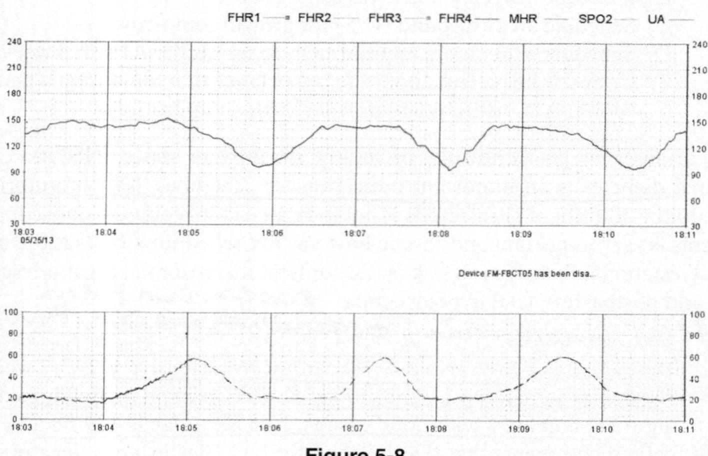

Figure 5-8

(A) Compression of the infant's head during contractions
(B) Prolapsed umbilical cord
(C) Oligohydramnios
(D) Uteroplacental insufficiency
(E) Polyhydramnios

The answer is D: Uteroplacental insufficiency. Late decelerations in the fetal heart rhythm strip are indicative of uteroplacental insufficiency.

CHAPTER

6

Obstetrics High Risk

1 An 18-year-old G1P0 with inadequate prenatal care presents to labor and delivery (L&D) in active labor at approximately 38 weeks by last menstrual period (LMP). Her admission history and physical examination are unremarkable and labor progresses with no complications. However, upon delivery the infant is in respiratory distress, has a protruding abdomen, and is covered in a bullous rash.

Which of the following tests performed on the mother might further clarify her infant's condition?

(A) Herpes simplex virus serum antibody screen
(B) Gonorrhea and chlamydia urine polymerase chain reaction
(C) Serologic testing for *Treponema pallidum*
(D) HIV serum antibody screen

The answer is C: Serologic testing for *Treponema pallidum* Given this presentation, it is possible that this infant has been born with congenital syphilis. The organism responsible for syphilis, *T. pallidum*, can cross the placenta and cause problems in development. The mnemonic TORCH can be used to organize the infections that can cross the placenta: (T)oxoplasma, (O)ther (syphilis, varicella zoster, HIV, parvovirus B-19), (R)ubella, (C)ytomegalovirus, and (H)erpes.

2 A pathologist is reviewing a placenta. She knows that the patient has had a prior Cesarean section and had to have an emergency hysterectomy with this pregnancy, hence, the placenta and uterus for her review. She reviews the slides and finds that the placenta invades through the myometrium to the uterine serosa.

What is the diagnosis?

(A) Placenta increta
(B) Placenta previa
(C) Placenta percreta
(D) Placenta accreta

The answer is C: Placenta percreta. In placenta accreta, placenta has abnormal adherence to the superficial lining of the uterus. In placenta increta, it penetrates into the muscle layer. And in percreta, there is complete invasion through the muscle to the serosal lining.

---

3 A 26-year-old G3P2002 with two previous Cesarean sections presents for her second-trimester ultrasound (U/S). The baby is growing appropriately and there are no markers for chromosomal anomalies. She is diagnosed with a placenta previa.

She is also at risk for which of the following?

(A) Gestational diabetes
(B) Preeclampsia
(C) Placenta accreta
(D) Vasa previa

The answer is C: Placenta accreta. Patients with prior Cesarean section and placenta previa are at high risk for other placental abnormalities such as placenta accreta. Vasa previa is vessels crossing the cervical os which would not be possible with placenta previa. Gestational diabetes and preeclampsia are independent of a placenta previa diagnosis.

---

4 A 36-year-old G2P1 presents in labor with a history of a prior Cesarean section and of placenta previa and accreta during this pregnancy diagnosed with magnetic resonance imaging (MRI). Her repeat Cesarean section is planned and you review the risks with her.

She is at high risk for which of the following?

(A) Anesthetic complications
(B) Emergency hysterectomy
(C) Difficulties with breastfeeding
(D) Hemolysis, Elevated Liver enzymes, Low Platelet count (HELLP) syndrome

The answer is B: Emergency hysterectomy. Patients with placenta previa and accreta are at high risk for needing hysterectomy at the time of Cesarean section (two-thirds of women). The risk of hemorrhage as well as abnormal placental separation often requires the placenta be left at its uterine attachment and the uterus removed.

---

5 A 22-year-old G1 at 20 week's gestation undergoes a routine screening ultrasound (U/S). During the procedure, several small areas of hypoechogenicity are seen within normal myometrial tissue. The fetus is developing normally and no other abnormalities are noted. The patient is very concerned about the changes in her myometrium. As her physician, what do you inform the patient?

(A) This is a normal benign physiologic change that occurs in all pregnancies
(B) Surgical intervention is warranted to protect the fetus from disruptions in blood flow
(C) These changes greatly increase the risk of postpartum uterine atony and hemorrhage
(D) These changes are usually asymptomatic and do not require therapy during pregnancy
(E) The pregnancy will likely not be affected but hysterectomy is needed after delivery

The answer is D: These changes are usually asymptomatic and do not require therapy during pregnancy. Based on the pelvic U/S, this patient most likely has uterine fibroids. Fibroid development is common during pregnancy since fibroids are hormonally responsive to estrogen. During pregnancy, they can develop and grow quickly when exposed to the high levels of estrogen. In pregnancy, most fibroids are asymptomatic and do not require treatment. Occasionally, fibroids may infarct, and contribute to intrauterine growth restriction (IUGR), malpresentation, preterm labor, and shoulder dystocia. As the physician of this asymptomatic patient, you should inform her that these findings typically require no intervention during pregnancy.

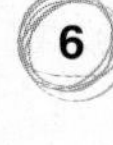

6 A 23-year-old, G2P1, presents to the emergency room with vaginal bleeding and cramping ultrasound (U/S) shows a 9-week intrauterine pregnancy without fetal cardiac activity. While getting the U/S, her bleeding and cramping increase and she spontaneously passes the products of conception.

What is the most likely etiology of her early pregnancy loss?

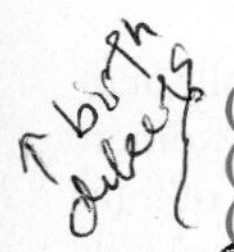

(A) Infectious disease
(B) Preexisting diabetes mellitus
(C) Teratogen-induced congenital abnormalities
(D) Fetal chromosomal abnormalities

The answer is D: Fetal chromosomal abnormalities. At least half of all first-trimester pregnancy losses result from fetal chromosomal abnormalities. Infectious disease, preexisting diabetes mellitus, and teratogen-induced congenital abnormalities have been linked to an increased risk of birth defects.

7 A 27-year-old, G1P0, is now at 18 week's gestation. Her first trimester was complicated by a false-positive result on first-trimester screening for trisomy 21. She had chorionic villus sampling (CVS) that revealed a fetal karyotype of 46, XY.

What additional screening test does she need at this time?

(A) No additional screening
(B) Quadruple screen
(C) Integrated screen
(D) Maternal serum α-fetoprotein (MSAFP)

The answer is D: Maternal serum α-fetoprotein (MSAFP). Neural tube defects (NTDs) are typically screened for in the second trimester with the triple or quadruple screen. MSAFP is the component of these screens which evaluates the risk of NTDs; women with an elevated MSAFP evaluation should receive an ultrasound (U/S) examination to detect identifiable causes of false-positive results (fetal death, multiple gestation, and underestimation of gestational age [GA]) and a targeted study of fetal anatomy for NTDs and other defects associated with elevated MSAFP. For women who have had first-trimester CVS, fetal karyotype has been determined, but screening for NTDs still needs to be performed. MSAFP is the most appropriate screening test; the remainder of the triple and quadruple screens is not needed because diagnostic genetic testing has already been performed by CVS.

---

8 A 37-year-old, G1P1, has an amniocentesis at 20 week's gestation for advanced maternal age. Amniotic α-fetoprotein (AFP) is 2.5 multiple of the median. A targeted study of fetal anatomy is performed by ultrasound (U/S) and an neural tube defects (NTD) is diagnosed.

Which of the following recommendations is the most appropriate recommendation for any future pregnancies this patient may have?

(A) Chorionic villus sampling (CVS) in the first trimester
(B) 4 mg of folic acid daily prior to conception
(C) Nuchal translucency measurement in the first trimester
(D) Genetic counseling prior to conception

The answer is B: 4 mg of folic acid daily prior to conception. Folic acid has been shown to prevent recurrence and occurrence of NTDs. For women who have previously had a child with an NTD, the recommended dose of folic acid is 4 mg daily prior to conception. Since most women at increased risk are not aware until they have an affected child, all women should take at least 0.4 mg of folic acid daily. CVS will diagnose chromosomal abnormalities, but cannot diagnose NTDs. Nuchal transparency (NT) measurement during the first trimester is an ultrasonographic marker for trisomy 21. Genetic counseling prior to conception may benefit this patient; however, the most important and appropriate recommendation is for the patient to be taking 4 mg of folic acid daily prior to conception.

9 A 55-year-old man and his 30-year-old wife present for preconception genetic counseling. A thorough family history shows no significant genetic disorders on either side. The couple is informed that advanced paternal age predisposes the fetus to an increased risk of the following:

(A) Autosomal recessive disorders
(B) X-linked recessive disorders
(C) Mitochondrial mutations
(D) X-linked dominant disorders

The answer is B: X-linked recessive disorders. Parental age of 50 or greater predisposes the fetus to an increase in gene mutations affecting X-linked recessive and autosomal dominant disorders (neurofibromatosis, achondroplasia, Apert syndrome, and Marfan syndrome). Advanced maternal age (≥35 years) also increases the risk of chromosomal abnormalities. The incidence of trisomy 21 among newborns of 35-year-old women is 1:385; the overall live birth incidence is 1:800. Although the risk increases with age, the majority of trisomy 21 cases occur in women younger than 35 years of age.

---

10 After undergoing the quadruple screening test at 16 weeks, a 24-year-old, G2P1, is notified that the fetus is at elevated risk for trisomy 18. She desires definitive diagnosis and plans to have an amniocentesis. During the preprocedure consent process, the risks of amniocentesis are discussed with her in detail.

What is the most likely outcome if amniotic fluid leakage occurs following midtrimester amniocentesis?

(A) Chorioamnionitis
(B) Pregnancy loss
(C) Heavy vaginal bleeding
(D) Rh sensitization
(E) Perinatal survival

The answer is E: Perinatal survival. Perinatal survival in cases of amniotic fluid leakage after midtrimester amniocentesis is greater than 90%. Pregnancy loss occurs in less than 1% of procedures. Heavy vaginal bleeding and Rh sensitization are rare. Patients who are Rh negative typically receive Rhogam prior to invasive diagnostic procedures such as amniocentesis, chorionic villus sampling (CVS), and cordocentesis.

---

11 A 25-year-old, G2P0010, and her husband present for a routine second-trimester ultrasound (U/S) at 20 week's gestation. She had previously declined both first- and second-trimester genetic screening. On U/S, a structural defect is discovered and an amniocentesis is offered to the patient.

Which of the following defects is most likely to be associated with aneuploidy?

(A) Gastroschisis
(B) Single umbilical artery
(C) Facial cleft
(D) Cystic hygroma
(E) Club foot

The answer is D: Cystic hygroma. The risk of aneuploidy with cystic hygroma is 60% to 75% (e.g., see *Figure 6-1*). The most common aneuploidy found is 45X (80%). There is a minimal risk of aneuploidy when gastroschisis or a single umbilical artery is seen. Facial clefts are associated with a 1% risk of aneuploidy and club food is associated with a 6% risk.

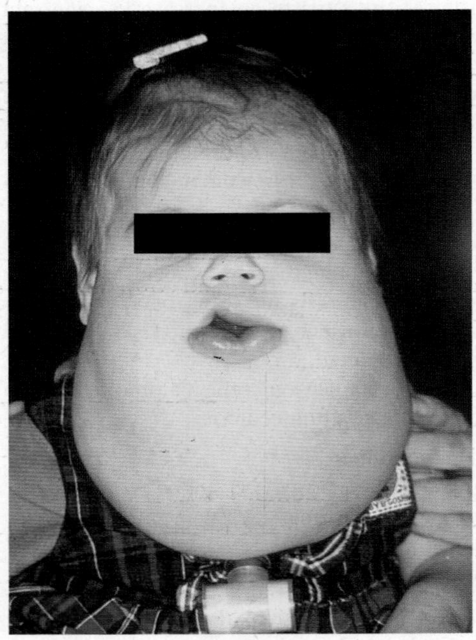

Figure 6-1

12 A 40-year-old, G4P3, presents with an unintended pregnancy at 10 week's gestation. She is concerned about her risk of Down syndrome and wishes to pursue the most effective genetic screening modality.

What screening test will have the highest detection rate for Down syndrome?

(A) First-trimester screening
(B) Second-trimester quadruple screening
(C) Stepwise sequential screening
(D) Serum integrated screening

The answer is C: Stepwise sequential screening. Stepwise sequential screening (Nuchal transparency [NT], pregnancy-associated plasma protein A [PAPP-A], and human chorionic gonadotropin [hCG] in the first-trimester followed by quadruple screen in the second-trimester; first report is available after first-trimester screening is completed; final report follows second-trimester screening) has a Down syndrome detection rate of 95%. The availability of first-trimester analysis allows for the option of fetal testing by chorionic villus sampling (CVS) for pregnancies identified to be at increased risk. Serum integrated screening (PAPP-A in the first trimester followed by quadruple screening in the second trimester) detects 85% to 88% of pregnancies with Down syndrome. The results are not reported until the second-trimester component is complete, making amniocentesis in the second trimester the recommended diagnostic option. First-trimester screening alone (NT, PAPP-A, and hCG) has a detection rate of 82% to 87%. Second-trimester screening (Maternal serum α-fetoprotein [MSAFP], hCG, unconjugated estriol, and inhibin A) has a detection rate of 81%. All of these screening tests have a 5% false-positive screen rate.

---

13 A 27-year-old, G1P0, is at 12 week's gestation. Her husband is affected with achondroplasia. They desire a first-trimester genetic diagnosis and are scheduled for chorionic villus sampling (CVS).

Which of the following ultrasound (U/S) findings will decrease the risk of pregnancy loss following the procedure?

(A) Breech fetal presentation
(B) Anterior placenta
(C) Short cervical length
(D) Uterine fibroids

The answer is B: Anterior placenta. CVS is performed after 10 week's gestation and consists of aspirating the immature placenta under U/S guidance. Transabdominal CVS has been demonstrated to have similar safety and accuracy rates to that of amniocentesis performed at or after 15 week's gestation (see *Figure 6-2*).

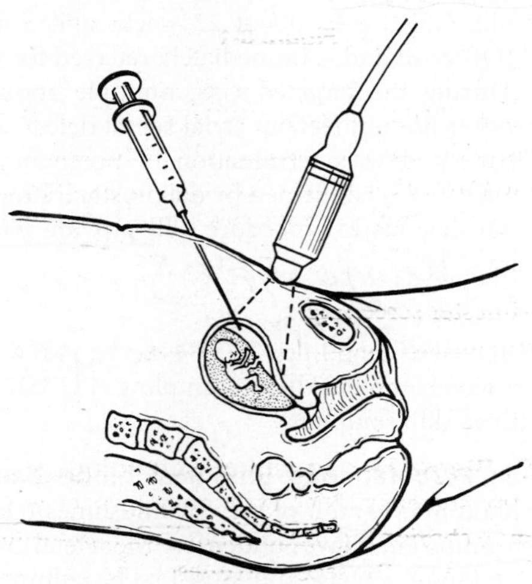

Figure 6-2

Transcervical CVS carries a higher risk of pregnancy loss (see *Figure 6-3*).

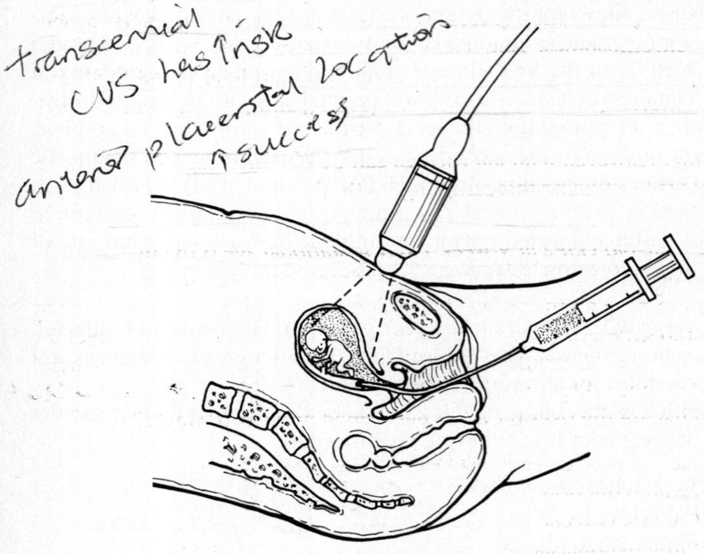

Figure 6-3

Anterior placental location will increase the likelihood that transabdominal CVS can be successfully performed. Fetal presentation, cervical length, and the presence of uterine fibroids may impact the performance of the procedure, but fetal loss has clearly been the route of CVS.

---

14 A 37-year-old, G5P4, presents at 22 weeks and 3 days for her first obstetrical (OB) visit and is immediately referred for ultrasound (U/S) screening. During the targeted U/S, multiple anomalies are noted, including rocker bottom feet, an atrial septal defect, and polyhydramnios. The patient desires termination of pregnancy if a significant genetic abnormality is confirmed by diagnostic testing.

What fetal diagnostic procedure will provide fetal DNA analysis most rapidly?

(A) Amniocentesis
(B) Chorionic villus sampling (CVS)
(C) Percutaneous umbilical blood sampling (PUBS)
(D) Fetal tissue skin sampling

The answer is C: Percutaneous umbilical blood sampling (PUBS). A karyotype is a photomicrograph of the chromosomes taken during metaphase, when the chromosomes have condensed. Most fetal cells obtained from amniocentesis are not in metaphase and must first be cultured in order to perform karyotype analysis. CVS allows for more rapid DNA analysis because the cells obtained from the placenta are more likely to be in metaphase. Fluorescence in situ hybridization (FISH) is a technique that labels genetic probes for specific chromosomes. Abnormalities in chromosome number can be identified by 48 hours. PUBS has been used to obtain fetal blood for blood component analysis (Rh status, hematocrit [HCT], and platelet count) as well as DNA analysis. With the advent of FISH, PUBS is not commonly used for genetic testing. However, fetal karyotypes can be obtained rapidly (within 18 to 24 hours) when utilizing this sampling method.

---

15 A 39-year-old G3P2 at 9-week 1-day gestational age (GA) by last menstrual period (LMP) undergoes first-trimester genetic screening. She is found to have an increased risk of Down syndrome and would like to undergo genetic testing to assess for genetic abnormalities. It is recommended that she should wait until at least 10-week GA before undergoing chorionic villus sampling (CVS).

What are the risks if CVS is performed prior to 10 weeks?

(A) Neural tube defects (NTDs)
(B) Limb reduction
(C) Cardiac defects
(D) Lung hypoplasia

The answer is B: Limb reduction. CVS performed prior to 10 weeks is associated with limb defects and oromandibular malformations. The ideal window for CVS testing is 10 to 12 weeks. After that time, it is recommended that patients undergo amniocentesis for genetic testing. CVS will not determine the presence of NTDs. If a patient undergoes CVS, she must undergo screening for NTDs later in pregnancy. The risk of NTDs can be greatly reduced with the administration of folic acid prior to conception and in the first few weeks of pregnancy. CVS is not known to have any effects on cardiac or lung formation.

---

16 A 29-year-old G2P0010 woman comes to see you at 6 weeks for her first prenatal visit. The patient had one previous pregnancy that ended in spontaneous abortion. The fetus had multiple congenital anomalies consistent with trisomy 18. The patient is now concerned that she could lose the current pregnancy and would like early prenatal testing. The patient read about chorionic villus sampling (CVS) and would like the procedure performed as soon as possible.

What is the mechanism of limb reduction in CVS before 9 weeks?

(A) Destruction of large areas of the chorionic villus
(B) Direct trauma to the growing fetus
(C) Vascular interruption to the growing fetus
(D) Leakage of amniotic fluid leading to oligohydramnios

The answer is C: Vascular interruption to the growing fetus. The mechanism of limb reduction due to CVS performed before 9 weeks is thought to be secondary to interruption of the vascular supply to the growing fetus. CVS can be used to obtain a fetal karyotype earlier than amniocentesis but should only be performed between 9 and 12 weeks to minimize the risk to the fetus. Even during this time period the risks with CVS are greater than with amniocentesis; however, CVS allows for earlier genetic diagnosis of potential abnormalities.

---

17 A recent immigrant from Nepal with no prenatal care delivers a female infant at 36-week gestational age (GA). Immediately upon delivery of the infant, the following features are apparent: protruding tongue, short arms and legs, large fontanelles, and poor muscle tone.

What is the most likely explanation for these findings?

(A) Maternal HIV
(B) Congenital rubella infection
(C) Gestational diabetes in the mother
(D) Congenital hypothyroidism

The answer is D: Congenital hypothyroidism. These are classic features of congenital hypothyroidism, or cretinism, which is most commonly caused by maternal hypothyroidism. Although hypothyroidism due to iodine deficiency is now rare in countries that regularly add iodine to salt, it is still seen in many developing nations. Congenital rubella syndrome is characterized by vision and hearing deficits and thrombocytopenic purpura (blueberry muffin rash) among other findings. Maternal gestational diabetes is a risk factor for various complications, including macrosomia, shoulder dystocia, and an increased risk of insulin resistance and diabetes mellitus type 2 later in life.

---

18 A 20-year-old G2P1001 with a history of depression, alcohol dependence, and cocaine abuse delivers a 2,046 g baby girl at 36-week gestational age (GA). She took fluoxetine throughout her pregnancy and admits to continued alcohol and cocaine use until 24 week's gestation. She also reveals that she has traded sex for cocaine in the past. On examination, the infant is found to have decreased muscle tone, slanted palpebral fissures, a highly arched palate, and a flattened nasal bridge.

Which of the following likely explains these findings?

(A) Young maternal age
(B) Fluoxetine use during pregnancy
(C) Alcohol use during pregnancy
(D) Cocaine use during pregnancy
(E) Congenital syphilis

The answer is C: Alcohol use during pregnancy. The above are classic findings for fetal alcohol syndrome, the prevalence of which is estimated to be between 0.2 and 2 per thousand live births. The risk is greatest with maternal alcohol consumption during early pregnancy and appears to increase with heavier use. Maternal age of 20 is not associated with increased risks to the fetus. Fluoxetine (Prozac) is currently a class C medication, but generally considered safe during pregnancy. Cocaine use during pregnancy is associated with premature birth, birth defects, and attention deficit disorder. Symptoms of congenital syphilis vary from poor feeding and rhinorrhea to organomegaly, skeletal abnormalities, and other findings.

---

19 A previously healthy, obese 26-year-old G1P0 has a positive glucose challenge test at 28 weeks gestational age (GA). Follow-up testing confirms the diagnosis of gestational diabetes mellitus (GDM). The patient asks what this diagnosis will mean for her baby.

Which of the following can be a significant consequence of poorly controlled GDM to the fetus?

(A) Hyperglycemia
(B) Macrosomia
(C) Cataracts
(D) Cerebral edema

The answer is B: Macrosomia. Macrosomia is a common finding in infants born to mothers with gestational diabetes. Other common findings include jaundice, transient hypoglycemia (not hyperglycemia), respiratory distress syndrome, and occasionally seizures and death. Cataracts are associated with adult diabetes, and cerebral edema is a known complication of diabetic ketoacidosis; these conditions are not commonly seen in infants born to mothers with gestational diabetes.

---

20 A routine prenatal examination for a 27-year-old G4P3003 at 27-week gestational age (GA) reveals a fundal height of only 22 cm. The patient is clinically underweight (body mass index [BMI] 18.1) and has a history of pregnancy-induced hypertension in two prior pregnancies; however, she has been normotensive during this pregnancy to date. Nonstress testing (NST) shows a fetal heart rate (HR) of 153 beats/min with moderate variability and no spontaneous decelerations.

What is the best next step in management?

(A) Immediate Cesarean section for fetal distress
(B) Scheduled induction at 37-week GA
(C) Ultrasound (U/S) biometry to verify diagnosis
(D) No action needed; fetal size is proportional to mother

The answer is C: Ultrasound (U/S) biometry to verify diagnosis. Intrauterine growth retardation (IUGR) is diagnosed when a pregnancy measures smaller than expected by prenatal U/S with reliable dating and is most commonly caused by nutritional deficits, either due to poor intake or due to metabolic disorders such as gestational diabetes mellitus (GDM). It may be symmetrical, in which growth is evenly delayed in all measurements, or asymmetrical, with the head disproportionately larger than the body. Perinatal morbidity and mortality are both significantly increased in IUGR. As NST in this case showed no evidence of fetal distress, there is no indication for either immediate Cesarean section or scheduled induction. That does not, however, mean that the condition is normal or that no further monitoring is warranted. U/S biometry is a more extensive set of prenatal measurements that are often performed in cases of suspected fetal abnormality. In this case, biometry may help to clarify the true extent of growth restriction in this fetus as well as whether the abnormality is symmetrical or asymmetrical.

---

21 A 37-year-old G3P1011 at 12-week gestational age (GA) presents to the high-risk maternity clinic for counseling after routine blood testing showed elevated levels of amniotic α-fetoprotein (AFP), estriol, and β-hCG. Ultrasound (U/S) shows increased nuchal translucency and echogenic intracardiac focus. Based on this history and these findings, the fetus is at greatest risk for which of the following?

(A) Duodenal atresia
(B) Omphalocele
(C) Micrognathia
(D) Absent thymus
(E) Hypogonadism
(F) Ambiguous genitalia

The answer is A: Duodenal atresia. Fetuses born to mothers of advanced maternal age, those with positive triple screen tests (AFP, estriol, and β-hCG), and those with prenatal U/S findings of increased nuchal translucency and cardiac abnormalities are at increased risk for trisomy 21 or Down syndrome. A postnatal finding of Down syndrome is duodenal atresia. Omphalocele and micrognathia can be seen in trisomies 13 and 18, respectively. Absent thymus is seen in DiGeorge syndrome (del22q11). Hypogonadism may be seen with multiple conditions but is commonly seen in Prader-Willi syndrome. Ambiguous genitalia may also be seen in many conditions, but generally not in trisomy 21.

---

22 Your patient is a 34-year-old G1 coming to see you for her first prenatal visit. Based on her last menstrual period (LMP), the patient is at 21 week's gestation. The patient is very excited about her pregnancy and wants to make sure she does everything to ensure a healthy baby. The patient's past medical history includes recurrent sinus infections and hypothyroidism. The patient's surgical history includes an appendectomy performed 3 years ago. The patient currently takes a prenatal vitamin and levothyroxine. The patient's blood pressure (BP) is 110/70 mmHg, HR 80 beats/min, respiratory rate (RR) 15 breaths/min, T 98, height 5′2″, and weight 129. Physical examination is normal with a fundal height of 20 cm and fetal heart tones (FHTs) of 150 to 160. Her thyroid-stimulating hormone (TSH) is slightly elevated. In addition to standard prenatal care, this patient should also:

(A) Increase levothyroxine by 25% at this appointment and again at 30 and 37 weeks

(B) Increase the levothyroxine until TSH is maintained below 2.5 mIU/L with frequent measurements of TSH and free thyroxine (T4)

(C) Increase the levothyroxine until the TSH is kept just below the normal range to prevent hyperthyroidism in the fetus

(D) Lower the TSH dosage by 25% now with frequent measurements of TSH and free T4 to ensure therapeutic levels

The answer is B: Increase the levothyroxine until TSH is maintained below 2.5 mIU/L with frequent measurements of TSH and free T4. The medical treatment of hypothyroidism in pregnancy is important to the health of the mother and the fetus. In pregnancy, the body's requirement for thyroid hormone increases secondary to increased volume of distribution, increased binding globulin, increased clearance, and increased metabolic rate. All pregnant women with hypothyroidism should have TSH and T4 levels checked at the initiation of prenatal care. Women with no reserve such as those with previous thyroidectomy or history of radioiodine ablation should have their levothyroxine increased by 25% to 30% at the initial visit. In addition, TSH and free T4 should be monitored throughout the pregnancy with increases in dose to maintain TSH below 2.5 mIU/L.

---

23 A 25-year-old G1 epileptic comes to see you for her first prenatal visit at 10 weeks. At the appointment, the patient informs you that she stopped taking her epileptic medication 2 months ago because she heard it could damage the fetus. The patient was first prescribed valproic acid 10 years ago and has not had a seizure in 5 years. The patient denies any complications since stopping the medication on her own. You inform your patient that there is an increased risk of fetal anomalies associated with epilepsy, even without medication.

What is the next best step in the management of this patient?

(A) Restart the patient on valproate but increase dosing to four times per day from two times per day, as the teratogenic risk is associated with high peak plasma levels

(B) Restart valproate only if the patient has a seizure and plan to use magnesium for management of any seizures during active labor

(C) Start the patient on lamotrigine for seizure prophylaxis, as the newer antiepileptic medications have not demonstrated the same increase in congenital anomalies as the older medications

(D) Restart the patient on valproate as the risk to the mother outweighs the risk to the fetus

(E) Allow the patient to continue without medication and perform an Maternal serum α-fetoprotein (MSAFP) at 16 weeks, level 2 fetal survey at 20 weeks, and use phenytoin at delivery if needed

The answer is E: **Allow the patient to continue without medication and perform an Maternal serum α-fetoprotein (MSAFP) at 16 weeks, level 2 fetal survey at 20 weeks, and use phenytoin at delivery if needed.** Since this patient has not had a seizure in 5 years, it is appropriate to allow the patient to discontinue all medications prior to conception. Guidelines indicate that a trial of complete withdrawal from antiepileptic drugs (AEDs) is possible if the patient has been seizure free for 2 to 5 years. Due to the increased risk of fetal anomalies associated with epilepsy, such as microcephaly, cleft lip with or without cleft palate, and congenital heart disease, a MSAFP at 16 weeks and a level 2 fetal survey at 20 weeks should be performed. In epileptic patients, the drug of choice for management of seizures during labor and delivery (L&D) is phenytoin, not magnesium. Choice A is incorrect since the patient should be tried without any AEDs. If, however, the patient did require AEDs for seizure prophylaxis, it is true that more frequent dosing is advisable to lower peak plasma levels. Choice C is also incorrect, but it is true that the newer AEDs have not demonstrated the same increase in congenital anomalies.

---

24 A 32-year-old, G2P1, presents for a prenatal visit at 42 weeks 3 days by last menstrual period (LMP) and 8-week ultrasound (U/S). Her previous child was delivered via low-transverse Cesarean section due to fetal distress during a prolonged second stage of labor. The patient has no complaints today, and her pregnancy has been uneventful to this point. The patient's vital signs are within normal limits, but the fetal nonstress testing (NST) is nonreactive. The patient's obstetrical (OB) informs her that they need to deliver the baby, and the patient says that she wishes to try vaginal birth. What is this patient's greatest risk if she undergoes induction?

(A) Placental abruption
(B) Uterine rupture
(C) Cord prolapse
(D) Eclampsia
(E) Pulmonary embolism

The answer is B: **Uterine rupture.** Indications for immediate delivery of a postterm fetus (greater than 42 week's gestation) include oligohydramnios and evidence of fetal distress, including a nonreactive NST. Studies indicate that vaginal birth after Cesarean section carries an increased risk of uterine rupture; the risk is increased when labor is induced or augmented. Prostaglandin analogues such as misoprostol pose a higher risk than oxytocin and are not used to induce or augment labor in patients with a history of Cesarean section.

---

25 A 33-year-old G1P0 at 13-week 1-day gestational age (GA) has elected to undergo amniocentesis secondary to results from her first-trimester genetic screen that indicated an increased risk of trisomy 18. She would like to have the test as soon as possible.

What is the earliest recommended time frame that amniocentesis can be performed safely?

(A) 12 weeks
(B) 13 weeks
(C) 14 weeks
(D) 15 weeks
(E) 16 weeks

The answer is C: 14 weeks. Early amniocentesis performed between 11- and 13 week's gestation has a higher risk of pregnancy loss and additional complications such as chorioamnionitis, amniotic fluid leakage, and vaginal spotting. It is therefore recommended that the earliest amniocentesis should be performed in 14 weeks. Prior to that, chorionic villus sampling (CVS) should be used for definitive genetic testing between 10 and 12 week's gestation.

---

26 A 29-year-old morbidly obese woman, G2P1 at 26 weeks gestational age (GA) presents to clinic for a routine obstetrical (OB) visit. Her previous pregnancy resulted in a term delivery and a third-degree laceration. Her current pregnancy has been complicated by placenta previa and gestational diabetes. Her past medical history is significant for a loop electrosurgical excision procedure (LEEP) 2 years ago secondary to cervical intraepithelial neoplasia II. She denies any abdominal pain or cramping at her visit today.

Which of the following are risk factors which make this patient at risk for cervical incompetence during this pregnancy?

(A) History of the LEEP procedure
(B) Morbid obesity
(C) Previous third-degree laceration of vagina
(D) Placenta previa

The answer is A: History of the LEEP procedure. Risk factors for cervical incompetence include a history of cervical surgery, cervical lacerations during vaginal delivery, uterine anomalies, and a history of drug-eluting stent exposure. Lacerations of the vagina are not a risk factor for incompetent cervix. While obesity has many adverse effects on outcomes, it does not increase the likelihood of patients having cervical incompetence. If the patient presents with short cervix, a cerclage may be beneficial.

---

27 A 34-year-old G1P0 at 18 week's gestation is incidentally found to have a cervical length 0.9 cm on a routine ultrasound (U/S). She denies any cervical trauma or prior cervical surgeries. She denies leakage of fluid, cramping, or abdominal pain. Membranes are not bulging on sterile speculum examination.

What is the next step in the management of this patient?

(A) Bed rest for the remainder of gestation
(B) Transvaginal progesterone cream
(C) Betamethasone injections
(D) Cervical cerclage

The answer is D: Cervical cerclage. Cervical length during pregnancy is usually between 2.5 and 4.5 cm. This patient presents with a shortened cervix and a previable pregnancy. Betamethasone and bed rest are recommended management options in patients with pregnancies that are greater than 24 week's gestation. Transvaginal progesterone cream may help to maintain cervical quiescence, but will not benefit the patient's shortened cervix. As this pregnancy is previable, the recommended next step in management would be placement of a cervical cerclage.

---

28 A 29-year-old G3P1011 patient has successfully delivered her second infant at term by a vaginal birth after Cesarean. After 45 minutes, the placenta has still not delivered. Currently the patient is stable with no excessive bleeding. Vital signs: BP 110/76 mmHg, P 105 beats/min. Given this patient's history, what is the most likely cause of retained placenta?

(A) Implantation site tumor
(B) Placenta accreta
(C) Succenturiate lobe
(D) Uterine atony
(E) Uterine rupture

The answer is B: Placenta accreta. Placenta accreta was formerly a rare complication of placental formation, but if a patient has had two or three Cesarean sections and has a low-lying anterior placenta or placenta previa, the risk of placenta accreta can be as high as 40%. A succenturiate lobe consists of accessory lobes that commonly are connected to the main placenta by blood vessels. It may present as a retained placenta typically when the history includes delivering the placenta normally. The patent does not have uterine atony which would present with bleeding of greater than 500 cc. The patient delivered successfully with a category 1 tracing. Uterine rupture is associated with, among other findings, abnormal fetal heart tones (FHTs).

---

29 A 28-year-old G2P1011 patient is currently postoperative day 2 after undergoing a Cesarean section for breech presentation at term. She is successfully breastfeeding exclusively. She was followed up in a high-risk clinic because of a long-standing diagnosis of bipolar disorder with no significant exacerbations during the pregnancy. The remainder of her prenatal course was unremarkable. With her last pregnancy, she experienced an episode of postpartum depression which she was told was exacerbated by not resuming lithium therapy. She requests a refill on her lithium prescription.

Which of the following is true regarding lithium and breastfeeding?

(A) It is the only mood stabilizer that does not require monitoring of breastfeeding infant serum levels
(B) It is the optimal choice of mood stabilizer for breastfeeding women
(C) It should be taken within 30 minutes of nursing to avoid high levels in breast milk
(D) Physical illness in the infant can increase its risk for lithium toxicity
(E) There is minimal excretion of lithium into the breast milk

The answer is D: **Physical illness in the infant can increase its risk for lithium toxicity.** Because of the very high risk of symptom recurrence postpartum, this patient should continue her lithium therapy. Although the most recent publication of the American Academy of Pediatrics classifies lithium as a drug that should be given to nursing mothers with caution, there is little evidence as to why. Moretti et al. looked at 11 mother–infant pairs and found lithium levels in the breast milk to be 0% to 30% that of the mother's serum levels, with no adverse effects reported. Lithium appears to be well tolerated by infants, with only minor and transient lab abnormalities after prolonged exposure. A patient with stable mood on lithium monotherapy who will present for infant monitoring is the best candidate.

---

30 A 27-year-old G1P0 at 15 week's gestation has a history of chronic hypertension. She presents for her first prenatal visit. Vital signs: T 98°F, P 66 beats/min, R 16 breaths/min, BP 146/98 mmHg. She stopped taking her BP medication 6 weeks ago when she found out that she was pregnant. Of the following medications, which is the best choice for treating chronic hypertension in pregnancy?

(A) Hydralazine
(B) Hydrochlorothiazide
(C) Labetalol
(D) Lisinopril
(E) Atenolol

The answer is C: **Labetalol.** Labetalol is a combined α-blocker and β-blocker. It has been extensively studied during pregnancy likely because of its overall low rate of adverse effects. Atenolol, a pure β-antagonist, is associated with growth restriction and not recommended in pregnancy. Lisinopril is an angiotensin-converting enzyme inhibitor and is contraindicated in pregnancy due to teratogenic effects. Hydralazine is given IV and used for acute BP management. Hydrochlorothiazide is a diuretic and is not recommended in pregnancy.

31 A 26-year-old G1 with no prenatal care presents to labor and delivery (L&D) because of bright red, painless vaginal bleeding that occurred with intercourse after her husband returned from a 6-month tour in Afghanistan. Ultrasound (U/S) in triage places her at 23 week's gestation which is within 1 week with her last menstrual period (LMP). It also reveals a complete placenta previa. There are no contractions and fetal heart tone (FHT) is reactive with average FHT of 140. The bleeding has subsided. Hemoglobin is 12.6 and platelets are 215K.

Management of this patient includes which of the following?

(A) Blood transfusion
(B) Double setup examination
(C) Hospitalization
(D) Immediate Cesarean section
(E) Immediate oxytocin induction of labor

The answer is C: Hospitalization. Conservative management with hospitalization in a stable, preterm patient is appropriate for mild preterm bleeding. Since this episode of vaginal bleeding is not life-threatening, aggressive expectant management is appropriate. Most episodes of vaginal bleeding are self-limited, but hospitalization is recommended after the initial episode of vaginal bleeding. The antepartum service is appropriate after the initial stabilization.

32 A 26-year-old G1P0 at 37 weeks presents with regular painful contractions for the past 6 hours of increasing intensity. Upon examination, there is a bulging bag with cervical dilation of 7 cm. No fetal part is detected. A bedside ultrasound (U/S) reveals a footling breech presentation. Fetal heart tracing reveals baseline of 130s with accelerations and no decelerations noted categorized as category I. The patient is taken for an immediate Cesarean section.

What would be the greatest risk for a vaginal delivery?

(A) Apnea associated due to prematurity
(B) Cord prolapse
(C) Entrapment of the aftercoming head
(D) Meconium aspiration
(E) Need for emergency Cesarean section

The answer is B: Cord prolapse. Although 37 week's gestation is not considered "term" it is also not considered preterm. The risk of apnea associated with prematurity is very small. While any breech delivery has a risk for entrapment of the aftercoming head, it is especially of concern in preterm infants. Meconium may or may not be present in this patient—there is no way of telling prior to rupturing membranes which in this scenario is not recommended. Any patient on labor and delivery (L&D) is at risk for an emergency Cesarean section. The alternative most specifically associated with footling breech presentation is that the cord can prolapse between the legs in a presentation that does not completely "block" the cervical opening—such as butt or head.

---

33 A 30-year-old G3P2 with a history of postpartum depression in each of her previous pregnancies presents at 6 weeks for prenatal care. She forgot her prescription bottle and there is no documentation in the medical record regarding the specific medication she has been taking recently. She requests a refill of her prescription which she says is an "SSRI" (selective serotonin reuptake inhibitor). She agrees to call the office with the name of the medication.

Which of the following medications would you advise discontinuing/ substituting immediately?

(A) Citalopram
(B) Fluoxetine
(C) Fluvoxamine
(D) Paroxetine
(E) Sertraline

The answer is D: Paroxetine. This particular SSRI is most suspected of teratogenic effects including reported cardiac defects. Of all SSRIs, fluoxetine has the most proven track record. You would not stop the SSRIs in this patient; you would simply substitute another of the same class. Paroxetine also has significant withdrawal effects, so stopping SSRIs completely would not be advised.

---

34 A 17-year-old G1P0 at 32 week's gestation arrives to the emergency room (ER) via ambulance after experiencing an eclamptic seizure at the mall. Upon arrival, her BP is 170/110 mmHg, P 110 beats/min, R 12 breaths/ min. She is drowsy but responsive and her airway is protected. Fetal heart tones (FHTs) are in the 130s with minimal variability. No contractions are present. Deep tendon reflexes are +4 with three beats of clonus.

What is your next step?

(A) Immediate induction of labor
(B) Intravenous (IV) magnesium
(C) IV valium
(D) Oxytocin
(E) STAT Cesarean delivery

The answer is B: Intravenous (IV) magnesium. IV magnesium is the treatment of choice for prevention and control of eclamptic seizures. Depending on how close to delivery the patient is, and the condition of the fetus, a decision will be made on the mode of delivery—since delivery is the cure for this condition. IV valium is not the treatment of choice when dealing with eclampsia. According to a recent Cochrane review, $MgSO_4$ is superior to valium in reducing the ratio of the risk of maternal death and recurrence of seizures.

---

35 A 30-year-old G1P0 with chronic hypertension presents at 33 week's gestation for an nonstress testing (NST) and routine prenatal visit. Her pregnancy has been characterized by well-controlled hypertension in the 110 to 120/70 to 80 range. She had an abnormal quad screen with a subsequent amniocentesis confirming a normal male fetus at 21 weeks. Upon arrival, her BP was 142/98. A repeat BP performed 15 minutes later during the NST was 152/102. The NST is reactive. She relates experiencing "heartburn" over the past 36 hours. Upon examination, she has mild right upper quadrant tenderness without rebound. DTRs are 3+ with clonus. You have the medical assistant accompany her over to labor and delivery (L&D) via wheelchair.

What is your immediate concern?

(A) Abruptio placenta
(B) Hepatic capsular rupture
(C) Impending eclampsia
(D) Intussusception of pregnancy
(E) Splenic aneurysm

The answer is C: Impending eclampsia. This patient is at risk for Hemolysis, Elevated Liver enzymes, Low Platelet count (HELLP) syndrome. Most likely she has chronic hypertension with superimposed preeclampsia. This places her at higher risk for placental abruption. If she does have HELLP syndrome, she is at an increased risk for hepatic capsular rupture, although her physical examination at this point in time is not suspicious for this condition. The most imminent concern is her risk of eclamptic seizures.

---

36 A 22-year-old G1 patient at 18 weeks presented 8 weeks ago with vaginal bleeding and a threatened abortion. Subsequently she had no further bleeding and the fundal height is appropriate for gestational age (GA) and fetal heart tones (FHTs) are present at 140 beats/min. Given her history in this pregnancy, which of the following factors is she at risk for developing?

(A) Fetal macrosomia
(B) Intrauterine infection
(C) Placental abruption
(D) Preeclampsia
(E) Preterm delivery

The answer is E: Preterm delivery. In fact, low birth weight, abnormal quad screen testing, preterm delivery, and fetal death are statistically more likely to occur in women with first-trimester bleeding.

37 A 39-year-old G1P1 is 7 days post-Cesarean section after a failed induction at term. She was diagnosed with endometritis on post-op day 2 and has remained febrile with elevated white blood cells (WBCs). Her antibiotic regimen initially was IV gentamicin and clindamycin. When she remained febrile on day 4, ampicillin was added to the regimen. She spiked a fever to 102.6 this morning. A complete blood count (CBC) revealed a WBC count of 15.3, hemoglobin of 11.4, and platelets at 252K.

What is the next step?

(A) Administration of fever-reducing drugs and rest
(B) Empiric treatment with heparin
(C) Placement of an inferior vena cava
(D) Switch from double- to triple-antibiotic therapy

The answer is B: Empiric treatment with heparin. This is because her most likely diagnosis is deep septic pelvic thrombophlebitis (DSPT). Patients with DSPT usually present within a few days after Cesarean section with fever that persists despite antibiotics. Typically, there is no radiographic evidence of thrombosis. The condition occurs in approximately 0.5% to 1% of Cesarean section patients. The best imaging tests to confirm the diagnosis of septic pelvic vein thrombophlebitis is a computed tomography scan where large clots in the ovarian vessels or vena cava can be observed. Often, the diagnosis is established by exclusion when the patient improves after an empirical trial of heparin.

---

38 A 26-year-old G3P2 at 38 weeks presents with spontaneous rupture of membrane (ROM) and regular contractions for the last 3 hours. On physical examination, two 1-cm "kissing lesions" are noted at 1 and 11 o'clock on the labia minora. She and her partner both have a history of "fever blisters." She denies a history of genital herpes.

Which question is most likely to help you with your management decision?

(A) Did she have this problem in any of her other pregnancies?
(B) Do she and her partner have vaginal, oral, or anal sex?
(C) Has she ever had the chickenpox?
(D) How long have the lesions been present?
(E) What are the current symptoms?

The answer is B: Do she and her partner have vaginal, oral, or anal sex? Herpes can be transmitted during oral sex in the presence of an active oral lesion. The first episode of a secondary infection is commonly not as symptomatic or generalized as a primary infection. Women with no history of genital herpes whose partner has a history of cold sores should avoid oral, vaginal, and anal sex during the last trimester of pregnancy. Condoms are recommended during the entire pregnancy. Suppression is recommended starting at 35 to 36 weeks.

39 A 24-year-old G1P0 at 40 4/7 weeks presents with a 3-day history of malaise, fatigue, and fever and a generalized extremely pruritic eruption of macules, blisters, and crusted lesions. She is contracting regularly and her cervical examination is 7/75/0.

Which of the following statements is true?

(A) Cesarean delivery is indicated
(B) No additional intervention is necessary
(C) The infant should be isolated from the mother after delivery
(D) Treatment with corticosteroids is indicated
(E) Ultrasound (U/S) examination of the fetus is necessary to make the diagnosis

The answer is C: The infant should be isolated from the mother after delivery. The rash described is classic for chickenpox. When this infection occurs 5 days prior to, through 2 days after delivery, the newborn is at high risk for developing neonatal varicella. Prior to the availability of antiviral drugs such as acyclovir, 20% to 30% of infants delivered in this situation developed varicella, and up to 30% of affected infants died.

40 A 23-year-old G2P1 who recently moved to the United States from Haiti presents at 32 week's gestation with limited prenatal care. Her previous birth was a normal spontaneous vaginal delivery at home in the Haitian countryside attended by a lay midwife.

Routine prenatal labs reveal maternal anemia with a hemoglobin of 7.6, sickle cell trait, and A-negative blood type with a positive antibody screen with a titer of 1/100. Upon (U/S) examination, fetal skin edema (7 mm), fetal ascites, polyhydramnios, and a thickened placenta are noted (see *Figure 6-4*).

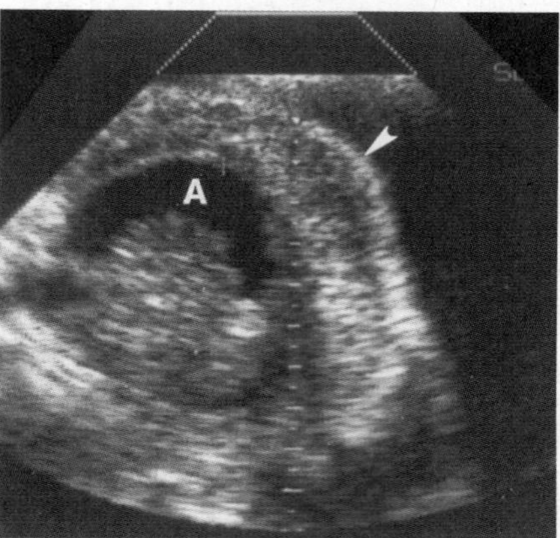

Figure 6-4

The fetus is suffering from intrauterine growth retardation (IUGR) measuring at 26 weeks.

What is the cause of this condition?

(A) Decreased fetal aldosterone secretion
(B) Irreversible carbohydrate metabolic failure
(C) Severe fluid retention due to renal failure in the fetus
(D) Sickling and clot formation at the uteroplacental junction
(E) Compensation for fetal anemia due to hemolysis

The answer is E: Compensation for fetal anemia due to hemolysis. This patient is RH sensitized and her immune system is currently attacking her fetus. The fetus is suffering from erythroblastosis fetalis where the hemolysis of Rh-positive fetal RBCs is a consequence of attack by maternal anti-D IgG antibody. Hemolysis causes fetal anemia. The fetal anemia promotes the production of erythropoietin. A cycle of events occur where erythropoiesis increases, and it is not possible for the fetal marrow to keep up with RBC production while simultaneously there is RBC destruction. As a result, extramedullary erythropoiesis in the spleen, liver, kidneys, and adrenals occurs. Hepatosplenomegaly is common. About 50% of fetuses destined to become hydropic do so after 18 week's gestation.

---

41 A 22-year-old G1 with last menstrual period (LMP) 18 weeks ago presents with a small amount of bright red bleeding overnight. On examination, her cervix is 2 cm dilated but she has not perceived any contractions. Fetal heart tones (FHTs) are 140s by Doppler.

What is the most likely diagnosis?

(A) Blighted ovum
(B) Cervical friability
(C) Incompetent cervix
(D) Molar pregnancy
(E) Normal pregnancy

The answer is C: Incompetent cervix. An incompetent cervix is otherwise known as cervical insufficiency. This presentation is usually between 18 and 22 weeks and includes painless dilation without contractions. It is not a normal pregnancy. The other conditions typically present in the first trimester.

---

42 A 26-year-old primigravida at term presented to labor and delivery (L&D) with painless vaginal bleeding in the absence of contractions. After a new intern panics at the amount of blood and performs a cervix check, she experienced profuse vaginal bleeding but fetal heart tones (FHTs) remain normal. The cervix is 2 to 3 cm dilated with an edge of placenta palpable. Her vital signs are currently stable with BP of 96/62 and pulse of 92 beats/min. You estimate she has lost 500 cc of blood since the cervical examination.

Which of the following is the most appropriate treatment?

(A) Voorhees bag
(B) Braxton-Hicks version
(C) Cesarean delivery
(D) Rupture of the fetal membranes to stimulate delivery
(E) Replace blood loss and await vaginal delivery

The answer is C: Cesarean delivery. The appropriate workup for third-trimester bleeding includes an ultrasound (US) localization of the placenta PRIOR to performing a digital examination. Performing a vaginal examination can cause an unacceptable increase in bleeding. This patient needs emergent delivery as well as resuscitation with blood products. Proceeding to Cesarean section is the most appropriate treatment. In the case of a low-lying placenta (not previa), the placenta will regress as the fetal head descends and a vaginal delivery may be possible.

---

43 A 34-year-old woman, G1P0, presents for her second prenatal visit at 9 week's gestation. A review of prenatal laboratory results reveals she is rubella nonimmune. The risk to the fetus should she contract rubella includes which constellation of findings:

(A) Blindness, deafness, and microcephaly
(B) Cerebral palsy, sensorineural hearing loss, and musculoskeletal deformity
(C) Chorioretinitis, hydrocephalus, and intracranial calcifications
(D) Ergogenic liver foci, microcephaly, ventriculomegaly, and deafness
(E) Nonimmune hydrops, placentamegaly, and anemia

The answer is A: Blindness, deafness, and microcephaly. The common triad of deformities associated with congenital rubella is blindness, deafness, and microcephaly. The vaccination for rubella should be administered immediately postpartum. Since this disease is spread through respiratory droplet and is infectious prior to other symptoms present in the infection, it is difficult for nonimmune women to avoid infection in endemic areas.

---

44 A 22-year-old G2P1 at 30 weeks presents to the emergency room (ER) with a history of fever, nausea, and recent onset of right flank pain. A urinalysis obtained by catheter is free of bacteria and negative for nitrites and leukocyte esterase. Appendicitis is considered.

Which of the following is true with respect to appendicitis in pregnancy?

(A) Abdominal pain, nausea, vomiting, and an elevated WBC count are helpful in establishing the diagnosis of appendicitis
(B) Acute appendicitis is a rare surgical emergency in pregnancy
(C) Appendectomies in the third trimester are associated with preterm labor
(D) Appendectomies in the first trimester have not been shown to adversely impact on pregnancy outcome
(E) Localization of pain in appendicitis varies depending on the gestational age (GA)

The answer is E: Localization of pain in appendicitis varies depending on the gestational age (GA). Pain in pregnancy is related to the position of the appendix which migrates cephalad and laterally during pregnancy. There are no signs, symptoms, or laboratory results that are considered diagnostic during pregnancy; therefore, a high level of suspicion is required. While appendectomies in the third trimester are not associated with preterm labor, those in the first and second trimesters are associated with miscarriage and preterm labor.

---

45 A 26-year-old G2P1 at 29 week's gestation with a history of severe allergies currently on maintenance allergy shots presents to the emergency room (ER) with wheezing, shortness of breath, and chest tightness. Her PO_2 is 89% on room air. Her medications include an inhaled corticosteroid and albuterol.

Which of the following is true regarding her obstetrical (OB) management?

(A) Begin biweekly nonstress testings (NSTs) immediately
(B) Begin ultrasound (U/S) at 32 weeks to monitor for fetal growth restriction
(C) Discontinue allergy shots
(D) Monitor with weekly spirometry
(E) Plan to bottle feed

The answer is B: Begin ultrasound (U/S) at 32 weeks to monitor for fetal growth restriction. Women with severe or uncontrolled asthma or significant asthma attacks are at increased risk for intrauterine growth retardation (IUGR). Maintenance allergy shots may be continued in pregnancy although there is an increased risk of anaphylaxis and death with the shots. Weekly spirometry in the absence of acute exacerbations is not indicated. Women who are taking asthma medications are candidates for breastfeeding. NSTs should begin as indicated but not routinely in the case of asthma at 29 weeks.

---

46 A 36-year-old woman, G4P3 at 34 week's gestation, presents with a 36-hour history or anorexia and vomiting that started soon after a dinner consisting of fried chicken, French fries and a milkshake. She describes stabbing pain that is localized to the right epigastric area.

Vital signs: T 38.6, P 110, R 18, BP 110/68. Her BMI is 38. Fetal evaluation includes a reactive nonstress testing (NST) and biophysical profile (BPP) of 10/10. Cervix is closed, thick, and high. An obstetrical (OB) ultrasound (U/S) reveals no evidence of intrauterine growth retardation (IUGR). A CBC reveals the following: WBC 16.6, hemoglobin 11.0, hematocrit (HCT) 32.8, and platelets 172,000.

What is the next step in the evaluation and management of this patient?

(A) Admit for induction of labor
(B) Betamethasone therapy
(C) Initiate magnesium sulfate intravenously
(D) U/S of the gallbladder
(E) Urine (24-hour specimen) for total protein and creatinine clearance

The answer is D: U/S of gallbladder. The presentation may appear similar to Hemolysis, Elevated Liver enzymes, Low Platelet count (HELLP) syndrome; however, this patient is normotensive with a normal platelet count. This patient is febrile with an elevated WBC count presenting with epigastric pain following a fat-ladened meal. The most likely etiology is gallbladder related.

---

47 A 32-year-old woman, G2P1, was discovered to have a complete placenta previa during a routine anatomy ultrasound (U/S) at 18 weeks. A repeat U/S today at 24 weeks confirms a complete placenta previa. She is concerned about complications associated with placenta previa and wants to know if it is safe to attend her grandfather's funeral approximately 2 hours away by car. In discussing the risks of bleeding due to placenta previa, you advise her the time most commonly associated with the first significant bleed due to placenta previa occurs:

(A) Before 20 weeks
(B) 23 to 25 weeks
(C) 26 to 28 weeks
(D) 29 to 31 weeks
(E) After 34 weeks

The answer is D: 29 to 31 weeks. The mean gestational age (GA) at the time of the first episode of vaginal bleeding is 29 to 32 weeks. While there is no guarantee that a bleed will not occur prior to this time, a short car trip at 24 weeks is unlikely to impose significant risk to the patient.

---

48 A 26-year-old G2P1 at 38 week's gestation presents to labor and delivery (L&D) with profuse vaginal bleeding. Her BP is 100/56 mmHg, pulse is 120 beats/min, and respirations are 20 breaths/min. fetal heart tones (FHTs) are in the 120s with no evidence of decelerations and moderate variability. An ultrasound (U/S) reveals a probable partial previa. Speculum exam reveals a visually closed cervix and active bleeding.

What is the most appropriate next step in the management of this patient?

(A) Cesarean delivery
(B) External version
(C) Placement of a B-Lynch suture
(D) Replace blood loss and await vaginal delivery
(E) Rupture of the fetal membranes to stimulate delivery

The answer is A: **Cesarean delivery.** This patient is remote from delivery and appears to have a partial placenta previa. A recent study concluded that more than two-thirds of women with a distance of more than 10 mm from the placental edge to cervical os have vaginal delivery without an increased risk of hemorrhage. In this case, this does not apply. A patient who presents in the third trimester with vaginal bleeding should not be examined digitally until an U/S is performed that rules out placenta previa.

External version is performed when the patient and fetus are stable in order to convert a breech or transverse lie to vertex to allow for a vaginal delivery. A B-Lynch suture is placed as a measure to control postpartum hemorrhage.

---

49 A 17-year-old, G1P0, currently at 22 week's gestation with no prenatal care is admitted to the antenatal floor after presenting to the emergency room (ER) with right flank pain, nausea, and a fever of 102.6°F. She has an elevated WBC count of 16.6, a hemoglobin of 10.3, a mucopurulent cervical discharge, and a urinalysis that is positive for nitrites and +2 glucose. This hospitalization could most likely have been prevented with earlier prenatal care that detected and instituted a management plan for which of the following?

(A) Allowed detection of glycosuria
(B) Identified and treated anemia
(C) Identified and treated asymptomatic bacteriuria (ASB)
(D) Identified and treated sexually transmitted infections
(E) Provided better dating criteria

The answer is C: **Identified and treated asymptomatic bacteriuria (ASB).** This patient could have been diagnosed with ASB. Ureteral dilation due to progesterone effect and obstruction by the enlarged uterus can lead to pyelonephritis 20-40% of the time if ASB is left untreated.

---

50 A 32-year-old woman, G2P2, at 32 weeks has just delivered via Cesarean section for severe preeclampsia . She received a 4 g bolus of magnesium sulfate followed by 2 g an hour. Her risk for magnesium toxicity associated with high magnesium plasma levels can best be explained by which of the following?

(A) Increased glomerular filtration rate (GFR) reducing effectiveness
(B) Postpartum third spacing
(C) Potentiation of seizure prophylaxis
(D) Pulmonary edema risks are increased
(E) Impaired renal function

The answer is E: Impaired renal function. According to American College of Obstetricians and Gynecologists (ACOG), vascular changes such as hemoconcentration and contraction of the intravascular space occur as well as renal changes due to vasospasm. The elevation in GFR commonly associated with normal pregnancy does not occur. Oliguria can occur. Third spacing is a normal fluid shift that occurs after delivery. Magnesium therapy can be associated with pulmonary edema but does not cause magnesium toxicity.

51 A 38-year-old G1P0 at 38 weeks who has had an uncomplicated course during this pregnancy presents for a routine 38-week prenatal visit. Her vital signs are P 72 beats/min, R 16 breaths/min, BP 180/110 mmHg.

Which of the following conditions provide support for a suspected diagnosis of severe preeclampsia?

(A) Acid reflux
(B) Peripheral edema
(C) Platelet count of 155,000
(D) Proteinuria of more than 3 g in a 24-hour collection
(E) Systolic BP of 160 mmHg or higher or diastolic BP of 110 mmHg or higher on two occasions at least 6 hours apart

The answer is E: Systolic BP of 160 mmHg or higher or diastolic BP of 110 mmHg or higher on two occasions at least 6 hours apart. According to the most recent Practice Bulletin from American College of Obstetricians and Gynecologists (ACOG), a diagnosis of severe preeclampsia requires at least one of the following criteria:

- Cerebral or visual disturbances
- Epigastric or right upper quadrant pain
- Fetal growth restriction
- Impaired liver function
- BP of 160 mmHg systolic or higher or 110 mmHg diastolic or higher on two occasions at least 6 hours apart while the patient is on bed rest
- Oliguria of less than 500 mL in 24 hours
- Proteinuria of 5 g or higher in a 24-hour urine specimen or 3+ or greater on two random urine samples collected at least 4 hours apart
- Pulmonary edema or cyanosis
- Thrombocytopenia

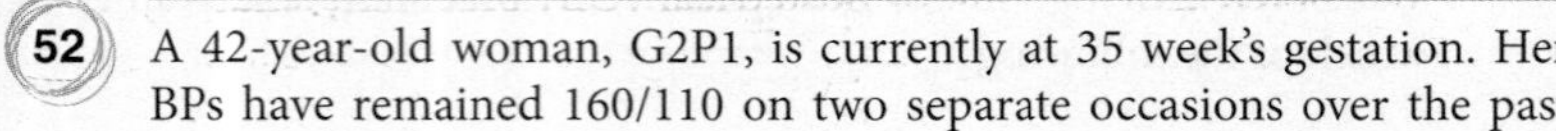

52 A 42-year-old woman, G2P1, is currently at 35 week's gestation. Her BPs have remained 160/110 on two separate occasions over the past

6 hours. Labetalol successfully normalizes the BP. She complains of a severe headache that improves slightly with acetaminophen. A CBC reveals a WBC count of 6.8, hemoglobin of 13.2, and platelet count of 150,000. Ultrasound (U/S) reveals a mildly growth-restricted fetus in vertex presentation with a biophysical profile (BPP) of 8/10.

Which statement is correct regarding management of this patient?

(A) Administer antenatal corticosteroids prior to delivery
(B) Assess cervix to determine if favorable for induction
(C) Begin magnesium prophylaxis when in active labor
(D) Due to fetal lung immaturity attempt to delay delivery until at least 37 weeks
(E) Immediately perform Cesarean section

The answer is B: Assess cervix to determine if favorable for induction. Candidates with favorable cervix and vertex presentation are good candidates for attempted vaginal delivery. $MgSO_4$ should begun when contemplating delivery. There is no indication for steroids in a patient at 35 week's gestation. There is no benefit to waiting 2 additional weeks in light of the diagnosis of severe preeclampsia when a patient is 35 week's gestation—the risk to the mother and the fetus for prolonged pregnancy is too high compared with the benefit gained at this point in pregnancy.

---

53 A 29-year-old G2P1 woman at 41 week's gestation with gestational diabetes presented 12 hours ago in active labor. The estimated fetal weight is 3,900 g. Her previous vaginal delivery was uncomplicated and her infant weighed 3,700 g. She progressed normally through labor and has pushed for 2 hours. She is exhausted and requesting "help" with the vacuum. During an informed consent discussion, shoulder dystocia is discussed.

Of the following complications associated with shoulder dystocia, which is the most common?

(A) Brachial plexus palsy
(B) Clavicle fracture
(C) Death
(D) Fetal asphyxia
(E) Humerus fracture

The answer is A: Brachial plexus palsy. Of this group of complications associated with shoulder dystocia, the most common is brachial plexus injury at 4% to 40% but less than 10% of these are permanent. When evaluating the impact of training on actual clinical outcomes in their hospital, Crofts and colleagues noted that the rate of obstetrical (OB) brachial plexus injury fell from 7.4% in a 4-year period prior to training, to 2.3% in a 4-year period after training.

54 A 39-year-old woman at 41 week's gestation G3P2 is delivering an infant with estimated fetal weight of 4,200 g. The second stage lasted 45 minutes and she is pushing effectively.

When the head crowns, you note a "turtle sign." What would be your first maneuver?

(A) Deliver the posterior arm
(B) Gaskin maneuver
(C) McRobert
(D) Woodscrew
(E) Zavanelli

The answer is C: McRobert. The "turtle sign" is indicative of a shoulder dystocia. Of these maneuvers, the correct choice is McRobert, although typically both a McRobert and suprapubic pressure are used together. The other choices are more advanced maneuvers reserved for shoulder dystocia not responding to McRobert.

55 A 23-year-old G2P0100 at 25 weeks presents with a complaint of loss of fluid vaginally. The fluid was copious and clear. Assessment by sterile speculum examination reveals vaginal pooling; ferning was noted under the microscope and nitrazine paper turned blue. She is very worried because she lost her first son about 4 weeks after he was born at 26 weeks due largely in part to severe respiratory distress. To reassure her, you discuss using antenatal corticosteroids.

Which of the following is the most correct statement with respect to antenatal corticosteroids?

(A) They are only helpful if given at least 24 hours prior to delivery
(B) Men have better outcomes than women
(C) Maternal infections are increased
(D) Surfactant alone is more effective than in combination with corticosteroids
(E) They are less effective in cases of ruptured compared with intact membranes

The answer is E: They are less effective in cases of ruptured compared with intact membranes. According to the consensus panel, "In the presence of preterm premature rupture of the membranes, antenatal corticosteroid therapy reduces the frequency of respiratory distress syndrome, intraventricular hemorrhage, and neonatal death, although to a lesser extent than with intact membranes." They are synergistic with surfactant. They reduce mortality, respiratory distress syndrome, and intraventricular hemorrhage in preterm infants between 24 and 34 week's gestation regardless of gender or race. Although benefits are greater after 24 hours, even a short period of time prior to delivery may also improve outcomes. Although the possibility of increased risk of neonatal or maternal infection is unclear, the risk of intraventricular hemorrhage and death from prematurity is greater than the risk from infection.

---

56 A 24-year-old primigravida is transferred from an outlying hospital because they do not have a neonatal intensive care unit. She is currently 26 weeks, 3 cm dilated, and contracting regularly. The transport will take 90 minutes. She will be accompanied by an EMT with little labor and delivery (L&D) experience.

Which tocolytic agent will be the safest for this person to manage?

(A) Terbutaline
(B) Indomethacin
(C) Magnesium sulfate
(D) Nifedipine

The answer is D: Nifedipine. Magnesium sulfate is generally considered to have the highest degree of safety; however, since the patient will be traveling with an inexperienced EMT, nifedipine is the safest choice if she is normotensive. Terbutaline is no longer recommended for tocolysis. The likelihood of this patient delivering in the near future makes indomethacin a poor choice. Nifedipine is the best choice for the trip.

---

57 A 26-year-old woman, G4P3021, is found to have a low-lying placenta during routine anatomy screen at 18 weeks. Her first child was stillborn at term due to a vasa previa. She is very concerned because the stillbirth was also associated with a low-lying placenta found at the second-trimester routine ultrasound (U/S).

Which of the following represents the best technique to evaluate this pregnancy for the presence of vasa previa?

(A) Biweekly biophysical profile (BPP) beginning at 28 weeks
(B) Color Doppler via transvaginal U/S
(C) Repeat U/S at 1-month interval
(D) Rule out funneling membranes on transvaginal U/S
(E) Sterile speculum examination

The answer is B: Color Doppler via transvaginal U/S. If the placenta is found to be low lying during a routine second-trimester U/S, evaluation for placental cord insertion is indicated. When vasa previa is suspected, transvaginal U/S color Doppler may be used to facilitate the diagnosis. However, vasa previa may be missed even when evaluated using transvaginal U/S color Doppler.

58 A 24-year-old G2P1001 at 38 4/7 presents to labor and delivery (L&D) with complaints of a steady amount of painless vaginal bleeding immediately following rupture of membrane (ROM) approximately 2 hours earlier. Since that time, she has not felt the baby move. Fetal heart tones (FHTs) cannot be detected via Doppler. A bedside ultrasound (U/S) reveals no cardiac activity. A formal U/S confirms a fetal demise.

Vital signs: BP 98/72 mmHg, P 78 beats/min, R 20 breaths/min. The physical examination is normal. Sterile speculum examination is fern, pooling, and nitrazine positive. CBC = WBC 10.3, Hgb 12.1, hematocrit (HCT) 35.2, platelets 350K.

What is the most likely finding upon delivery of the placenta?

(A) Perifunicular calcifications
(B) Retroplacental clot affecting 50% of the surface
(C) Succenturiate lobe
(D) True knot in the cord
(E) Two-vessel cord

The answer is C: Succenturiate lobe. The etiology of this fetal demise is a classic presentation of vasa previa with painless vaginal bleeding on spontaneous ROM or artificial ROM. Of the findings listed, a succenturiate lobe of the placenta has been implicated most often in vasa previa. Retroplacental clot is associated with abruptio placenta.

---

59 A G3P2 at term was just checked and found to be 7 cm. At that point, amniotomy was performed, and bright red bleeding was noted. The fetal heart tracing that had been reactive until this point dropped to 60 immediately after artificial rupture of membrane (ROM) and then decreased to 40 beats/min verified by internal scalp electrode.

What is the most important intervention?

(A) Begin O_2
(B) Fluid resuscitation
(C) Positional changes
(D) STAT Cesarean section
(E) Stop oxytocin

The answer is D: STAT Cesarean section. This patient has classic signs of a vasa previa and there is little time for delivery prior to fetal exsanguination and death.

---

60 A primigravid patient from your clinic presents to the hospital with excessive vomiting. She is 14-week gestational age (GA) dated by last menstrual period (LMP) and has lost 15 lb since becoming pregnant. On physical examination, you note a dry oral mucosa and poor capillary refill. You decide to admit her to the hospital, and she is started on IV fluids and antiemetics. Her blood sugar and other vitals are stable.

Which of the following tests should be included in your evaluation of her condition?

(A) MRI to rule out brain tumor
(B) 24-Hour urine total protein
(C) Transvaginal ultrasound (U/S)
(D) Tuberculin (TB) skin test

The answer is C: Transvaginal ultrasound (U/S). An intrauterine pregnancy should always be confirmed by U/S in a patient with hyperemesis. Molar pregnancies as well as multiple pregnancies are associated with hyperemesis and should be ruled out as part of the workup in a patient with severe symptoms. Thyroid studies should also be performed.

---

61 A 24-year-old G2P1 at 24 weeks presents to the hospital with a fever of 102.1, severe right flank pain, and urine dip positive for nitrates.

What is your plan for this patient?

(A) Start on Keflex and have her follow up in the office in 1 week
(B) Obtain surgical consult for appendicitis
(C) Plan for induction due to chorioamnionitis
(D) Admit for IV antibiotics and observation

The answer is D: Admit for IV antibiotics and observation. Pyelonephritis has potentially serious complications such as septic shock and acute respiratory distress syndrome. Therefore, in pregnancy pyelonephritis is treated with inpatient hospitalization and IV antibiotics. Although chorioamnionitis and appendicitis may be on the differential diagnosis with fever in pregnancy, positive nitrates are associated with urinary tract infections.

---

62 A patient is being discharged to home after inpatient treatment of pyelonephritis. She will continue oral antibiotics for a total of 10 to 14 days to complete her treatment of the infection.

What will you advise after her follow-up visit?

(A) We should start prophylactic daily antibiotic for the rest of her pregnancy
(B) We should start a 24-hour urine collection for total protein
(C) We should treat her for group B strep during labor
(D) No further treatment needed

The answer is A: We should start prophylactic daily antibiotic for the rest of her pregnancy. Patients with pyelonephritis or two or more episodes of asymptomatic bacteria (ASB) and/or cystitis are placed on prophylaxis for the rest of pregnancy due to potential risks of further infections.

63 A 33-year-old G3P1102 presents to the prenatal clinic for her 37-week appointment. She denies any medical complaints but states that she wants this pregnancy to be over. Her BP is 122/75 with a pulse of 66 beats/min and a fundal height of 38 cm. Her last ultrasound (U/S) showed that the fetus was in the frank breech position with an amniotic fluid index (AFI) of 15 cm. Leopold maneuvers today confirm the same position.

What is the next step in the management of this patient?

(A) Encourage her to do stretches and exercises and hope that the baby rotates to the vertex position
(B) Tell the patient that she needs a Cesarean section at 39 weeks
(C) Discuss an external cephalic version for subsequent vaginal delivery
(D) Reassure her that her baby will flip if she waits and lies on her side
(E) Admit the patient to the hospital for a Cesarean section after clinic today

The answer is C: **Discuss an external cephalic version for subsequent vaginal delivery.** This patient is a suitable candidate for external cephalic version based on her dates. An ECV is indicated when the fetus is in breech presentation at a gestation of at least 36 weeks and labor has not begun. She has adequate amniotic fluid and the baby is in frank breech position. Breech presentation is not an absolute indication for Cesarean section.

64 A 22-year-old G1P0 at 32 weeks presents to the obstetrical (OB) clinic complaining of malodorous vaginal discharge for the past 18 hours. The patient denies fever, abdominal cramping, vaginal bleeding, or dysuria. Vaginal examination shows a copious amount of fluid in the vaginal vault. Laboratory examination reveals a clear to whitish, mildly odorous fluid with 0 to 5 WBCs/high power field, 0 to 5 RBCs, and a few budding yeast. Ferning is noted in the report.

What is the next step in the management of this patient?

(A) Admit to the hospital to begin latency antibiotic therapy
(B) Reassure her that some fluid discharge is normal and that you will see her in clinic again in 2 weeks
(C) Send the patient to the ultrasound (US) clinic to have an amniotic fluid index (AFI) study performed
(D) Perform an urgent Cesarean section
(E) Start oxytocin induction after confirming vertex presentation

The answer is A: **Admit to the hospital to begin latency antibiotic therapy.** This patient presents with preterm premature rupture of membranes (PPROM) without overt signs of infection. The patient needs to be treated as an inpatient with prophylactic antibiotics to prevent infection. If this patient manifested signs of infection, fever, tachycardia, cramping, etc., prompt delivery would be indicated. Ordering an U/S to determine the AFI would not be indicated at this early stage of evaluation treatment.

---

65 A 38-year-old G5P3013 woman presents to clinic at 19 weeks. You are concerned due to fundal height of 23 cm. In-office ultrasound (U/S) reveals an active fetus with measurements consistent with 19 weeks. The fetal HR is in the 140s and multiple small echodense areas are noted in the uterine wall.

What is the most effective treatment of this patient's condition?

(A) Uterine wall biopsy
(B) Immediate admission with delivery by Cesarean section at 34 weeks
(C) Expectant management
(D) Cesarean hysterectomy at term
(E) Termination of pregnancy

The answer is C: Expectant management. This patient has a fibroid uterus as manifested by the U/S findings. This accounts for the size/dates discrepancy. Uterine leiomyomas provide a small increase in risk to the mother but do not necessitate any immediate intervention. If myomectomy is elected, it should be deferred until after the postpartum period.

---

66 A 35-year-old G2P0101 Hispanic woman at 34 weeks presents for a prenatal visit. The patient is dated by last menstrual period (LMP) as this is her first visit to the clinic. She complains of swollen feet and difficulty sitting. Her BP is 110/65 with a pulse of 85 beats/min. Fetal HR is 135 mmHg, and fundal height is 44 cm.

What would you expect to find on ultrasound (US)?

(A) Normal pregnancy
(B) Uteroplacental insufficiency
(C) Esophageal atresia
(D) Potter syndrome
(E) Trisomy 13

The answer is C: Esophageal atresia. Amniotic fluid is generated by the fetal kidneys and passed into the amnioticsac by fetal micturition. The fetus then swallows the amniotic fluid and absorbed in the fetal gastrointestinal tract and returned to the mother as waste through the umbilical vein. If this cycle is interrupted, oligohydramnios or polyhydramnios may result. This patient is manifesting signs of polyhydramnios as her fundal height is well above what would be expected in the normal fetus. Esophageal atresia interrupts the swallowing/reabsorption phase of the cycle. When this happens, the amniotic fluid continues to accumulate resulting in polyhydramnios. Potter syndrome manifests with a marked oligohydramnios beginning in the second trimester. Uteroplacental insufficiency is associated with moderate oligohydramnios in the third trimester. Trisomy 13 is not associated with polyhydramnios.

67 A 15-year-old G1P0 at 41 weeks presents to triage in active labor and is admitted to labor and delivery (L&D). On examination, it is noted that her membranes are intact and her cervix is 5 cm dilated, 90% effaced, and at –1 station. Upon review of her chart, it is noted that her last ultrasound (U/S) showed an amniotic fluid index (AFI) of 4 cm. Fetal heart tracing is reactive with intermittent accelerations and variable decelerations.

What is the next step in the management of this patient?

(A) Amnioinfusion
(B) Expectant management
(C) Emergent Cesarean section
(D) Augment labor with oxytocin
(E) Forceps delivery

oligohydramnios

The answer is B: Expectant management. Expectant management is the appropriate course of action in this patient. Even in the case of oligohydramnios, if there is no immediate risk to the mother or baby, expectant management is appropriate. Amnioinfusion is not indicated in oligohydramnios. Augmentation of labor would put unnecessary stress on the baby due to the insufficient quantity of amniotic fluid.

68 A 31-year-old G2P1001 presents to the emergency room (ER) at 8 week's gestation complaining of heavy vaginal bleeding over the past week and is concerned about the well-being of her baby. As part of her workup, the ER draws a quantitative β-hCG that is reported as 1,850 IU/L. You are consulted to see the patient on the obstetrical (OB) or gynecologic team. After interviewing the patient, the physical examination is performed and reveals a closed cervix, 10 to 15 mL of blood, and no tissue in the vaginal vault.

What is the next step in the management of this patient?

(A) Inform the patient that she is no longer pregnant due to a low β-hCG test for 8 weeks and express condolences
(B) Order an abdominal ultrasound (U/S) in the radiology department
(C) Perform a transvaginal U/S in the ER
(D) Perform a Doppler study to look for fetal heart tones (FHTs)
(E) Reassurance

1,000–2,000 IU/dL
transabdominal 6,500 IU/dL

The answer is C: Perform a transvaginal U/S in the ER. The minimal threshold for visualization in transvaginal U/S is approximately 1,000 to 2,000 IU/dL, while the threshold for transabdominal is 6,500 IU/dL. Doppler study would be inappropriate because it is too early in the pregnancy to detect a fetal heartbeat by Doppler. Reassurance and expressing condolences are inappropriate as no definitive diagnosis has been made.

69 A 20-year-old G3P0111 with no prenatal care presents with bleeding and abdominal pain. She is uncooperative but appears to be in good health. You obtain her obstetrical (OB) history remarkable for previous preterm birth at 34 weeks for preeclampsia and a spontaneous abortion. Her vital signs are as follows: BP 150/105, P 100, R 18, T 99. She appears to be in moderate pain. Fetal heart tones (FHTs) are noted in *Figure 6-5*.

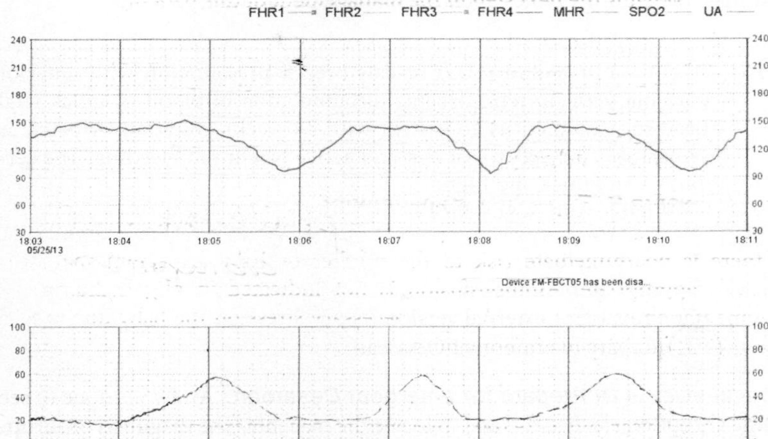

Figure 6-5

The monitor strip can be described as:

(A) Baseline 140; minimal variability; late decelerations
(B) Baseline 140; moderate variability; late decelerations
(C) Negative contraction stress test
(D) Reactive nonstress testing (NST)

The answer is A: Baseline 140; minimal variability; late decelerations.

70 The nurse notes that the fundus is tender when the monitors were applied. Fundal height is 35 cm. She denies trauma, recent intercourse, and cocaine or other drug use.

What is the most urgent clinical question you must make answer?

(A) Is it vertex or breech?
(B) Is it placenta previa or is it abruptio placenta?
(C) Is it placenta accreta or is it placenta increta?
(D) What is the gestational age (GA)?
(E) What is the blood type and Rh?

The answer is B: Is it placenta previa or is it abruptio placenta? Any woman presenting with third-trimester bleeding must be evaluated for placenta previa versus abruption. Generally previa is painless and abruption is painful bleeding. In this care, the patient is in severe pain so abruption is at the top of our list. If there is no previous imaging an ultrasound (U/S) must be done before digital examination. The other questions are not as critical and can be quickly assessed with the U/S (quick measurement for GA or only an estimate depending on the urgency). Blood type can wait.

---

71 A quick ultrasound (U/S) reveals breech presentation with anterior placenta with no retroplacental accumulation of blood. A quick fetal head measurement is consistent with 34 week's gestation. A pelvic is remarkable for 200 mL of clot and active bright red bleeding. The cervix is 1 cm, thick and high.

What is your next step?

(A) Start oxytocin
(B) Start amnioinfusion
(C) Prepare for external version
(D) Prepare for emergent Cesarean

The answer is D: Prepare for emergent Cesarean. An U/S is done to see if the abruption can be seen and to locate the placenta. The diagnosis of abruption is not made by U/S, though. It is a clinical diagnosis. The vaginal examination and late decelerations make this a medical emergency.

---

72 The patient undergoes emergency Cesarean section and is delivered of a viable male Apgar score of 2/4/8 weighing 2,100 g. Estimated blood loss is 1,500 mL. She is transfused 4 units of blood.

What blood work would you order intraoperatively?

(A) Sexually transmitted disease panel
(B) Coagulation panel
(C) Toxicology screen
(D) Hepatitis panel

The answer is B: Coagulation panel. Abruption is the most common cause of coagulopathy in pregnancy.

---

73 You are shadowing the genetic counselor who is seeing a young couple with abnormal quad screen at 17 weeks dated by last menstrual period (LMP) and ultrasound (U/S). The patient is a 24-year-old Latin American woman G2P0010 now at 19 weeks with a negative history except for a previous spontaneous abortion at 8 weeks and normal prenatal course thus far. The quad screen risk factor for Down syndrome is 1 in 8.

What would you recommend to this couple?

(A) Termination of pregnancy
(B) Amniocentesis
(C) Chorionic villus sampling (CVS)
(D) Repeat quad screen

The answer is B: **Amniocentesis.** Although the screen shows a risk of 1 in 8, it is not diagnostic; therefore, termination based on the quad would be unwarranted. CVS is done in the first trimester. Repeating the quad screen is not indicated unless there is an issue of gestational dating in which case a dating U/S would be performed and the quad recalculated based on the new gestational age (GA). The quad would be redrawn if it was felt to be drawn too early. In this scenario, the dates by LMP are confirmed by U/S.

74 You are following up A.G., a 34-year-old G3P1102 at 35 weeks who had a previous classical Cesarean at 29 weeks with her last pregnancy for breech presentation with preterm premature rupture of membranes (PPROM) and labor at 26 weeks. The maternal fetal medicine specialist recommends delivery before the onset of labor because of her uterine scar. She is a gestational diabetic on insulin and is having twice weekly nonstress testings (NSTs) and weekly biophysical profiles (BPPs) and you are called because of a score of 2 on her BPP and a nonreactive NST.

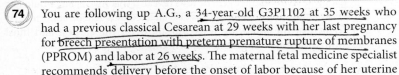

What is your next step?

(A) Perform an amnio for fetal lung maturity
(B) Start oxytocin induction of labor
(C) Perform an emergency Cesarean section
(D) Admit her and repeat the NST and BPP in the am

The answer is C: **Perform an emergency Cesarean section.** An amnio would not be warranted since the patient has an indication for delivery. Induction of labor is contraindicated due to the classical scar. Observation is not warranted in a BPP of 2.

75 A 23-year-old G1P0 presents to the emergency room (ER) complaining of contractions and fluid loss. She has had no prenatal care, but her gestational age (GA) is around 36 to 38 weeks by her last menstrual period (LMP). Her fundal height is 34 cm. She labors for several hours and gives birth to a male infant weighing 2,200 g who has small palpebral fissures, a thin lip, and head circumference less than the 10th percentile.

What substance is the most likely cause of this infant's appearance?

(A) Alcohol
(B) Cocaine
(C) Nonsteroidal anti-inflammatory drugs
(D) Narcotics
(E) Lithium

The answer is A: Alcohol. The infant is born with characteristics consistent with fetal alcohol syndrome. Fetal alcohol syndrome is characterized by dysmorphic facial features, including small palpebral fissures, thin vermillion border, and a smooth philtrum. The infant's weight is classified as low birth weight and his head circumference is consistent with intrauterine growth retardation (IUGR). Alcohol is the most common nongenetic cause of mental retardation and the leading cause of preventable birth defects.

76 A 40-year-old G2P0010 at 10 week's gestation presents to your clinic to discuss her options for genetic testing. She previously had an elective termination at 17 weeks after genetic tests revealed trisomy 18. She would like to know if the current pregnancy is also affected by a genetic abnormality.

Which of the following tests will allow for the earliest and most definitive diagnosis of genetic abnormalities?

(A) hCG, plasma protein A (PAPP-A)
(B) Amniocentesis
(C) Integrated screening
(D) Chorionic villus sampling (CVS)
(E) Amniotic α-fetoprotein (AFP), hCG, estriol, inhibin A

The answer is D: CVS. CVS is a procedure performed at 10 to 13 week's gestation that allows for the earliest detection and confirmation of fetal genetic abnormalities. CVS directly samples fetal tissue from the placenta and therefore the results are diagnostic. Amniocentesis is another definitive diagnostic test, but it is not performed until the second trimester. First-trimester screening for aneuploidy includes the serum markers hCG and PAPP-A. The quad screen performed in the second trimester includes AFP, hCG, estriol, and inhibin A. The integrated screening test incorporates results from both the first- and second-trimester screening test and has the highest detection rate for aneuploidy; however, the results are not available until the second trimester. It is important to understand that the first-trimester, second-trimester, and integrated screening tests only assess the risk of genetic abnormalities and are not diagnostic.

77 A 37-year-old G4P2012 at 18 week's gestation presents to your clinic to discuss the results of her recent quadruple screen. The results of the quad screen are as follows: decreased Amniotic α-fetoprotein (AFP), increased hCG, decreased estriol, increased inhibin A. She is concerned about the results and would like further evaluation.

What is the next step in evaluating this patient's risk of aneuploidy?

(A) Ultrasound (U/S)
(B) Amniocentesis
(C) Repeat quadruple screen
(D) Chorionic villus sampling (CVS)
(E) Nuchal translucency measurement

The answer is A: Ultrasound (U/S). Incorrect gestational age (GA) and a multiple-gestation pregnancy can lead to incorrect interpretation of quad screen results; therefore, the next best step in evaluating an abnormal quad screen is to perform an U/S to accurately determine the GA and the number of fetuses. Amniocentesis can be used at 16 to 20 week's gestation to collect fetal DNA for karyotyping; however, it is important to first confirm the GA with U/S in order to prevent unnecessary risks to the fetus. CVS must be performed during the first trimester, specifically at 10 to 12 weeks. Measurement of nuchal translucency is utilized during the first trimester to determine the risk of aneuploidy.

---

78 A 29-year-old G1P0 at 24 week's gestation presents for routine prenatal care. She had a prepregnancy BMI of 32 kg/m^2 and has gained 18 lb since her first visit at 8 week's gestation. Her pregnancy has been uncomplicated so far and a 20-week ultrasound (U/S) revealed normal fetal anatomy.

What is the patient's most likely complication this pregnancy?

(A) Gestational diabetes
(B) Preeclampsia
(C) Macrosomia
(D) Postterm pregnancy
(E) Postpartum hemorrhage

The answer is A: Gestational diabetes. Obese women were 3.6 times more likely to develop gestational diabetes than nonobese women. They are also at a higher risk for preeclampsia, fetal macrosomia, postterm pregnancy, and postpartum hemorrhage, but the risk of gestational diabetes is highest. The risk of gestational diabetes is high because of the effect of insulin resistance that occurs in both pregnancy and obesity.

79 A 34-year-old G2P1001 at 12 week's gestation presents to your clinic following an abnormal first-trimester screen. She desires genetic testing for further evaluation. You explain the risks and benefits and she decides to have an amniocentesis performed during the second trimester.

Had the patient chosen chorionic villus sampling (CVS) before 10 weeks, which of the risks would be of specific concern?

(A) Fetal loss
(B) Vaginal spotting
(C) Chorioamnionitis
(D) Amniotic fluid leakage
(E) Fetal limb-reduction defects

The answer is E: Fetal limb-reduction defects. Birth defects resulting from fetal limb-reduction are associated with CVS when performed at less than 10 week's gestation. This risk necessitates obtaining an accurate gestational age (GA) prior to performing the test. CVS performed at 10 to 13 week's gestation is safe, and the risk of adverse effects is similar to that of amniocentesis. Fetal loss, vaginal spotting, infection, and amniotic fluid leakage can occur with both CVS and amniocentesis.

---

80 A 24-year-old G1P0 at 18 week's gestation presents for initiation of prenatal care. Her past medical history is significant for asthma for which she occasionally uses an albuterol inhaler. Her last Pap smear revealed atypical cells of undetermined significance. She reports drinking four alcoholic beverages per week prior to pregnancy. She has smoked for 8 years.

How is this pregnancy most likely to be affected by her history?

(A) Cervical abnormality
(B) Congenital malformation
(C) Small for gestational age (GA) fetus
(D) Fetal chromosomal abnormality
(E) Abnormal placental implantation

The answer is C: Small for gestational age (GA) fetus. This patient's most significant risk factor is her current smoking status. Tobacco use in pregnancy is associated with fetal growth restriction, premature rupture of membranes (ROMs), placenta previa, and low birth weight. Atypical cells of undetermined significance would not result in cervical abnormalities that would impact this pregnancy. Congenital malformations and fetal chromosomal abnormalities are not associated with tobacco use. Tobacco use can impact the placental vasculature by causing uteroplacental insufficiency or placental abruption but does not impact the initial formation and implantation of the placenta.

---

81 A 22-year-old G1P0 at 19 weeks presents to discuss the results of her recent quad screen. She was diagnosed with epilepsy as a child and was taking valproic acid until she discovered that she was pregnant at 12 week's gestation. Assuming that the pregnancy has been affected by valproic acid, you expect her quad screen results will mirror the results seen with which of the following disorders?

(A) Trisomy 13
(B) Trisomy 18
(C) Trisomy 21
(D) Anencephaly
(E) Holoprosencephaly

The answer is D: Anencephaly. Valproic acid is associated with spina bifida which is an neural tube defects (NTD). Anencephaly is also an NTD which will be associated with elevated Maternal serum α-fetoprotein (MSAFP). The majority of cases of holoprosencephaly are sporadic and occur in fetuses with a normal karyotype. In the prenatal period, holoprosencephaly is diagnosed by characteristic ultrasound (U/S) findings. Trisomies 13, 18, and 21 are all aneuploidy genetic disorders that can be screened for by first- and second-trimester screening and diagnosis can be confirmed with direct analysis of fetal DNA from an amniocentesis. In trisomy 21, a second-trimester quad screen will show decreased amniotic α-fetoprotein (AFP), increased hCG, decreased estriol, and increased inhibin A. Trisomy 18 will show all four analytes to be decreased. Trisomy 13 will show normal AFP and decreased β-hCG.

---

82 A couple has just learned by a third-trimester ultrasound (U/S) that their baby has a decreased femur length compared with biparietal diameter as well as other findings highly suspicious for dwarfism. Both parents are of normal height and deny any dwarfism in their family. The mother is 34 years old and otherwise healthy. She reports compliance with prenatal vitamins, takes no other medications, and has had no complications throughout the pregnancy. The father is 42 years old and is otherwise healthy.

What is the most likely interpretation of these results?

- **(A)** This most likely resulted from a new mutation
- **(B)** The fetus is most likely homozygous for this allele
- **(C)** The father should request a paternity test
- **(D)** The mother most likely did not take prenatal vitamins as recommended
- **(E)** The fibroblast growth factor (FGF) receptor is under active in this fetus and will result in achondroplasia

The answer is A: This most likely resulted from a new mutation. Cases of achondroplasia in unaffected parents are the result of a spontaneous new mutation. This is an autosomal dominant mutation but can occur spontaneously (80% of cases). If the fetus is homozygous, this is lethal. The result is an overactive FGF receptor that results in defective cell signaling. It is also associated with advanced paternal age (over 35).

---

83 A 28-year-old woman G3P2 at 25 weeks has just moved to the United States from Eastern Europe. As part of her routine health screening she received a purified protein derivative (PPD) test and now presents to the clinic for her results. She currently denies any fever, shortness of breath, cough, wheezing, or chest pain. She denies any previous vaccinations or regular medical care previously. Her injection site shows 10-mm induration.

What is the next best step in management?

Table 6-1 Estimated Fetal Exposure from Some Common Radiologic Procedures

Procedure	Fetal Exposure
Chest x-ray (two views)	0.02–0.07 mrad
Abdominal film (single view)	100 mrad
Intravenous pyelography	≥1 rad
Hip film (single view)	200 mrad
Mammography	7–20 mrad
Barium enema or small-bowel series	2–4 rad
CT scan of head or chest	<1 rad
CT scan of abdomen and lumbar spine	3.5 rad
CT pelvimetry	250 mrad

CT, computed tomography.

(A) Chest x-ray now
(B) Chest x-ray after delivery
(C) Begin treatment for tuberculosis
(D) Close follow-up as PPD skin testing is contraindicated in pregnancy
(E) Obtain further history of exposure

The answer is A: Chest x-ray now. The chest x-ray should be performed before delivery with the fetus properly shielded. The risk of active TB infection to a neonate far outweighs the risk of x-ray now. PPD is not contraindicated in pregnancy. A single diagnostic x-ray does not result in exposure adequate to threaten the well-being of the embryo or fetus and is not an indication for abortion. If indications suggest the need for multiple diagnostic images, MRI or ultrasound (U/S) should be considered as they do not result in exposure to ionizing radiation. The use of radioactive isotopes of iodine is contraindicated for therapeutic use during pregnancy. Exposure to less than 5 rad cumulatively has not been associated with an increase in fetal anomalies or abortion (*Table 6-1*).

84 A 34-year-old woman presents to the emergency room (ER) after experiencing intense vaginal bleeding, abdominal pain, and passage of clots and possibly tissue. She is uncertain of when her last menstrual period

(LMP) occurred. She has had three previous term pregnancies. She says that she had not suspected pregnancy because of a history of irregular periods. Earlier in the day, she had intense abdominal cramping following episodes of bleeding and passage of clots. The bleeding and cramping increased over the next few hours. She reports continued cramping and bleeding. She is afraid and tearful. She says she has never experienced anything like this. Her vital signs are BP 135/75 mmHg, HR 80 beats/min, RR 18 breaths/min, T 98.9. Pelvic examination reveals an 8-week sized boggy uterus with an open cervical os and brisk active bleeding. There is no adnexal fullness or tenderness. Your transvaginal probe is broken.

What is the next best step in management?

(A) Perform a dilation and curettage
(B) Discharge patient home after explaining that she has had a complete abortion
(C) Obtain an abdominal ultrasound (U/S)
(D) Administer methotrexate
(E) Admit for observation

The answer is A: Perform a dilation and curettage. The history of bleeding, abdominal cramping, and passage of tissue vaginally all suggest abortion, but an open cervical os with continued bleeding and cramping are likely due to an incomplete abortion. A transvaginal U/S would likely show retained products. A history of possible passage of tissue does not confirm all products have been expelled. This patient requires a dilation and curettage to clear the uterus of all retained tissue to prevent infection and hemorrhage. Abdominal U/S would unlikely be helpful at this stage of her pregnancy. A complete abortion would result in a resolution of bleeding and cramping with a closed cervical os.

---

85 An African American married couple has met with a genetic counselor in order to discuss pregnancy. The man reports that he has never been genetically tested but does not have sickle cell disease. He reports that his father had sickle cell disease. His mother did not have the disease. The woman was adopted and does not know her family history but has never been diagnosed with the disease. They want to know the risk of their baby having sickle cell disease. You decide to do further testing to ascertain the carrier status of the woman. Testing reveals she is a carrier.

What would be the risk of their child developing sickle cell disease?

(A) 0
(B) 1/8
(C) 1/4
(D) 1/2

The answer is C: 1/4. The mother does not know her family history but testing reveals she is a carrier. The father must be a carrier since he does not have the disease (he had a ½ or 50% chance of having sickle cell or carrying the trait). Since they are both carriers, there is a ¼ chance their baby will have sickle cell disease.

---

86 A 29-year-old G1P0010 patient comes to see you for the first time in clinic to establish routine care. She mentions to you that she is not using any contraception methods and that she and her husband are hoping to have children someday soon. She has no known medical conditions or surgical history and takes no medications. The noted vitals are within normal ranges and she has a BMI of 24. Her family history is unremarkable and she has no gynecologic complaints at this time. She has questions about attempting pregnancy. You learn that her previous abortion was spontaneous and within the first trimester. The most common genetic anomaly associated with first-trimester pregnancy loss is:

(A) Trisomy 21
(B) Trisomy 13
(C) Trisomy 18
(D) Trisomy 16
(E) Trisomy 11

The answer is D: Trisomy 16. An estimated 60% to 80% of first-trimester abortions are associated with chromosomal abnormalities. Trisomy 16 is the most common genetic anomaly associated with first-trimester abortion. It is a lethal anomaly when it is a full trisomy resulting most often from nondisjunction. Trisomy 21 results in Down syndrome. Trisomy 13 results in Patau syndrome and few infants live past the first year of life due to multiple medical conditions including congenital heart defects. Trisomy 18, Edward syndrome, can result in stillbirths as well as many medical complications with few babies living past a year old. Trisomy 11 is associated with other syndromes not often associated with spontaneous abortion.

---

87 A 23-year-old woman G1 last menstrual period (LMP) 6 weeks ago comes into the emergency room (ER) with vaginal bleeding and cramping abdominal pain. Pregnancy is confirmed by β-hCG of 4,200 mIU/mL. She is surprised by the news of pregnancy. She denies any use of illicit substances, tobacco, or alcohol. She reports a diagnosis of chlamydia 2 years ago that was treated. Her last Pap smear was 7 months ago. She is sexually active and lives with her boyfriend. She works at a bar in the evenings and attends community college. She reports diffuse lower abdominal pain as a 5/10 with cramping. BP is 125/73 mmHg, HR 75 beats/min, RR 16 breaths/min, T 98.8. Pelvic examination reveals a closed cervical os, mild active bleeding, 6-week sized boggy uterus, and no adnexal masses.

What is the best next step in management?

(A) Give methotrexate
(B) Obtain a transvaginal ultrasound (U/S) to rule out an ectopic pregnancy
(C) Repeat hCG in 48 hours to determine viable uterine pregnancy
(D) Prescribe pain medication and discharge home
(E) Obtain an abdominal U/S to rule out ectopic pregnancy

The answer is B: Obtain a transvaginal ultrasound (U/S) to rule out an ectopic pregnancy. The β-hCG is high enough to visualize a pregnancy by a transvaginal U/S (1,500 to 2,000 β-hCG) but not an abdominal U/S (>6,500 β-hCG). As this patient does not report any passage of tissue at this time and continues to have abdominal cramping, it is likely a threatened abortion. There is also the possibility that this is an ectopic pregnancy, which should be ruled out by U/S as this can be a surgical emergency if the ectopic ruptures. The patient has stable vitals at this time which does not suggest urgent action such as taking the patient to the operating room (OR). Passage of tissue, a closed os, and resolution of bleeding would suggest clinically that the patient has undergone a complete abortion.

---

88 A 28-year-old G2P1 is seen in your clinic for her initial obstetrical (OB) visit. Vitals today are BP 110/72 mmHg, HR 75 beats/min, RR 15 breaths/min, T 98.0. Her last menstrual period (LMP) was 8 weeks ago. She denies any spotting or discharge. She reports a weight gain of about 5 lb over the past 2 months. She reports taking prenatal vitamins and continuing her exercise regimen. She delivered a 7 lb 2 oz baby vaginally 3 years ago without any complications. She has no family history of any genetic disorders. She reports to you that she adheres to a diet rich in fish and vegetables. Upon further questioning, she tells you that she mostly eats canned albacore tuna.

What are the best recommendations you can give her about how much she should consume weekly?

(A) None, she should stop eating any canned fish
(B) 3 oz/wk
(C) 6 oz/wk
(D) 10 oz/wk
(E) 12 oz/wk

The answer is C: 6 oz/wk. The Food and Drug Administration recommendations are that pregnant women should limit ingestion of albacore tuna to 6 oz/wk, or 12 oz/wk of a mixed variety of low mercury fish and shellfish. Women who eat fish store high levels of mercury. Exposure to mercury can lead to damage to the fetus. Neurologic effects are the most prominent, including affecting cognitive thinking, memory, attention, language skills, and visual spatial skills. The nervous system seems to be the most vulnerable to toxic levels of mercury.

89 A 25-year-old primigravida with gestational hypertension presents to your clinic for routine prenatal care. She is now at 37-week gestational age (GA) with dates confirmed by first-trimester ultrasound (U/S). In clinic, she has a BP of 150/85 and you are considering delivering her early due to potential complications from her disease. Her urine protein is negative and she denies any headache, vision changes, or abdominal pain.

Which of the following test results would be most reassuring that the fetus would not have respiratory distress after birth?

(A) Lamellar body count of 55,000
(B) Lecithin:sphingomyelin of 1.2:1
(C) Phosphatidylglycerol of 0.3
(D) Good diaphragmatic movement on biophysical profile (BPP)
(E) Surfactant:albumin of 25

The answer is A: Lamellar body count of 55,000. Lamellar body count is currently the most commonly used test in the United States to assess fetal lung maturity. A value >50,000 strongly suggests fetal lung maturity. All of the other answers give values that are not reassuring for fetal lung maturity.

CHAPTER

7

Obstetrics Postpartum

1 A 38-year-old woman presents to labor and delivery in the first stage of labor. She has had an uncomplicated pregnancy and has attended all of her prenatal care visits. After complete cervical dilation and effacement, she is ready to give birth. The baby arrives and is given 1- and 5-minute Apgar scores of 6 and 9, respectively.

Which of the following is an appropriate use of the Apgar score?

(A) To define the degree of birth asphyxia
(B) To score the infant's neuromuscular maturity
(C) To grade the overall health of the infant
(D) To evaluate the need for neonatal resuscitation

The answer is D: To evaluate the need for neonatal resuscitation. The Apgar scoring system is an objective way for health-care providers to quickly assess an infant's need for and responsiveness to neonatal resuscitation. An assessment is done at both 1 and 5 minutes following birth. There is no correlation between Apgar score, neonatal outcome, maturity, and overall health, and it cannot be used to determine the cause of neonatal distress or to define birth asphyxia. Typically, Apgar scores of 7 to 10 indicate no need for resuscitation, scores between 4 and 7 suggest mild-to-moderate depression, and a score less than 4 suggests severe depression.

2 A G1P1 you have been following for her entire pregnancy has just given birth. The birth was uncomplicated; the baby, born at term, received Apgar scores of 7 and 10; and the placenta has just arrived, full and intact. If you have not done so already, which of the following is the most appropriate next step?

(A) Place the infant on the mother with skin-to-skin contact
(B) Transfer the infant to the neonatal nursery and allow the mother to rest
(C) Perform a uterine sweep for occult placental remnants
(D) Evaluate the newborn for appropriate neonatal reflexes

The answer is A: Place the infant on the mother with skin-to-skin contact. Maintaining an appropriate body temperature is difficult for all infants. If resuscitation is not needed, routine care should include thoroughly drying the infant and placing the newborn on its mother's chest with skin-to-skin contact. This can also assist with maternal–infant bonding and breastfeeding.

---

3 A 31-year-old gives birth via a forceps-assisted vaginal delivery to a 6-lb 2-oz girl. In the process of delivery, she sustains a second-degree perineal laceration, and during inspection prior to repair, a nonenlarging, solid swelling of clotted blood 3 cm in diameter is noted adjacent to the tear within the submucosa. After repairing the laceration, what is the next step in management of this patient?

(A) Manage expectantly with frequent evaluation
(B) Surgically open the area of clotted blood at its most dependent portion and drain
(C) Apply drains and vaginal packs to the area of clotted blood
(D) Apply heat packs to the affected area

The answer is A: Manage expectantly with frequent evaluation. Hematomas that are <5 cm in diameter and are not enlarging can usually be managed expectantly by frequent evaluation of the size of the hematoma and close monitoring of vital signs and urinary output. Ice packs applied to the affected area can be helpful, but heat should be avoided. For hematomas greater than 5 cm, surgical management is indicated which involves opening and draining the area and then applying drains and vaginal packs to prevent reaccumulation of blood.

---

4 A 22-year-old woman gives birth at 39 weeks 3 days by normal spontaneous vaginal delivery (NSVD) to a 6-lb 12-oz boy. After delivery of the baby, the placenta is delivered within 10 minutes and inspected to determine whether it is intact. After confirmation that the entire placenta has been removed, the uterus is palpated abdominally and noted to be soft and boggy.

What is the next step in the management of this patient?

(A) Manual massage of the uterus
(B) Wait 10 minutes and reassess
(C) Blood type and screen the patient
(D) Apply uterine compression sutures

The answer is A: Manual massage of the uterus. This patient has uterine atony. The first step in management is to begin uterine massage. This should be done while preparing other treatments including uterotonics such as oxytocin, methylergonovine maleate, and misoprostol. Uterine atony should be assessed and managed immediately. By waiting any amount of time and reassessing, one increases the risk of significant postpartum hemorrhage (PPH). The patient should be typed and screened for blood prior to her delivery in preparation for a potential blood transfusion. Uterine compression sutures should only be employed if initial treatments of uterine atony are unsuccessful.

5 A 24-year-old G2P1 at term has precipitously delivered a viable female infant. The tracing had been category 1 and reassuring until the membranes ruptured spontaneously approximately 15 minutes before delivery. At that point, the fetal heart rate decreased and never rose above 85 beats per minute (BPM). The newborn has a heart rate of less than 100, a slow respiratory rate, flaccid muscle tone, a grimace, and blue coloring. The appropriate Apgar assignment is:

(A) 1
(B) 2
(C) 3
(D) 4
(E) 5

The answer is D: 4. See *Table 7-1*.

Table 7-1 Apgar Score

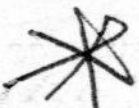

Sign	Score = 0	Score = 1	Score = 2
Heart rate (beats/minute)	Absent	Below 100/min	Above 100/min
Respiratory effort	Absent	Weak, irregular, or gasping	Good, crying
Muscle tone	Flaccid	Some flexion of arms and legs	Well flexed or active movements of extremities
Reflex/irritability	No response	Grimace or weak cry	Good cry
Color	Blue all over or pale	Body pink; hands and feet blue	Pink all over

6 A 26-year-old G2P1 has just delivered a 3,245-g term male infant after a 65-minute second stage of labor that was characterized by repetitive severe variable decelerations over the last 20 minutes of labor. Amniotic fluid remained clear. Upon delivery, a double nuchal cord was noted. At 1 minute, the newborn has a heart rate of 60, slow and irregular respiratory rate, minimal flexion of arms and legs with stimulation, a grimace, and blue color centrally. The correct Apgar assignment is:

(A) 1
(B) 2
(C) 3
(D) 4
(E) 5

The answer is D: 4. See *Table 7-1.*

---

7 A 34-year-old G3P2 at 30 week's gestation in vertex presentation undergoes induction of labor for a diagnosis of severe preeclampsia. Symptoms include a severe headache, right upper quadrant pain, and a blood pressure (BP) of 176/105 mmHg. Her platelet count, which was initially normal at 185K 6 hours ago, recently decreased to 100K. A 24-hour urine revealed 1,200 mg protein. She has responded favorably to induction of labor with and is currently 7 cm with a category 1 tracing. A vaginal delivery is anticipated.

Which current medication is most commonly associated with uterine atony?

(A) Ampicillin
(B) Betamethasone
(C) Meperidine
(D) Magnesium sulfate
(E) Misoprostol

The answer is D: Magnesium sulfate. Magnesium sulfate causes vascular dilation which is in part responsible for its effectiveness in preventing eclamptic seizures. This also increases the risk of bleeding since the major mechanism for prevention of postpartum hemorrhage (PPH) is contraction of the gravid uterus after delivery of the placenta.

---

8 A 32-year-old G2P2 now 8 days postpartum from a labor complicated by prolonged rupture of membranes presents with shaking chills and general malaise. Examination reveals moderate uterine tenderness with guarding in the lower abdomen, a fever of 39.2, and foul-smelling lochia. A culture is performed prior to beginning antibiotic therapy.

Which bacteria are the least likely isolate in this case?

(A) *Enterococcus*
(B) Group B beta strep
(C) *Neisseria gonorrhoeae*
(D) *Peptostreptococcus*
(E) *Ureaplasma urealyticum*

The answer is A: *Enterococcus*. This patient has endomyometritis; 25% of women who have received cephalosporin prophylaxis at Cesarean section will have *Enterococcus* identified on culture. All other bacteria are present in the vagina and have been identified as causing ascending infections in the case of prolonged rupture of membranes.

---

9 A 24-year-old G1P1 breastfeeding mother is now post-op day 2 from a primary low transverse Cesarean section for failure to progress and arrest of dilation at 7 cm. Within the past 36 hours, she has had two fevers over 38°C. A complete blood count (CBC) reveals WBC 16.3K and hemoglobin 8.6/hematocrit (HCT) 25. A urinalysis (UA) per catheter is leukocyte esterase and nitrite negative. She complains of abdominal pain and generalized malaise. Examination reveals the following: breast examination: no redness, inflammation, or nipple cracks; no costovertebral angle (CVA) tenderness; lungs are clear to auscultation. Homan sign is negative. Incision is clean, dry, and intact. Bowel sounds are present. There is exquisite uterine tenderness with guarding but no rebound in the lower abdomen. Lochia is moderate. The appropriate initial intravenous antibiotic regimen for this patient is:

(A) Cefazolin
(B) Doxycycline
(C) Gentamicin and clindamycin
(D) Gentamicin and ampicillin
(E) Metronidazole and ampicillin

The answer is B: Doxycycline. Doxycycline can cause problems with stippling of the infant's teeth and should not be given to nursing mothers. Cefazolin had most likely already been given as prophylaxis prior to Cesarean section and would not be a good choice since the patient developed the infection despite prophylactic antibiotic therapy.

---

10 A 29-year-old G2P1 is now 4 days post-op from a primary low transverse Cesarean section for failure to progress complicated by chorioamnionitis. She had been diagnosed with endometritis and started on intravenous gentamicin and clindamycin on postpartum day 2. She has continued to spike fevers above 38°C despite 48 hours on the antibiotic regimen. A complete blood count (CBC) reveals white blood cell (WBC) count of 18.2K and hemoglobin 11/hematocrit (HCT) 33. A urinalysis (UA) per catheter is leukocyte esterase and nitrite negative. Homan sign is negative. She complains of abdominal pain. Examination reveals the following: breast examination: no redness, inflammation, or nipple cracks; no costovertebral angle (CVA) tenderness; lungs are clear to auscultation. Incision is clean, dry, and intact. Bowel sounds are present. There is exquisite uterine tenderness with guarding but no rebound in the lower abdomen. Lochia is moderate and foul smelling. The addition of what antibiotic should be considered at this time:

(A) Ampicillin
(B) Cefazolin
(C) Cefotetan
(D) Doxycycline
(E) Metronidazole

The answer is A: Ampicillin. Over 25% of cases of endometritis after Cesarean section with cephalosporin prophylaxis will be caused by *Enterococcus*. In order to cover these bacteria, ampicillin should be added to the current gentamicin and clindamycin regimen. If the patient does not respond within 24 hours, imaging and additional evaluation should be considered to determine whether she has septic pelvic thrombophlebitis.

---

11 A G2P1 delivered a preterm 32-week infant precipitously via spontaneous vaginal delivery (SVD). Although the neonatal team had been called, they did not arrive until 4 minutes after the delivery. Upon delivery, the infant cried spontaneously and received an Apgar score of 7 at 1 minute. The most effective method to keep this infant warm after initially drying it until the neonatal team arrives would be:

(A) Move to the warmer immediately
(B) Cover the infant's head with a stocking net
(C) Swaddle the infant
(D) Place in a plastic bag
(E) Place the baby skin-to-skin with the mother

The answer is E: Place the baby skin-to-skin with the mother. This comes from the Cochrane database "Interventions to prevent hypothermia is preterm and/or low birthweight infants" March 2010.

---

12 A 24-year-old G1P1 has just delivered a 3,250-g term infant by spontaneous vaginal delivery (SVD) without complications. The

fetal heart tracing remained category 1 throughout the entire labor. When the infant is being resuscitated, the nurses offered the blow by oxygen. Select the statement that best reflects the current evidence related to oxygen use in neonatal resuscitation.

(A) Mortality of babies at 1 month seems to be reduced by the use of room air
(B) Mortality of babies at 1 month seems to be reduced by the use of 100% oxygen
(C) Mortality of babies at 1 month seems to be reduced by the use of blow by oxygen
(D) Mortality of babies at 1 month seems to be reduced when no ventilatory assistance is offered routinely

The answer is A: **Mortality of babies at 1 month seems to be reduced by the use of room air.** There was no evidence of differences in other adverse outcomes when comparing 100% O_2 with room air.

---

13 A 24-year-old G2P1011 just delivered a 29-week infant via primary low vertical Cesarean section with an estimated blood loss of 1,200 cc. She was initially admitted 28 hours ago with threatened preterm labor and was undergoing a preterm labor protocol including a preterm antenatal corticosteroid regimen but was noted approximately 45 minutes ago to be 8 cm in footling breech presentation. A STAT Cesarean section was performed, and the infant had Apgar scores of 6/8/9 and was transferred to the neonatal intensive care unit.

Which of the medications she has been recently administered is most likely responsible for the postpartum hemorrhage (PPH)?

(A) Ampicillin
(B) Betamethasone
(C) Fentanyl
(D) Magnesium sulfate
(E) Cefazolin

The answer is D: **Magnesium sulfate.** In this case, the patient was receiving magnesium sulfate for neuroprophylaxis based on fetal age. She received ampicillin and betamethasone as part of a preterm labor protocol. She received cefazolin as prophylaxis at the time of Cesarean section. Fentanyl was used in the spinal. Of these medications, magnesium sulfate is implicated in uterine atony. Uterine atony is the most common cause of PPH. A blood loss of greater than 1,000 cc at Cesarean section is considered a PPH.

14 A 23-year-old G2P2 just delivered a 3,120-g infant via spontaneous vaginal delivery (SVD) and has lost approximately 800 cc. Her medical history is significant for seasonal allergies and asthma.

Which of the following should be avoided when treating a postpartum hemorrhage (PPH) in this patient?

(A) Carboprost tromethamine
(B) Methylergonovine
(C) Misoprostol
(D) Oxytocin
(E) Prostaglandin E1

The answer is A: Carboprost tromethamine. Carboprost tromethamine should be used with caution in patients with asthma.

15 A 24-year-old woman, G2P2, delivered a 3,400-g male infant via repeat Cesarean section for breech presentation just after midnight today. Prior to delivery, her vital signs were normal. Six hours after delivery, the nurse reports a fever of 38.2°C. Upon evaluation, there is no fundal tenderness, incision is intact, lungs are clear to auscultation, and there is no Homan sign.

Which of the alternatives below best describes an appropriate management strategy for this patient?

(A) Order lower extremity Doppler
(B) Reassure the nurese and patient and manage expectantly
(C) At the next scheduled blood draw obtain complete blood count (CBC) with differential
(D) Obtain a catheterized specimen for urine culture in 12 hours if the fever continues
(E) Request blood cultures to be drawn immediately

The answer is B: Reassure the nurese and patient and manage expectantly. By definition, this is not a postpartum fever. The definition of postpartum fever is an oral temperature of 38°C or above twice in the first 10 days postpartum exclusive of the first 24 hours.

16 A 26-year-old is ready to go home after an uneventful spontaneous vaginal delivery (SVD). Her pregnancy, though, was complicated by severe anxiety that did not respond to nonpharmacologic measure. After extensive discussion and failed trials of other medications, she was placed on lorazepam with good results. You discuss the pros and cons of stopping the medication versus continuing postpartum. She is uncomfortable stopping at this time.

What instructions should be given with regard to breastfeeding?

(A) Compared with diazepam, lorazepam has a more adverse risk profile for nursing newborns
(B) Lorazepam effects on nursing newborns are unknown but may be of concern
(C) Lorazepam is a short-acting benzodiazepine; therefore, it is less likely to be concentrated in the breast milk
(D) Lorazepam should be taken immediately before nursing so that there will be no opportunity for it to concentrate in the milk the neonate receives at that feeding
(E) No adverse effects on neonates have been reported with lorazepam while breastfeeding

The answer is B: Lorazepam effects on nursing newborns are unknown but may be of concern. Lorazepam is a high-potency, intermediate-duration benzodiazepine. It is considered contraindicated in pregnancy, but apparently this patient tried other medications without success. The American Academy of Pediatrics warns that the effects on breastfeeding are unknown but may be of concern.

---

17 A 31-year-old G3P3 delivered a 4,160-g boy via spontaneous vaginal delivery (SVD) 30 minutes ago. Which of the following is a recommendation for exclusively breastfeeding mothers in the puerperium?

(A) Early supplementation with formula will help extend the time between night feedings
(B) Establish a feeding schedule as soon as possible
(C) Lactational amenorrhea can be an acceptable form of contraception until 6 months postpartum
(D) Use of combination oral contraceptives is recommended after the 6th postpartum week

The answer is C: Lactational amenorrhea can be an acceptable form of contraception until 6 months postpartum. Lactational amenorrhea is an acceptable form of contraception up to 6 months postpartum. Combination oral contraceptives are generally not used in breastfeeding as they may decrease the milk supply. Early supplementation is not recommended, and demand feeding is preferred over an early feeding schedule.

---

18 A 24-year-old G2P2 presents for a 2-week wound check after an uncomplicated repeat Cesarean delivery. An Edinburgh Postnatal Depression Scale was positive for postpartum depression.

Which element of her history would increase her risk of this condition?

(A) Absence of breastfeeding
(B) Cesarean delivery
(C) High school dropout
(D) Recent move from out of state
(E) Unplanned pregnancy

The answer is D: **Recent move from out of state.** Any highly stressful life event can cause an increased risk of depression. A move is considered a major life event and is known to increase stress substantially. All of the rest of the choices have not been linked to causing postpartum depression. A history of postpartum depression would increase the risk to 25%.

---

19 A 33-year-old G3P1021 is now 10 days postpartum. During her hospital admission, she had a fever of 38.2°C 12 hours after delivery, but the remainder of her hospital course was unremarkable. She presents with the following:

On arrival to the emergency room, vital signs are T 39.2, P 120 beats/min, and R 16 breaths/min. A complete blood count (CBC) reveals WBC 15.2K and hemoglobin 11.6/ hematocrit (HCT) 33. A voided midstream urinalysis (UA) is leukocyte esterase positive and nitrite negative. There are 15 WBC per high power fields with WBC casts present. Homan sign is negative. Breast examination is normal, nonengorged. costovertebral angle (CVA) tenderness is positive on the right.

What is the most likely organism?

(A) *Enterococci*
(B) *Escherichia coli*
(C) *Klebsiella* spp.
(D) *Pseudomonas aeruginosa*
(E) *Staphylococcus saprophyticus*

The answer is E: ***Staphylococcus saprophyticus.*** In this case, the most likely etiology is a coagulase-negative *Staphylococcus* which can be present in up to 10% of urinary tract infections (UTIs) in women. *S. saprophyticus* does not reduce nitrates to nitrites; hence, this is the only listed organism that would meet this criterion. The presence of greater than 10 leukocytes/μL in an unspun voided midstream urine specimen is considered abnormal, and WBC casts are considered diagnostic of an upper UTI.

---

20 A 26-year-old G6P5015 has precipitously delivered a 4,520-g male infant via normal spontaneous vaginal delivery (NSVD). Following the delivery, she has a period of uterine atony and the resident estimates that her blood loss was 650 cc.

Which most correctly characterizes her postpartum blood loss?

(A) Less than typical for a vaginal delivery
(B) Typical for a vaginal delivery
(C) More than normal for a vaginal delivery
(D) More than normal for a Cesarean section

The answer is C: More than normal for a vaginal delivery. A postpartum hemorrhage (PPH) is greater than 500 cc for a vaginal delivery and more than 1,000 cc for a Cesarean section. This patient has several risk factors for a PPH: she is a grand multipara, she delivered precipitously, and she had a macrosomic infant.

---

21 A 29-year-old G3P1112 with severe preeclampsia on magnesium sulfate therapy has just delivered a preterm infant at 31 weeks via Cesarean section for breech presentation. During the surgery, the uterus remained flaccid and unresponsive to uterine massage. Of the uterotonics below, which one is contraindicated in women with this presentation?

(A) Carboprost tromethamine
(B) Methylergonovine
(C) Misoprostol
(D) Oxytocin
(E) Prostaglandin E2

The answer is B: Methylergonovine. Methylergonovine is contraindicated in the hypertensive patient. Oxytocin given rapidly intravenously can cause hypotension. Carboprost should be avoided in asthmatic patients and may be associated with diarrhea, fever, and tachycardia. Prostin E2 should be avoided if the patient is hypotensive. Misoprostol can cause temperature elevation and diarrhea in high doses.

---

22 A normotensive 28-year-old G2P1001 completes the third stage of labor 27 minutes after delivery of a 3,280-g male infant. The labor was spontaneous and lasted 8 hours. The second stage of labor lasts 35 minutes. The nurse reports that the uterus is boggy and 6 cm above the umbilicus. When massaged, a clot of approximately 125 mL is expressed. In the prevention of postpartum hemorrhage (PPH), the medication employed as the first-line therapy is:

(A) Carboprost tromethamine
(B) Methylergonovine
(C) Misoprostol
(D) Oxytocin
(E) Prostaglandin E1

The answer is D: Oxytocin. The choice of other uterotonic agents after uterine massage and oxytocin are not effective including all other medications listed as alternatives. Use depends on patient condition, sensitivities, and in the face of no contraindication for the medication, provider preference.

---

23 A 26-year-old woman, G3P3, had an uneventful normal spontaneous vaginal delivery (NSVD) approximately 6 hours ago. The postpartum nurse requested an evaluation due to excessive vaginal bleeding. She describes saturation of three chux pads in the past 60 minutes. The patient's most recent vital signs are BP 70/36 mmHg, P 128 beats/min, and R 18 breaths/min.

Which of the following is the most likely cause of the bleeding this patient is experiencing?

(A) Blood clotting abnormalities
(B) Lacerations of the genital tract
(C) Retained fragments of placental tissue
(D) Uterine atony
(E) Uterine inversion

The answer is D: Uterine atony. While the patient should be evaluated for genital tract lacerations and the placenta should be inspected for missing pieces, uterine atony is the most likely cause of bleeding. The contraction of the uterus that effectively closes the placental bed (blood vessels) is the most significant physiologic mechanism for controlling postpartum bleeding. Approximately 80% of cases of early postpartum hemorrhage (PPH) are related to uterine atony.

---

24 A 27-year-old G2P2 delivered a 3,750-g infant spontaneously 1 hour ago. Her labor was complicated by induction for gestational diabetes at 39 weeks with 3.5-hour second stage of labor. The blood loss during delivery was estimated to be less than 500 cc, but when called by the nurse to evaluate the patient's bleeding, you express several fist-sized clots. That in addition to the blood on the chux pad is estimated to be 400 cc, making the total blood loss 900 cc.

Which of the following is not a strategy to reduce postpartum hemorrhage (PPH)?

(A) Administration of a uterotonic agent immediately after delivery of the infant
(B) Early cord clamping and cutting
(C) Gentle cord traction with uterine countertraction when the uterus is well contracted
(D) Immediate skin-to-skin contact
(E) Uterine massage

The answer is D: Immediate skin-to-skin contact. The other actions are part of a management strategy called active management of the second stage. Although immediate skin-to-skin contact is an excellent method to cause uterine contraction and prevent PPH, it is not part of the active management protocol.

---

25 A 17-year-old G1P0 at 37 week's gestation with diet-controlled gestational diabetes presents for a prenatal visit accompanied by her mother. A sonogram that was performed today reveals a singleton gestation with estimated fetal weight of 3,100 g consistent with last menstrual period, vertex presentation, anterior grade 2 placenta, amniotic fluid index of 12.6. A cervical examination today is cl/th/−3. The plan is induction at 39 weeks due to her gestational diabetes. The mother expresses concern because she had a postpartum hemorrhage (PPH) after delivering her daughter. She received 3 units of packed RBCs and subsequently developed hepatitis C. She wants to know whether there are ways to prevent PPH and thus avoid blood products during her daughter's delivery. You tell them that the daughter's risk factors include:

(A) A family history of PPH
(B) A possible induction of labor at 39 weeks
(C) Developing macrosomia
(D) Polyhydramnios
(E) There are no increased risks based on history

The answer is B: A possible induction of labor at 39 weeks. A nulliparous patient undergoing an induction of labor with an unfavorable cervix is at risk for a prolonged labor. Prolonged labor and induction have been linked to increased risk of PPH.

26 After the delivery of the placenta of a preeclamptic patient on magnesium therapy you become concerned that her bleeding is excessive. The maneuvers to control the bleeding are guided by the fact that immediate postpartum uterine hemostasis is a result of:

(A) Coagulation of the uterine vascular bed
(B) Mechanical obstruction of vessels
(C) Muscular contraction of the uterus
(D) Sludging effect of the postpartum state
(E) Tamponade effect of clots

The answer is C: Muscular contraction of the uterus. The major mechanism for prevention of PPH is contraction of the gravid uterus after delivery of the placenta.

27 A 26-year-old G2P2 with an uncomplicated pregnancy and delivery is now 12 hours postpartum. You are called to evaluate her on the postpartum floor due to excessive bleeding. She had previously received 0.2 mg of methergine and is currently on Oxytocin with 40 mEq/L running at 150 mL/h. Upon arrival, her BP is 98/58 mmHg and her pulse is 90 beats/min. Upon examination, her uterus is boggy and is felt vaguely felt and soft at 4 cm above the umbilicus. You note about 400 cc of blood clots on the chux pad.

Which of the following interventions is appropriate at this point in time?

(A) Methergine
(B) Oxytocin
(C) Prostaglandin
(D) Misoprostol
(E) Bimanual uterine massage

The answer is E: Bimanual uterine massage. The patient is currently bleeding with a uterus that is larger than expected. Immediately after delivery, the uterine fundus is located approximately at the umbilicus. The fact that this uterus is larger is concerning for blood clots that are preventing the uterus from contracting down normally. If a patient does not respond to one dose of Methergine, she is unlikely to respond to a second dose. While Cytotec and Carboprost Tromethamine are good considerations, the initial management at this point should be placing one hand in the vagina in the posterior cul-de-sac and palpating the uterine fundus exteriorly. This will allow direct determination of uterine response and also allow determination of clots present at the cervical opening.

28 An 18-year-old G1P1 had a prolonged induction of labor and after a 3-hour second stage delivered a 3,900-g male infant but had brief shoulder dystocia. During the last 1 hour of labor, the nurse noted her temperature to be 38.2°C. Antibiotics were administered. After delivery, the uterus was boggy and the nursing notes indicated a postpartum hemorrhage (PPH). Proper documentation of this condition requires a blood loss of greater than:

(A) 250 cc
(B) 500 cc
(C) 750 cc
(D) 1,000 cc
(E) 1,250 cc

The answer is B: 500 cc. A PPH in a vaginal delivery is greater than 500 mL and 1,000 cc for a Cesarean section.

CHAPTER

8

Breast and Lactation

1 A 25-year-old G1P1001 woman is seen on the postpartum service 6 hours after her normal vaginal delivery. She has no medical conditions and takes no medication. She wishes to breastfeed but begins crying when you enter the room. She tells you that her mother is encouraging her to begin feeding the baby formula because she seems to be fussy, and no milk is really coming out of her nipples anyway. She is considering asking for the nurse to bring her some formula. You reassure the patient by informing her about the benefits of colostrum and inform her that milk production usually begins on which postpartum day:

(A) 1
(B) 2
(C) 3
(D) 4
(E) 5

The answer is B: 2. The second stage of lactogenesis (the first 2 to 4 days after birth) begins following the delivery of the placenta, as the progesterone levels fall. Stage 2 includes dramatic increases in mammary blood flow and oxygen/glucose uptake by the breast. At 2 to 5 days postpartum, the secretion of milk is copious and "the milk comes in." This is the most common time for engorgement if the breasts are not drained by efficient, frequent nursing.

2 A 23-year-old G0P0 of Ashkenazi descent presents with a 3-week history of a painful right breast lump that is about the size of a golf ball. Her last menstrual period (LMP) was 2 weeks ago. She has no medical problems. Family history is positive for premenopausal breast cancer in her mother and a maternal aunt who were diagnosed at 39 and 42, respectively. Her maternal grandmother died from ovarian cancer at age 62. What imaging should you order?

(A) Diagnostic mammogram
(B) Helical computed tomography scan
(C) Magnetic resonance imaging
(D) Screening mammogram
(E) Ultrasound

The answer is E: Ultrasound. This study is most appropriate because breasts in this age are dense and mammography is less sensitive. Although this patient is at risk for a genetically transmitted breast cancer, breast imaging is generally started 10 years prior to the onset in the youngest affected relative. A diagnostic mammogram is performed when a dominant mass is identified; however, due to the resolution issues associated with dense breasts, an ultrasound would be indicated in a young woman. Additionally, the onset of her complaint is most consistent with a cyst (rapid onset), related to menses and painful. Regardless of age, the imaging of choice to diagnose a cyst is the ultrasound.

---

3 A 50-year-old G3P2101 with last menstrual period (LMP) 3 months ago presents with a thick green nipple discharge associated with breast tenderness and nipple discomfort. On examination, no masses or nipple changes were noted. A mammogram 4 months ago was classified as Breast Imaging Reporting and Data System (BI-RADS) 2. What is the most likely diagnosis?

(A) Candidiasis
(B) Ductal ectasia
(C) Fibroadenoma
(D) Intraductal papilloma
(E) Papillary carcinoma

The answer is B: Ductal ectasia. Ductal ectasia is a benign inflammatory condition typically diagnosed in perimenopausal women. The condition occurs when milk ducts become dilated and the walls thicken and become blocked with a cheesy-like substance. The condition often causes no symptoms, but some women may have nipple discharge, breast tenderness, or inflammation of the clogged duct. Advanced cases may cause nipple inversion and characteristic annular mammographic findings. It is most often managed by treating symptomatically.

---

4 A 42-year-old G1P1001 with an last menstrual period (LMP) 2 weeks ago presents with a firm, nontender mass in her right breast that she discovered in the shower 2 weeks ago. Cytology from a fine needle aspiration (FNA) of the lesion was verbally reported as negative for malignancy, but the written report classified the specimen as inadequate. What is the next step?

(A) Immediate mammography
(B) Mammography in 6 months
(C) Open biopsy
(D) Reassurance and mammography as per routine
(E) Repeat FNA

The answer is C: Open biopsy. The triple evaluation for a dominant mass includes examination, imaging, and tissue. While an immediate mammogram can further characterize the lesion, this patient will need to have more tissue tested to determine whether a malignancy exists. The decision to perform an FNA prior to other evaluation was reasonable since it can often hasten a diagnosis. Regarding FNA biopsy, samples categorized as inadequate are not sensitive enough to rule out malignancy. In these cases, further invasive procedures including core biopsies or open surgical biopsy are indicated in order to minimize the chance of missed diagnosis of breast cancer. Both choices B and D could delay a diagnosis of breast cancer, resulting in adverse impact on survival rates; therefore, they are unacceptable alternatives. Delay in the diagnosis of breast cancer is one of the most common medical malpractice claims resulting in payouts.

5 A 25-year-old G2P1011 delivered a term infant via spontaneous vaginal delivery without complication 7 weeks ago. At 6 weeks postpartum visit last week, her examination was unremarkable and she was successfully breastfeeding exclusively. She calls the office today complaining of a 101.8 body temperature and flu-like symptoms. Additional information reveals that she has an area on her right breast that is hard, red, and inflamed. The most appropriate management plan is:

(A) Push fluids get rest and stop breastfeeding on the affected side
(B) Keep breastfeeding and come to the office in a week if not better
(C) Take Tylenol to lower the fever because the breast is probably engorged
(D) Breastfeed more frequently on the affected side and start antibiotics
(E) Continue breastfeeding on the left side, pump on the affected right side, and throw out the expressed milk

The answer is D: Breastfeed more frequently on the affected side and start antibiotics. This presentation is diagnostic for mastitis. In order to reduce the bacterial load most effectively, the breast should be emptied since any milk left in the breast provides a culture medium. The most effective mechanism for removing milk from the affected breast is a nursing infant. Fever and hard red area on the breast differentiate engorgement from mastitis.

6 A 34-year-old G2P2002 is ready for discharge from the hospital. She had a prenatal course complicated by asthma, rheumatoid arthritis, seizure disorder, diabetes, and reflux. She also had a history of gallbladder disease and intermittent pain. The workup was delayed until after delivery. You review her medications and recommended diagnostic studies. Which one of the following medications is contraindicated in breastfeeding?

(A) Intravenous contrast
(B) Lansoprazole
(C) Metformin
(D) Methotrexate

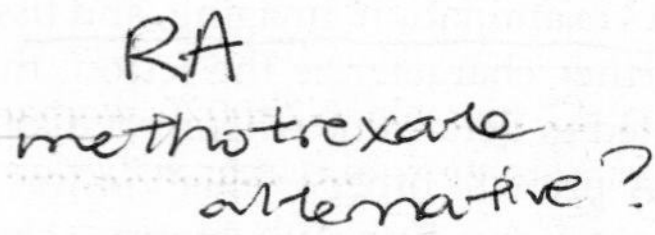

The answer is D: Methotrexate. The high-dose therapy that is used to treat rheumatoid arthritis is considered by the American Academy of Pediatrics to be contraindicated during breastfeeding. The rest of the medications are not contraindicated during lactation. It is important to consult a reliable reference when making decisions about medication use during lactation. Often women are discouraged from breastfeeding not because the information is available but because of a fear that a medication or intervention might possibly be a problem. Many medications are safe to use when breastfeeding. It is advisable to have the patient consult her rheumatologist prior to filling the methotrexate prescription as there may be a safer alternative that will allow her to continue exclusive breastfeeding. A better option would be to have a consult prior to delivery that addressed postpartum plans and the possibility of breastfeeding.

7 A 25-year-old G0P0 woman presents for an annual examination. Her last menstrual period (LMP) was 3 weeks ago. She expresses a concern over a maternal great aunt who died recently from breast cancer at age 85. There is no other family history of cancer. She experiences breast tenderness 2 to 3 days prior to menses. Breast examination reveals mild nodularity with a single, 1-cm, mobile mass in the right breast at 10 o'clock. The patient denies noting the mass that is painful to palpation. No lymphadenopathy or nipple discharge is noted. The remainder of her history, review of systems, and physical examination are unremarkable. The most appropriate management plan for this patient is:

(A) Ultrasound
(B) Biopsy
(C) Mammogram
(D) Re-examine after the next menses
(E) Routine follow-up in 1 year

cyclic fibrocystic breast changes

The answer is D: Re-examine after the next menses. The most appropriate follow-up for this patient who gives a history consistent with cyclic fibrocystic breast changes is choice D, to re-examine the patient after the next menstrual cycle. An ultrasound is the preferred imaging technique for a patient aged 20 to 30 with a dominant, persistent mass. Ultrasound can differentiate between cystic and solid lesions. A mammogram is more appropriate later in life when the breast parenchyma contains a higher percentage of adipose tissue. Any solid dominant mass requires a biopsy regardless of age. From a medical–legal perspective, it is inappropriate to commit any patient to routine follow-up when a dominant mass has been identified.

---

8 A 48-year-old G2P0020 woman presents 3 months after her annual examination and mammogram complaining of a spontaneous clear discharge from the nipple of her left breast. Her recent mammogram was Breast Imaging Reporting and Data System (BI-RADS) 2. Breast examination reveals mild nodularity without dominant mass and no nipple changes. A clear serous discharge was expressed by pressure on a point at 6 o'clock on the subareolar region. The most likely diagnosis is:

(A) Ductal ectasia
(B) Fibrocystic hyperplasia
(C) Galactorrhea
(D) Intraductal papilloma
(E) Plasma cell mastitis

The answer is D: Intraductal papilloma. Solitary intraductal papillomas are benign lesions that most typically occur in women in their late reproductive or postmenopausal years. The average age at presentation is 48 years. Breast examinations in this condition typically reveal no palpable mass. The discharge may be clear or bloody. Mammograms of women with a solitary papilloma are most frequently normal. Although this is a benign condition, it confers a 1.5 to 2 times relative risk of developing invasive breast carcinoma at some point in the future.

---

9 A 5-day-old neonate, born via spontaneous vaginal delivery to a G1P0 mother at 38 week's gestation, presents to the clinic with a 7% weight loss from birth. He is quite sleepy and breastfeeding every 4 to 5 hours. You are counseling the mother about building her milk supply and making sure that her baby is adequately breastfed. You recommend the mother:

(A) Give the infant a bottle of formula after each feeding to make certain he is getting enough nutrition
(B) Breastfeed the infant only as often as he demands, allowing him to sleep as he will wake to feed when he is hungry
(C) Breastfeed every 2 to 3 hours; a minimum of 8 to 12 times per day, waking the sleepy infant to feed if necessary
(D) Sleep through the night to get enough rest in order to care for her infant and protect against postpartum depression

The answer is C: **Breastfeed every 2 to 3 hours; a minimum of 8 to 12 times per day, waking the sleepy infant to feed if necessary.** The recommended feeding pattern for sufficient milk production is to feed on demand a minimum of 8 times daily.

---

10 A 30-year-old G2P1 at 16 weeks presents for routine prenatal care. She did not breastfeed her first child, but she describes a pamphlet she read about the benefits of breastfeeding. You review her past medical history and see that she has a long history of iron deficiency anemia due to heavy periods. You tell her breastfeeding could help minimize her anemia problems by which of the following in the postpartum period?

(A) Early return to ovulatory status
(B) Increased fertility
(C) Increased risk of postpartum bleeding
(D) Rapid uterine involution
(E) Sequestering of iron in the breast milk

The answer is D: **Rapid uterine involution.** Full-time breastfeeding is associated with a delay in ovulation and therefore provides natural childbirth spacing. A more rapid postpartum uterine inversion is associated with a decreased risk of postpartum hemorrhage.

---

11 A 36-year-old G2P2 patient presents for a 1-week incision check after a primary Cesarian section for breech presentation. She has no complaints and her incision is healing well. She is exclusively breastfeeding and it is going well. She relates a recent outbreak of rotavirus in her oldest child's preschool. She is concerned that her 3-year-old will bring the infection home to the baby. Which of the following should best help reassure her?

(A) Antibodies are readily demonstrable in colostrum
(B) Colostrum contains less sugar and fat than breast milk
(C) Colostrum contains more protein and minerals than breast milk
(D) Immunoglobulin A content is protective against enteric infection
(E) Secretion of colostrum persists for at least 2 weeks

The answer is D: **Immunoglobulin A content is protective against enteric infection.** While antibodies are readily demonstrable in colostrum, and alternatives B and C correctly describe elements of colostrum content, it is the immunoglobulin A content that has been demonstrated to be effective in enteric infections. The passive immunity conferred by colostrum lasts between 8 and 12 weeks.

---

12 A 58-year-old postmenopausal woman presents to the emergency room because she says that she has been hearing voices that are telling her to kill herself. Based on her history, the on-call psychiatrist decides to admit her to the inpatient psychiatric unit. After 2 weeks in the hospital, the patient is released with a medication to help with her hallucinations. Six months later, this patient presents to your clinic complaining of a milky white discharge from both breasts that began soon after she started the psychiatric medication. Her recent mammogram was normal. Which hormone is the medication most likely blocking?

(A) Androstenedione
(B) Dopamine
(C) Gonadotropin releasing hormone
(D) Estrogen
(E) Luteinizing hormone

The answer is B: Dopamine. Dopamine is required in order to suppress prolactin release. Antipsychotics act by blocking dopamine in multiple areas in the brain. Unfortunately, it may also interfere with dopamine in the tuberoinfundibular pathway.

---

13 A 36-year-old G3P0212 initially presents 8 weeks after delivery and is treated for mastitis. You evaluate and treat her in the usual manner. She returns 7 days later with exquisite pain and a flocculent 4-cm mass in the same breast. The most likely pathogen associated with this condition is:

(A) *Escherichia coli*
(B) *Gardnerella*
(C) *Pneumococcus*
(D) *Staphylococcus aureus*
(E) *Streptococcus pyogenes*

The answer is D: *Staphylococcus aureus*. Mastitis occurs most frequently in the first 2 to 4 weeks postpartum and at times of marked reduction in nursing frequency. Risk factors include maternal fatigue, poor nursing technique, nipple trauma, and epidemic *S. aureus*. The most common organisms associated with mastitis are *S. aureus, S. epidermidis, Streptococci*, and occasionally, gram-negative rods. The treatment for mastitis is dicloxacillin in the nonallergic patient.

---

14 The most appropriate step in treating the condition described in the previous question is:

(A) Aggressive pumping of infected breast
(B) Biopsy
(C) Change in antibiotic coverage
(D) Fine needle aspiration (FNA)
(E) Referral to general surgeon

The answer is E: Referral to general surgeon. This patient has a breast abscess. The goal of treatment for mastitis is to provide prompt and appropriate management to prevent complications such as a breast abscess. An FNA may be considered for abscesses less than 3 cm in size. In practice, these are most often performed by a general surgeon. For abscesses greater than 3 cm, a breast surgeon should always be consulted for definitive management (incision and drainage). One reason for trying to prevent the development of breast abscesses in lactating women is that when the breast is incised to drain the abscess, it disrupts the glands that store milk and they drain out of the incision site making continued nursing very difficult for patients. Antibiotics typically do not penetrate well into the interior of abscesses. Pumping will not relieve symptoms or definitively treat an abscess which has typically infiltrated surrounding tissue beyond the ducts.

---

15 A 30-year-old G2P2 lactating patient who is currently 6 weeks postpartum presents with a fever of 101.6, right-sided breast pain that has increased in the past 24 hours. On examination, a red, indurated wedge of the breast between 9 and 11 o'clock is exquisitely sensitive to palpation.

What is the most likely source of the infection causing organism?

(A) Poor personal hygiene
(B) Contaminated nursing bra
(C) The hospital environment
(D) The baby's mouth

The answer is D: The baby's mouth. The source of the infection is the baby's mouth through small disruptions in the skin around the nipples. Often it is a consequence of inappropriate latch that predisposes this delicate tissue to tear and become a mechanism for infection. Often there is a tendency to believe it is bad for the infant to drink this milk. However, the bacteria came from the baby and will be destroyed by the acids in its stomach. Since the nursing infant is the most effective means of emptying the breast and reducing the culture medium (milk), this mother should be encouraged to continue aggressively feeding on that affected side.

The treatment of this organism in the nonallergic patient is dicloxacillin which takes into account the possibility of resistance to penicillins.

---

16 A 26-year-old G3P2012 presents with fever and chills 5 weeks postpartum. She complains of flu-like symptoms and a very sore area on the left breast. Vital signs are P 110 beats/min, R 16 breaths/min, and T 39°C. Her pelvic and abdominal examinations are completely benign. Uterus is small, perineum intact, vagina with mild atrophic changes, no adnexal masses, and normal physiologic discharge. Breast examination: Right reveals an engorged breast approximately 3 hours from the last feeding, nipples without lesion or abrasion. Left breast is also engorged, a small 2-mm crack on the nipple with a bright red indurated area above it on the breast. This area is tender to palpation. The remainder of the breast examination is normal. The most appropriate recommendation and treatment is:

(A) Doxycycline: Continue nursing on both sides
(B) Amoxicillin: Continue nursing on both sides
(C) Dicloxacillin: Continue nursing on both sides
(D) Doxycycline: Pump affected side and discard
(E) Amoxicillin: Pump affected side and discard
(F) Dicloxacillin: Pump affected side and discard

The answer is C: Dicloxacillin: Continue nursing on both sides. Treat with dicloxacillin and continue nursing on both sides. Dicloxacillin is the treatment of choice because it treats Streptococcus and Staphylococcus bacteria from the baby's mouth that may be resistant to penicillins or cephalosporins. Doxycycline can cause permanent tooth deformities and is not appropriate for nursing mothers who can transmit this to their infants through the breast milk. Mastitis is caused when bacteria overgrow in the rich culture media of collected breast milk. The best and most efficient method to remove the breast milk is through continued nursing. The bacteria that have caused the infection are from the baby's mouth. They will be destroyed when they enter the stomach.

17 A 35-year-old G1P1001 calls stating she is very concerned that her milk production is inadequate. She has been exclusively breastfeeding since her son was born 5 weeks ago. Until today, the infant has fed regularly, not been fussy, and wetted sufficient diapers. He has also had normal checkups with the pediatrician. But today, he has cried nonstop and wants to nurse what seems like incessantly. He has plenty of wet diapers, normal stools, no vomiting and distended abdomen, and does not have a fever. She is frantic that her milk supply is dwindling prematurely and his actions indicate he is not getting enough nutrition. The best explanation of cluster feeding phenomenon is:

(A) Oxytocin is the hormone associated with increased milk production along with chronic hunger
(B) Oxytocin is the hormone associated with increased milk production along with growth spurts
(C) Prolactin is the hormone associated with increased milk production along with chronic hunger
(D) Prolactin is the hormone associated with increased milk production along with growth spurts

The answer is D: Prolactin is the hormone associated with increased milk production along with growth spurts. Infants commonly go through a growth spurt as they approach 6 weeks. At this point, their metabolic needs increase and they are temporarily "fussy," and try to nurse more. This stimulates milk production mediated by prolactin. Since the cycle requires about 1 day to affect the amount of breast milk produced, the infant is temporarily more hungry until the following day. In this case, the infant has no physical signs of concerns, including adequate number of wet diapers. It is most appropriate to reassure these mothers that a normal physiologic process is functioning exactly as would be expected and that no pathology exists. Oxytocin causes contraction of the myoepithelial unit in the breast and is related to letdown of milk already stored in the breast. Oxytocin does not stimulate the production of breast milk.

CHAPTER

9

Gynecology

1 A 29-year-old G1P1 comes to see you concerned about recent changes in her menses. The patient reports having regular periods until her pregnancy at age 24. After her child was born, the patient's periods returned to normal after 10 months and remained regular until 12 months ago. The patient does not take any medications and denies any other health concerns. The patient is worried about these changes because her mother had cervical cancer at age 35. The patient tells you that for the first 4 months of this year her periods increased from 5 days in duration to 9 days but otherwise remained unchanged. The pattern of bleeding that best describes her symptoms during the first 4 months of this year is:

(A) Normal menses
(B) Dysfunctional uterine bleeding
(C) Polymenorrhea
(D) Heavy menstrual bleeding (HMB)

The answer is D: Heavy menstrual bleeding (HMB). The classification of abnormal bleeding was changed in 2012 (see *Figure 9-1*). The often confusing terms menorrhagia, metrorrhagia, and menometrorrhagia have been replaced by the PALM-COEIN classification system that includes etiology wherever possible. For example, the term "menorrhagia" (bleeding greater than 80 mL per cycle) has been replaced with HMB, any amount of bleeding that disrupts the patient's daily function.

If an underlying etiology is identified, treatment is directed at correcting the inciting abnormality. If no causative abnormalities can be identified, treatment will be directed toward symptom reduction.

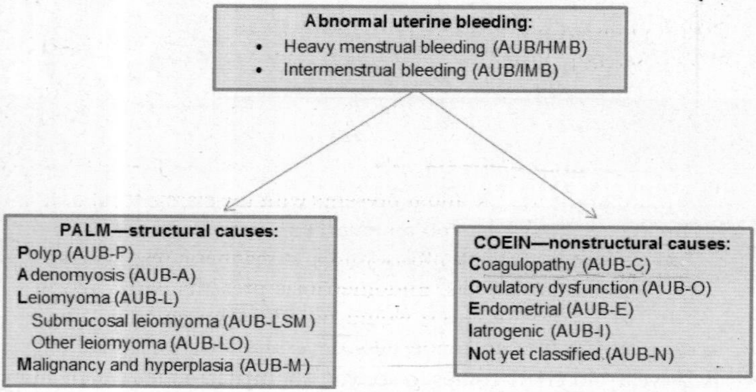

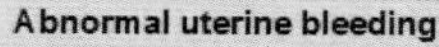

Figure 9-1

---

2 Refer to the patient in Question 1. On a follow-up visit, the patient states that her menses are still at regular intervals but are now settling in at only 5 days. What is worrying her is that she now has up to 3 days of bleeding 1 to 2 weeks after her period stops. How would you classify this bleeding pattern?

(A) Polymenorrhea
(B) Menometrorrhagia
(C) Abnormal uterine bleeding (AUB)-I
(D) AUB/intermenstrual bleeding (IMB)
(E) Metrorrhagia

The answer is D: AUB/intermenstrual bleeding (IMB).

---

3 A 30-year-old G1P1001 presents with pelvic pain persisting for several months. The pain does not change with her menstrual cycles. She mentions that she has been feeling fatigued and occasionally dizzy recently. On examination, she is afebrile, her pulse is 90 beats/min, and her blood pressure (BP) is 110/65 mmHg. She is pale-appearing, and her uterus is nontender and palpated midway between her pelvic symphysis and umbilicus. A pregnancy test is negative, a complete blood count (CBC) reveals microcytic anemia, and transvaginal ultrasound shows a thickened junctional zone. Which of the following is the most likely diagnosis?

(A) Adenomyosis
(B) Endometriosis
(C) Pelvic inflammatory disease
(D) Ectopic pregnancy
(E) Endometrial carcinoma

The answer is A: Adenomyosis. Adenomyosis is an endometrial tissue in the myometrium of the uterus, and it presents with the classic triad of noncyclical pelvic pain, menorrhagia, and an enlarged uterus. Diagnosis is made by hysterectomy pathology, though ultrasound and magnetic resonance imaging (MRI) can suggest adenomyosis. Endometriosis presents with cyclical pain. Pelvic inflammatory disease (PID) would not cause an enlarged uterus and would cause cervical motion tenderness on examination. A pregnancy test would be positive with ectopic pregnancy. Endometrial carcinoma would be rare in a 30-year-old, though adenomyosis can rarely progress to endometrial carcinoma.

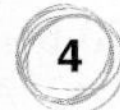
4 A 26-year-old G0 presents with a 2-week history of right lower quadrant sharp abdominal pain. She has noticed intermittent spotting, but has not had her normal menstruation in 8 weeks. She is currently sexually active with two partners. She only uses condoms for contraception, but mentions she occasionally forgets. On examination, she is afebrile, and her abdomen is mildly tender to palpation in the right lower quadrant. What is the next most appropriate step in the evaluation?

(A) Computed tomography (CT) of the abdomen and pelvis
(B) Urinalysis + chlamydia/gonorrhea testing
(C) Quantitative beta-human chorionic gonadotropin (β-hCG)
(D) Transvaginal ultrasound

The answer is C: Quantitative beta-human chorionic gonadotropin (α-hCG). The patient may have an ectopic pregnancy, which can become an obstetric emergency. The best screening test is a pregnancy test. The other options are important to pursue once it is confirmed that the patient is not pregnant.

5 A 40-year-old G2P2002 presents to the emergency department (ED) with a 2-hour history of severe left lower quadrant (LLQ) pain. The pain began suddenly and has stayed constant since. On examination, her pulse is 85 beats/min, her BP is 145/80 mmHg, and her abdomen is diffusely tender without rebound or guarding. On ultrasound, the left ovary is larger than the right, and blood flow is diminished. What is the next best step in the management of this patient?

(A) MRI of the abdomen and pelvis
(B) Emergent surgery
(C) Left ovary biopsy
(D) Obtain CA-125, α-fetoprotein, and β-hCG levels
(E) CT of the abdomen and pelvis
(F) Intravenous (IV) antibiotics

The answer is B: Emergent surgery. The most likely diagnosis of this patient is ovarian torsion, especially considering she has decreased blood flow to the left ovary. Emergent laparoscopy is indicated to evaluate the viability of the ovary and treat the probably torsion. An MRI can help evaluate for torsion if findings on ultrasound are equivocal, but that is not the case in this situation. Furthermore, an MRI wastes time and resources, and surgery is warranted without further imaging if the clinical picture is convincing for torsion. Answers C and D might be appropriate if an ovarian mass is visualized while the torsion is reduced, as ovarian mass is the main risk factor for torsion. Choice E would be indicated for an acute abdomen where the ultrasound was inconclusive. Ovarian torsion is a clinical diagnosis. IV antibiotics would be indicated for a severe infection.

6 A 32-year-old G0 presents for an infertility workup. She and her partner have been trying to conceive for 2 years without success. She has regular menstruation, though she mentions she has severe cramping during her cycles. She also notes she experiences pelvic pain during sex. On examination, she is a thin, well-developed woman. She is afebrile, and she experiences a great deal of pain during the pelvic examination. You do not note discharge on examination. Which of the following tests is required for diagnosis of the patient's infertility?

(A) Ultrasound
(B) β-hCG level
(C) Pap smear
(D) Laparoscopy
(E) Hysterosalpingogram

The answer is D: Laparoscopy. The cause of this patient's infertility is most likely endometriosis, the most common cause of infertility among menstruating woman >30 years old. Diagnosis of endometriosis requires direct visualization of the blue-black or dark brown lesions via laparoscopy or laparotomy. The other answer choices are helpful in diagnosing other causes of infertility and pelvic pain.

7 A 39-year-old G3P3 presents to the clinic complaining of a fever of 100.7 and reports pelvic pain. She is post-op day 3 from a total abdominal hysterectomy and was discharged on post-op day 2 without any concerns after a normal early post-op course. She denies nausea, vomiting, diarrhea, constipation, chest pain, or shortness of breath. The patient has no allergies and has no other medical conditions. What is the next step in the management of this patient?

(A) Reassure the patient
(B) Begin antibiotics
(C) Perform a urinalysis
(D) Order a CT angiogram
(E) Order a chest X-ray

The answer is C: Perform a urinalysis. Postoperative fever is diagnosed as a core body temperature greater than 100.4. The most likely etiology of a fever 3 to 5 days post-op is a urinary tract infection (UTI). Surgical site infection is a common cause of a post-op fever; however, surgical site infections generally occur later in the recovery course, around days 5 to 7.

8 A 46-year-old woman who is 1 day postoperative from a vaginal hysterectomy due to fibroids is complaining of dizziness when she sits up or tries to walk. She had heavy menstrual bleeding (HMB) and multiple 3- to 5-cm fibroids. The surgery was uncomplicated but took longer than expected due to the enlarged uterus. The most likely diagnosis for her dizziness is:

(A) Medication reaction
(B) Anemia
(C) Fluid overload from the long surgery
(D) Transient dizziness that is self-limited
(E) Atelectasis

The answer is B: Anemia. The patient was having heavy periods before surgery so may have been anemic even before the surgery. Given the large uterus and long surgery, the blood loss may have been higher than normal. The diagnosis of anemia would be confirmed by low hemoglobin and hematocrit measurements.

9 A 68-year-old G0 patient is postoperative day 0 from a vaginal hysterectomy with anterior and posterior repair of pelvic organ prolapse. The nurse calls to review her vital signs with you and states that the patient has a BP of 142/84 mmHg, a heart rate (HR) of 67 beats/min, a respiratory rate (RR) of 22 breaths/min, and a urine output of 120 cc/6 hours. What is the next step in the management of this patient?

(A) Begin a β-blocker
(B) Give her a fluid bolus
(C) Initiate incentive spirometry
(D) Begin antibiotics

The answer is B: **Give her a fluid bolus.** This patient has decreased urine output. The lowest normal urine output is 30 cc/h. In a patient with low urine output, who is otherwise healthy, the first line of treatment is to give a fluid bolus. If the patient is hypovolemic, a fluid bolus will remedy the decreased urine output. Patients are often dehydrated secondary to not eating for many hours in preparation for surgery or receiving a bowel prep. However, it should be noted that preoperative dehydrated status is remedied intraoperatively by anesthesiology as they manage the patient.

---

10 A 48-year-old G3P3003 with a history of chronic hypertension and type 2 diabetes mellitus underwent a total vaginal hysterectomy today. Her body mass index (BMI) is 35. Her surgery took longer than average 2 hours, and she had an estimated blood loss of 400 cc. She had appropriate prophylactic antibiotics preoperatively. Which of the following is this patient's most significant risk factor for postoperative infection?

(A) Hypertension
(B) Obesity
(C) Diabetes mellitus
(D) Vaginal surgery
(E) Foley placement

The answer is C: **Diabetes mellitus.** Risk factors for infection for this patient include diabetes, length of surgery, and elevated blood loss. Vaginal surgery, BMI, and BPs are not independent risk factors for infection.

---

11 A 53-year-old patient who is 7 days post-op from a laparoscopic hysterectomy presents to the clinic with abdominal pain. She has a body temperature of 100.8; other vitals are within normal limits. She has normal bowel movements, urinary function, and appetite. She denies any other complaints. Her incisions are examined, and the infraumbilical incision is erythematous and tender to palpation. What is the next step in the management of this patient?

(A) Reassure the patient
(B) Order CT abdomen/pelvis
(C) Initiate antibiotics
(D) Plan surgical repair for umbilical hernia
(E) Wound debridement

The answer is C: Initiate antibiotics. Postoperative cellulitis is a common complication. Although pelvic abscess and umbilical hernia are possible complications, they would have other symptoms or problems associated with them.

---

12 A 45-year-old patient post-op day 6 from total abdominal hysterectomy presents to the emergency room (ER) complaining of serous fluid that is oozing from her incision. The patient's BMI is 33. She has diabetes and required an open laparotomy for her surgery. On her examination, the skin incision is separated, and a Q-tip can be placed past the fascial layer. What is the most likely cause of this patient's condition?

(A) Fascial dehiscence
(B) Hematoma formation
(C) Normal healing
(D) Infection development
(E) Seroma formation

The answer is A: Fascial dehiscence. Fascial dehiscence is a rare, but serious complication that requires surgical repair. Being able to pass a Q-tip past the fascial layer is suggestive of an opening in the fascial layer. The serous discharge is the peritoneal fluid that is extruding from the wound opening. Hematoma would have a bloody discharge, and infection would cause a purulent discharge.

---

13 A 27-year-old G2P1102 presents to the infertility clinic after 20 months of unsuccessful attempts at conception. The patient states that her previous children took a long time to conceive. Her periods began at age 14 lasted for 5 days and occurred regularly each month; however, they are very painful and she has taken birth control pills since her early teens to control the pain. Which of the following does not increase the risk of this patient's condition?

(A) Müllerian anomalies
(B) First-degree relative with endometriosis
(C) Short menstrual cycles
(D) Multiparity

The answer is D: Multiparity. Multiparity has not been demonstrated to be a risk factor for endometriosis.

---

14 A 32-year-old G0 presents to the clinic with worsening pelvic pain for the last several years. Physical examination is grossly benign with the exception of some mild diffuse lower abdomen tenderness on deep palpation. Which of the following is the most common gynecologic diagnosis associated with chronic pelvic pain (CPP)?

(A) Pelvic inflammatory disease (PID)
(B) Adhesions
(C) Gynecologic malignancy
(D) Dysmenorrhea
(E) Endometriosis

The answer is E: Endometriosis. CPP refers to the pain of at least 6-month duration that occurs below the umbilicus and causes functional disability or requires treatment. The etiologies are numerous and can include all of the above, individually, or in combination. The relative frequency is influenced by patient population and practice specialties, though over one-third of patients who undergo laparoscopy for CPP are diagnosed with endometriosis. In private practice settings, irritable bowel syndrome (IBS) is the most common associated diagnosis.

---

15 A 29-year-old G2P2002 complains of pelvic pain since the delivery of her second child 8 months ago. She notices it most when sitting, though it is relieved when she sits on the toilet. She also reports leaking urine more often since the delivery. As a part of the evaluation, her practitioner evaluates her pelvic floor musculature and notices tenderness at the sacrospinous ligament. What nerve is most likely responsible for the patient's symptoms?

(A) Genitofemoral
(B) Pudendal
(C) Iliohypogastric
(D) Lateral femoral
(E) Ilioinguinal nerve

The answer is B: Pudendal. The pudendal nerve comprised the anterior branches of the ventral rami from S2 to S4. It exits the pelvis through the greater sciatic foramen and reenters the pelvis through the lesser sciatic foramen, passing between the sacrospinous ligament anteriorly and sacrotuberous ligament posteriorly, while wrapping behind the ischial spine. The pudendal nerve can be traumatized during labor. A prolonged second stage of labor during vaginal delivery, a third-degree tear through the perineal body, and a high neonatal birthweight have been reported to traumatize the nerve. Surgical pudendal nerve injuries have been reported with sacrospinous vaginal vault suspension, vaginal laceration repairs, and various types of episiotomies. Other patients have developed pudendal neuropathy after straddle injuries, prolonged motorcycle or bicycle riding, and laser treatment to the vulva and perineum.

The typical presentation of pudendal neuralgia is pain in the labia, perineum, or anorectal regions when sitting that resolves when standing or when sitting on a surface that removes pressure from the ischial tuberosity (like a toilet seat).

16 A 62-year-old G6P5106 presents to the clinic complaining of intermittent resting pelvic pain after eating certain foods and pain with urination. She states that it has persisted for several months and denies overt urine leakage but does admit to urgency, frequency, and nocturia. She went through menopause when 48 years old. She has six children that were delivered vaginally without complication. A urine culture is negative. Which therapy would be of least therapeutic benefit to this patient?

(A) Nonsteroidal anti-inflammatory drugs (NSAIDs)
(B) Dietary restrictions
(C) Antibiotics
(D) Tricyclic antidepressants
(E) Sacral neuromodulation

The answer is C: Antibiotics. The patient history is suspicious for interstitial cystitis. Antibiotics are not indicated. Interstitial cystitis/bladder pain syndrome is not well understood. It is characterized by bladder discomfort associated with bladder filling and the exclusion of other etiologies for symptoms. Many therapeutic approaches have been attempted with none helpful for all patients.

Stepwise approach includes:

(1) Education, self-care, behavioral modification, and other psychosocial support
(2) Physical therapy/oral medications—amitriptyline, antihistamines, etc.
(3) Hydrodistention/dimethylsulfoxide
(4) Neuromodulation
(5) Botulinum toxin/cyclosporine
(6) Urinary diversion

NSAIDs and other analgesics can be used at any point to manage symptoms.

17 A 24-year-old nonpregnant woman is seen for recurrent diarrhea and dysmenorrhea. She also complains of pain with intercourse. She has a history of depression but has otherwise been healthy with no other concerns. She states that these symptoms have been present for more than 3 years. What would be the most appropriate question to accurately ascertain her diagnosis?

(A) "Are your menses regular?"
(B) "Does the pain improve after a bout of diarrhea?"
(C) "Have you ever been pregnant before?"
(D) "What surgeries have you had in the past?"
(E) "What medications are you taking currently?"

The answer is B: "Does the pain improve after a bout of diarrhea?" The other questions are helpful in gathering the pertinent historical data but answer B is an indicator of irritable bowel syndrome (IBS).

ROME III criteria classify the functional gastrointestinal disorders into six major domains: esophageal, gastroduodenal, bowel, functional abdominal pain syndrome, biliary, and anorectal. It has evolved from the initial criteria set forth in 1989, which now includes "recurrent abdominal pain or discomfort at least 3 days per month in the last 3 months associated with 2 or more of the following:

1) Improvement with defecation
2) Onset associated with change in frequency of stool
3) Onset associated with a change in form (appearance) of stool"

---

18 A 37-year-old waitress, G3P3003, is seen for increasing pelvic pain over the last 2 years. She describes the pain as a dull, constant ache and finds that it is worse after a long day waiting tables. It is also worse right before her periods. She has tried ibuprofen and acupuncture with little relief. On physical examination, you notice varicose veins along her thighs. The remainder of her examination is benign. You order a transvaginal ultrasound and find a slightly enlarged uterus and thickened endometrium. Ovaries are normal. What is the most accurate test to identify this patient's problem?

(A) MRI
(B) CT scan
(C) β-hCG
(D) Venogram
(E) CA-125

The answer is D: Venogram. The best test for diagnosing pelvic congestion syndrome (PCS) is a venogram. Ultrasound is typically the initial examination. It is useful, primarily, in ruling out other causes of pelvic pain. An MRI and CT are also frequent first-line modalities to rule out other causes, though they are often performed with the patient lying down and may not rule out PCS.

The diagnosis of PCS is confirmed with the following venographic findings: ovarian vein diameter >6 mm, retrograde ovarian or pelvic venous flow, the presence of several tortuous collateral pelvic venous pathways, and delayed or stagnant clearance of contrast at the end of injection.

---

19 A 20-year-old woman presents to the emergency room (ER) around midnight after being sexually assaulted earlier in the evening as she walked to her car from the grocery store. What is the risk to the patient of developing chronic pelvic pain (CPP) following this event?

(A) 10%
(B) 25%
(C) 50%
(D) 75%
(E) 90%

The answer is C: 50%. Multiple studies have shown an increased association between CPP and a history of sexual or physical abuse. Between 40% and 50% of patients diagnosed with CPP have a history of abuse, indicating the importance of thorough history taking and evaluation by mental health professionals to optimally care for these patients.

---

20 A 70-year-old woman presents with complaints of leaking of urine with a cough, sneeze, or while walking daily. It is significantly impacting her life. Medical history is complicated by hypertension controlled on hydrochlorothiazide. Vital signs are BP 149/90 mmHg and P 87 beats/min. Physical examination is remarkable for loss of her mid-urethral angle and minimal cystocele. There is no uterine prolapse or rectocele. The patient undergoes urodynamic testing confirming your suspected diagnosis of her urinary incontinence. What is the next best step in therapy for this patient?

(A) Oxybutynin
(B) Mid-urethral sling
(C) Trimethoprim/sulfamethoxazole
(D) Tolterodine

The answer is B: Mid-urethral sling. In this case, the next best step in her management is a mid-urethral sling. This patient suffers from stress incontinence, and her physical examination confirms an anatomic defect. Although muscle training is the first step in therapy for these patients, if symptoms persist, surgical treatment via mid-urethral sling or urethropexy can be of significant benefit. Medications for detrusor overactivity is not helpful in stress incontinence, and the patient has no proven urinary tract infection (UTI).

---

21 An 80-year-old woman presents to the office with complaints of leaking large amounts of urine when she hears running water. Her symptoms began about 1 month ago and have gotten progressively worse. She denies any abdominal or pelvic pain. Medical history is complicated by hypertension treated with hydrochlorothiazide and lisinopril. BP today is 150/99 mmHg with a pulse of 65 beats/min. What is the next best step in her workup?

(A) Urinalysis
(B) Urine cytology
(C) Urine culture
(D) Basic metabolic panel

The answer is A: Urinalysis. The first step in any workup for urinary incontinence is ruling out reversible causes. Although this patient's presentation is likely detrusor overactivity, it is important to address any reversible causes. A urinalysis is the first step and may lead to performing further testing such as urine cytology and urine culture.

---

22 A 64-year-old woman presents with complaints of leaking a large amount of urine after a cough or sneeze. She has no significant past medical history. During examination, you have the patient stand or cough. The patient begins to leak a large amount of urine a few seconds after a deep cough. From this examination, what is the most likely type of incontinence this patient suffers from?

(A) Stress urinary incontinence
(B) Detrusor overactivity
(C) Mixed urinary incontinence
(D) Neurogenic bladder

The answer is B: Detrusor overactivity. Although this patient does have symptoms after a stress, the delayed response is classic for detrusor overactivity.

---

23 A 65-year-old woman presents with complaints of leaking of a large amount of urine along with a sudden urge to urinate several times a week. She has no significant past medical history. Your clinical diagnosis based on the history is confirmed by cystometrics. What is the first step in therapy for this patient?

(A) Oxybutynin
(B) Mid-urethral sling
(C) Trimethoprim/sulfamethoxazole
(D) Prazosin

The answer is A: Oxybutynin. She suffers from detrusor overactivity, and the anticholinergic effects on the smooth muscle of the bladder help prevent these occurrences. She does not have a clearly diagnosed urinary tract infection (UTI), and surgical correction would not help her detrusor overactivity. Prazosin is an α-adrenergic blocker sometimes used for urinary hesitancy associated with prostatic hyperplasia.

---

24 A 70-year-old woman presents with complaints of leaking a small amount of urine multiple times per day. She states over the last several weeks she has had worsening difficulty voiding along with a small amount of leaking throughout the day. Her past medical history is significant for type 2 diabetes mellitus, chronic obstructive pulmonary disease, congestive heart failure, hypertension, and hyperlipidemia. Medications include hydrochlorothiazide, lisinopril, metformin, ipratropium, lasix, and pravastatin. Of the patient's medications, which one is likely to cause the patient's complaint?

(A) Hydrochlorothiazide
(B) Lisinopril
(C) Metformin
(D) Ipratropium
(E) Furosemide
(F) Pravastatin

The answer is D: Ipratropium. The patient presents with complaints classic for urinary retention. Of the medications listed, only the anticholinergic properties of ipratropium can produce this clinical finding. Patients on Furosemide will often complain of urinary frequency and nocturia but not difficulty voiding.

---

25 An 85-year-old woman presents to the emergency department (ED) with new-onset pelvic pain and leaking of urine. Her medical history is complicated by congestive heart failure, hypertension, diabetes mellitus, and osteoarthritis. On evaluation, her BP is 161/105 mmHg, P 102 beats/min, T 99.7°F, and RR 18 breaths/min. Blood count shows a white blood cell (WBC) count of 12.5 and a red blood cell count of 10.2. Urinalysis shows negative leukocytes, negative nitrites, and moderate blood. What is the next best step in her workup?

(A) Basic metabolic panel
(B) Urodynamics
(C) Urine culture
(D) Urine cytology

The answer is D: Urine cytology. In this case, the next best step would be urine cytology. This patient presents with new-onset pelvic pain and blood on urinalysis without an evidence of infection; this is concerning for a malignant cause for her urinary incontinence. Of the choices, the best step to evaluate that is urine cytology.

---

26 A 59-year-old woman presents to the office with complaints of leaking urine whenever she coughs. Symptoms began recently and have been getting progressively worse. She does not complain of any significant suprapubic pain since onset. The patient smokes one half pack per day and drinks three beers nightly. She has no significant past medical history. Urinalysis shows moderate leukocytes with positive nitrites and trace blood. Urodynamics reveal stress urinary incontinence. What is the next best step in the treatment for this patient?

(A) Oxybutynin
(B) Mid-urethral sling
(C) Trimethoprim/sulfamethoxazole
(D) Tolterodine
(E) Retropubic urethropexy

The answer is C: Trimethoprim/sulfamethoxazole. This patient does have stress incontinence so choices mid-urethral sling and retropubic urethropexy are reasonable surgical options, but given the patient has an active urinary tract infection (UTI), these recent symptoms may be from a reversible cause. If there may be a reversible cause of incontinence that must be addressed first. Therefore, trimethoprim/sulfamethoxazole is the best answer. Oxybutynin and tolterodine are medications best used in detrusor overactivity.

---

27 A 31-year-old P0 woman complains of pelvic pain that increases with menstrual cycles. She also admits to dyspareunia. What would be the most probable findings of a diagnostic laparoscopy?

(A) Black pinpoint lesions on the appendix
(B) Erythema in the posterior cul-de-sac
(C) Red, white, or blue lesions on the ovaries
(D) Abscess adjacent to the uterosacral ligaments

The answer is C: Red, white, or blue lesions on the ovaries. The ovaries are involved in two-thirds of women with endometriosis, often bilaterally. The anterior and posterior cul-de-sacs, uterosacral, round, and broad ligaments are also commonly involved, though not as frequently as the ovaries.

---

28 A 23-year-old G0 presents for her annual well-woman examination complaining that she is unable to get pregnant after trying for more than 1 year. She notes severe pain with her menses and heavy vaginal bleeding. A clinical diagnosis of endometriosis is made. What are the expected pathologic findings if tissue biopsies were collected during a diagnostic laparoscopy?

(A) Ectopic endometrial glands, neutrophil invasion of glandular tissue, rete pegs
(B) Ectopic endometrial glands, hemorrhage, and ectopic endometrial stroma
(C) Ectopic endometrial stroma, neutrophil invasion of glandular tissue, and hemorrhage
(D) Hemorrhage, neutrophil invasion, and rete pegs

The answer is B: Ectopic endometrial glands, hemorrhage, and ectopic endometrial stroma. The glandular and stromal tissues respond cyclically to progesterone and estrogen. Hemorrhage may be identified by the presence of large macrophages filled with hemosiderin (see *Figure 9-2*).

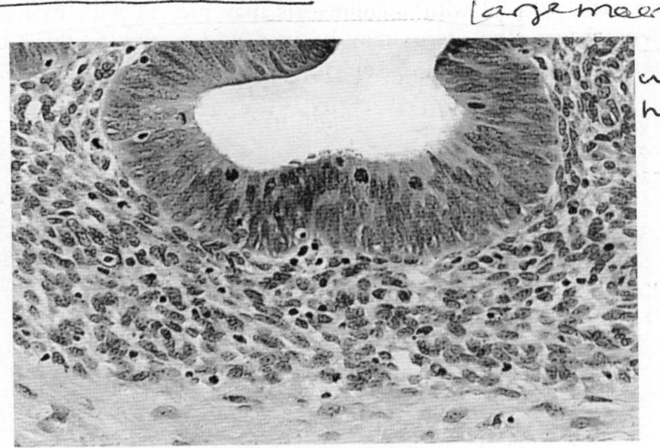

Figure 9-2

---

29 A 45-year-old G2P1102 complains of worsening pelvic pain that coincides with menses. What is the mechanism of action of the empirical drug of choice for endometriosis?

(A) Activates androgen and progesterone receptors
(B) Acts as a gonadotropin-releasing hormone (GnRH) antagonist
(C) Decreases sex hormone binding globulin
(D) Acts as a GnRH agonist

The answer is D: Acts as a GnRH agonist. Leuprolide acetate is a GnRH agonist that works by continuously binding GnRH receptors to produce downregulation of gonadotropin secretion and secondary downregulation of ovarian steroidogenesis.

---

30 A 37-year-old woman, G3P3003, presents to your office complaining of gradually worsening dysmenorrhea and menorrhagia, though her cycles remain regular. Bimanual examination reveals a mildly tender, 14-week-sized globular uterus. Abdominal ultrasound reveals a globally enlarged uterus without evidence of discrete masses. What is the most likely diagnosis?

(A) Adenomyosis
(B) Leiomyomata
(C) Endometriosis
(D) Endometrial hyperplasia
(E) Leiomyosarcomata

The answer is A: Adenomyosis. Adenomyosis is the presence of endometrial glands and stroma in the myometrium (see *Figure 9-3*). Though usually asymptomatic, women with adenomyosis may present with dysmenorrhea and menorrhagia. The uterus may be increased to two to three times its normal size.

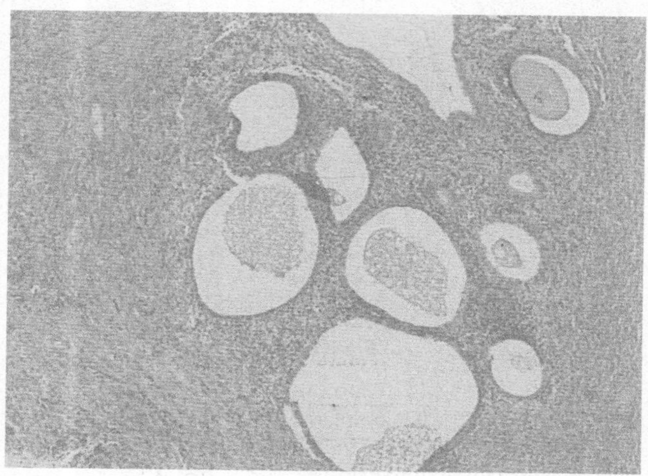

Figure 9-3

---

31 A 26-year-old woman complains of a golf ball–sized mass at the entrance of her vagina. She says that this area is "sore all the time" and began hurting "about 3 days ago." On examination, the patient has a tender 4-cm mass on the lateral aspect of the labia minora at the 5 o'clock position. There is erythema and edema, and the area is very tender and fluctuant. No cellulitis is noted. What is the most appropriate treatment for this condition?

(A) Trimethoprim/sulfamethoxazole
(B) Azithromycin for the patient and any sexual partners
(C) Incision and drainage of the mass followed by a course of trimethoprim/sulfamethoxazole
(D) Incision and drainage of the mass
(E) Incision and drainage of the mass with placement of a Word catheter

The answer is E: Incision and drainage of the mass with placement of a Word catheter. The patient has a Bartholin gland abscess. This condition may be treated by incising the abscess and creating a tract for it to drain facilitated by placement of the Word catheter. In the absence of cellulitis, antibiotics are not required (see *Figures 9-4* to *9-6*).

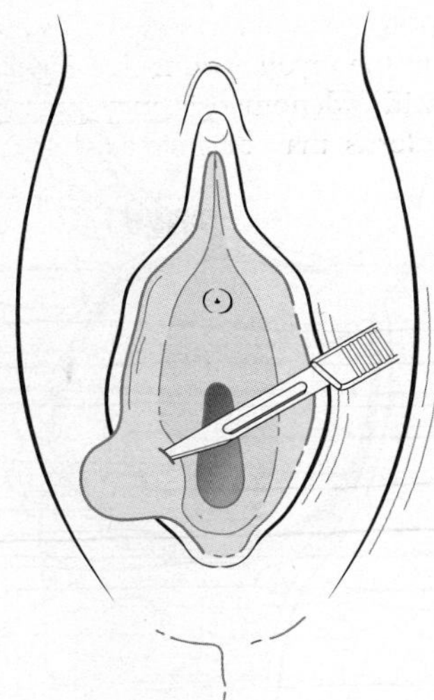

Figure 9-4

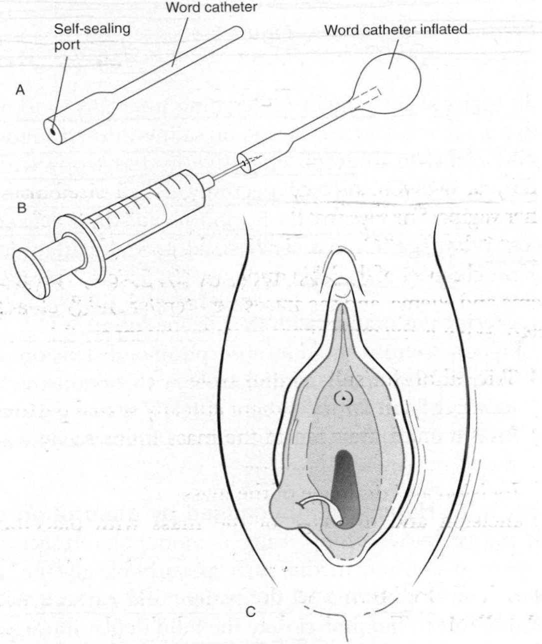

Figure 9-5

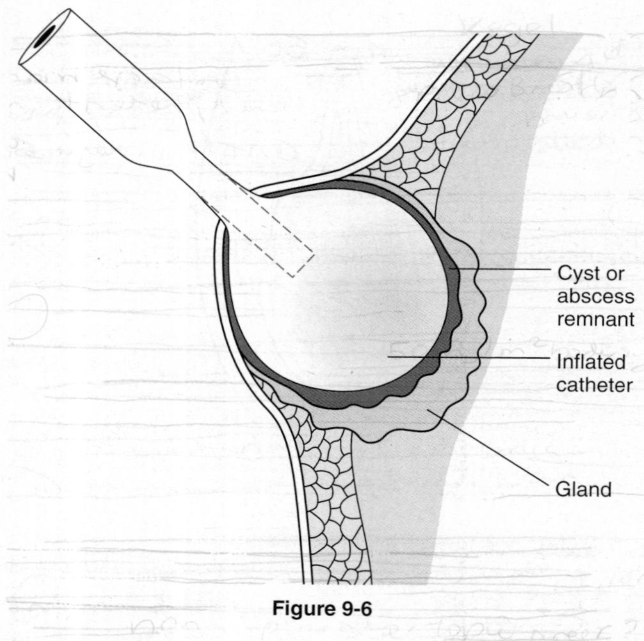

Figure 9-6

32 A 39-year-old P0 woman undergoing infertility workup is diagnosed with a small intracavitary lesion on saline-infused sonography.

She elects to undergo operative hysteroscopy with dilation and curettage (D&C) and polypectomy using monopolar cautery. She has a history of chlamydia 5 months ago that was treated in your office. What is the most serious risk to this patient associated with this procedure?

(A) Uterine perforation with the uterine sound
(B) Hyponatremia caused by absorption of distension media
(C) Seeding the upper genital tract with organisms likely to cause pelvic inflammatory disease (PID)
(D) Risk of anesthesia causing uterine atony and subsequent hemorrhage

The answer is B: Hyponatremia caused by absorption of distension media. Operative hysteroscopy using a monopolar resectoscope requires electrolyte-poor distension media such as sorbitol, glycine, and mannitol. These media may be absorbed by the patient and cause hyponatremia. It is therefore important to monitor closely the fluid deficit intraoperatively when using these media. *Figure 9-7* indicates polyp visualized with saline infusion hysterogram.

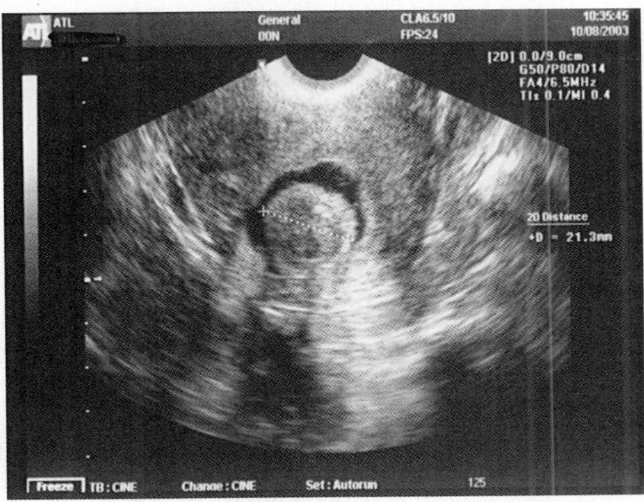

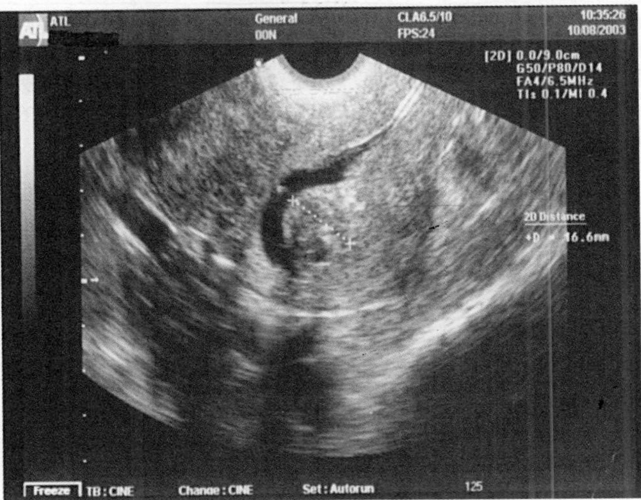

Figure 9-7

---

33 A 21-year-old woman presents to the emergency room (ER) complaining of gradually worsening left lower quadrant (LLQ) pain and vaginal spotting. Her quantitative β-hCG is 3,761. On examination, her abdomen is tender to palpation in the LLQ but is without rebound or guarding. No intrauterine pregnancy is seen on transvaginal ultrasound, but a fetus with positive cardiac activity is noted in the patient's left adnexa. The patient is frightened of anesthesia and declines surgery. What is the best course of management?

(A) Urge the patient to reconsider surgery, as she is not a candidate for expectant or medical management for a presumed ectopic pregnancy
(B) Recommend expectant management with precautions and in-office follow-up for a quantitative β-hCG in 3 and 6 days
(C) Admit the patient for a 3-day course of intravenous (IV) cyclophosphamide
(D) Administer intramuscular methotrexate and follow up for a quantitative β-hCG in 3 and 6 days
(E) Consult psychiatrist to determine the patient's mental competency to make decisions regarding her health

The answer is D: **Administer intramuscular methotrexate and follow up for a quantitative β-hCG in 3 and 6 days.** A nonruptured ectopic pregnancy may be managed medically with intramuscular methotrexate in the amount of 50 mg/m^2 of calculated body surface area. Quantitative β-hCG levels are drawn on days 4 and 7 to ensure a 15% drop in the level of this hormone between these days. Cardiac activity is a relative contraindication as is ectopic >3.5 cm.

---

34 A 49-year-old G5P5 woman comes to see you because of intermittent pelvic pain and constipation. The patient saw her primary care physician 1 month ago for the same complaints. A colonoscopy performed at that time showed no abnormalities. Today, the patient also confides that she has experienced increasing postcoital spotting over the past year. The patient is afebrile with a BP of 125/85 mmHg and an HR of 90 beats/min. Cardiac, pulmonary, and abdominal examinations are unremarkable. Bimanual pelvic examination reveals a nontender, 15-week-sized uterus with several dense cobblestone-like protrusions. Pelvic ultrasound shows at least seven 2- to 5-cm areas of hypogenicity. What is the next best step in the care of this patient?

(A) Saline infusion sonogram
(B) Endometrial biopsy
(C) Medroxyprogesterone
(D) Hysterectomy
(E) MRI-guided thermoablation

The answer is D: **Hysterectomy.** This patient can be diagnosed with uterine leiomyomas based on the pelvic ultrasound findings. Since this patient is experiencing pain, constipation, and abnormal bleeding, a hysterectomy is warranted. Other treatment options for uterine leiomyomas include medroxyprogesterone, which works to shrink fibroids by decreasing estrogen and MRI-guided thermoablation. These treatments are not appropriate for this patient due to her symptoms and age. The patient is likely perimenopausal and is most likely past her childbearing years, and therefore, preservation of fertility is not a primary concern. Therefore, the next best step in the care of this patient would be a hysterectomy.

---

35 A 68-year-old woman presents to clinic complaining of lower abdominal "heaviness," which worsens and localizes to the vagina when she lifts her 5-year-old grandson. She also admits to some stress urinary incontinence, as well as the need to urinate two to three times during the night. She has not been sexually active since the death of her husband 2 years ago. Pelvic examination reveals poorly estrogenized vaginal mucosa with a herniation of the anterior vaginal wall; when the patient is asked to bear down, this herniation extends to the level of the introitus. What is the likely diagnosis?

(A) Grade 2 enterocele
(B) Grade 3 enterocele
(C) Grade 2 cystocele
(D) Grade 3 cystocele
(E) Grade 2 rectocele
(F) Grade 3 rectocele

The answer is C: Grade 2 cystocele. This description is consistent with a cystocele, in which a weakening of the anterior vaginal wall allows the urinary bladder to prolapse into the vagina. Enterocele is diagnosed with the prolapse of a segment into the vagina, and a rectocele involves prolapse of the rectum through a weakened portion of the posterior vaginal wall. All of these, as well as uterine prolapse, are diagnosed by the position of the defect; in grade 1, the defect is fully contained within the vagina; in grade 2, the defect extends to the level of the introitus (as in this case); and in grade 3, the prolapsed portion extends outside of the introitus.

---

36 A 58-year-old postmenopausal woman is seen in clinic for a routine examination. At the end of the visit, she sheepishly admits to mild urinary incontinence over the past several years. She is G4P4; all her children were normal spontaneous vaginal deliveries, and the largest weighed 8 lb 7 oz. She has hypertension treated with metoprolol and has been using a topical estrogen cream for vaginal dryness since menopause at age 54. Further questioning reveals that she occasionally leaks small amounts of urine, particularly with laughing, sneezing, or coughing. She denies large volume loss, increased urinary frequency, or nocturia. Based upon this history, which of the following is a good initial treatment option for this woman's urinary incontinence?

(A) Pelvic floor strengthening exercises
(B) Urethral bulking injections
(C) Imipramine
(D) Discontinue topical estrogen cream
(E) Urethral sling procedure

The answer is A: Pelvic floor strengthening exercises. This woman's history is consistent with stress urinary incontinence, likely caused by a weakening of the pelvic floor muscles. Multiple vaginal deliveries and postmenopausal state are both associated with higher rates of stress incontinence. Pelvic floor strengthening exercises (Kegel exercises) are the least invasive means of addressing this issue and should be tried prior to other interventions. Imipramine is a tricyclic antidepressant used to treat mixed stress and urge incontinence. Topical estrogen cream is used as a treatment for stress incontinence; discontinuing it would likely worsen this woman's incontinence. Urethral bulking injections and urethral slings are both surgical procedures that may be reasonable for this woman if less invasive methods fail.

---

37 A 72-year-old nursing home resident with mild cognitive impairment is brought to clinic with complaints of constant "dribbling" of urine during the day and increased urinary urgency, both during the day and at night. When she does urinate, her stream is weak and hesitant, occasionally stopping and starting several times. In addition, she has occasional episodes of large-volume urinary incontinence. A postvoid residual in the clinic shows urinary retention of 225 mL. What is the likely diagnosis?

(A) Stress incontinence
(B) Urge incontinence
(C) Mixed incontinence
(D) Functional incontinence
(E) Overflow incontinence

The answer is E: Overflow incontinence. Overflow incontinence is characterized by continuous dribbling or leakage of urine and increased residual volume, with or without increased urgency. The increased pressure caused by residual urine volumes can lead to sudden large-volume loss, as in this case. It is caused by poor contractility of the detrusor muscle and/or bladder outflow obstruction; true outflow obstruction is more common in men. Stress incontinence is precipitated by activities such as sneezing, coughing, and lifting and is caused by weakened pelvic floor muscles. Urge incontinence is characterized by increased urgency accompanied by large-volume leakages and is caused by detrusor hyperactivity. Mixed incontinence refers to coexisting symptoms of stress and urge incontinence. Functional incontinence refers to a lack of behavioral control (intentional or otherwise) over bowel or bladder function in the absence of physiologic explanations. It can be seen in individuals with cognitive impairment, but the constant leakage described by this patient is not consistent with functional incontinence.

---

38 A 74-year-old woman with Alzheimer dementia is brought to clinic for a medical examination prior to admission to a nursing facility. She is healthy and has had little medical care since the birth of her last child 46 years ago. Menopause occurred at age 53. Speculum and bimanual examination reveal uterine prolapse to the level of the introitus. Surgery to correct this patient's condition involves plication of which of the following structures?

(A) Uterosacral ligaments
(B) Rectal fascia
(C) Endopelvic fascia
(D) Rectovaginal fascia and posterior abdominal wall

The answer is A: **Uterosacral ligaments.** Plication of the uterosacral ligaments is the McCall culdoplasty, performed along with a vaginal hysterectomy as definitive surgical correction of uterine prolapse. Posterior colporrhaphy is the surgical treatment for rectocele and involves removal of excess (posterior) vaginal mucosa and plication of the rectal fascia. Surgical correction of a cystocele is done by anterior colporrhaphy, which involves removal of excess anterior vaginal mucosa and plication of the endopelvic fascia. Enteroceles can be surgically corrected via plication of the rectovaginal fascia and the posterior abdominal wall.

---

39 A 37-year-old G0 with a history of irregular periods comes to see you to discuss her bleeding pattern. The patient reports that she menstruates 9 to 10 times per year and she has felt that her bleeding has gotten heavier over the years. She also has occasional spotting between periods. The patient's P is 80 beats/min, R 18 breaths/min, BP 126/88 mmHg, weight 180, and height 5′2″. The most important next step in the management of this patient is:

(A) Prescribe oral contraceptive pills (OCPs) to regulate bleeding
(B) Perform an endometrial biopsy
(C) Measure complete blood count (CBC), prothrombin time/partial thromboplastin time, factor VIII, and von Willebrand factor antigen and activity
(D) Perform a pelvic ultrasound
(E) Administer intravenous (IV) estrogen 25 mg every 4 hours for 24 hours

The answer is B: **Perform an endometrial biopsy.** The patient in the question presents with abnormal uterine bleeding (AUB). Woman over the age of 35 with AUB should undergo an endometrial biopsy to rule out endometrial hyperplasia and cancer. Obesity, which this patient has, is also a risk factor for hyperplasia. Pelvic ultrasound may identify structural etiologies, such as endometrial polyps and fibroids; however, this patient still requires an endometrial biopsy.

---

40 A 27-year-old G3P2 at 32 week's gestation comes to see you for a routine prenatal appointment. The patient has had an uncomplicated pregnancy so far. Today, the patient reports increased fatigue and weakness. The patient takes no medications other than a prenatal vitamin. Lately, however, the prenatal vitamin has caused nausea, and the patient is unable to tolerate it. On examination, the patient is pale, afebrile with a BP of 100/60 mmHg and an HR of 90 beats/min. Heart and lung examinations are unremarkable. Fundal height is 31.5, and fetal heart tones are in the 150s. Laboratories show a hemoglobin of 9 g/dL with a mean corpuscular volume (MCV) of 70. What is the most likely cause of the patient's anemia?

(A) Iron deficiency
(B) Folate deficiency
(C) β-Thalassemia minor
(D) Hemolytic anemia
(E) Glucose-6-phosphate dehydrogenase deficiency

The answer is A: Iron deficiency. The patient presents with a mild microcytic anemia as evidenced by a low hemoglobin and a low MCV. The most common cause of microcytic anemia is iron deficiency. This is especially true in pregnant patients. In pregnancy, there is an increased demand for iron due to the increasing needs of the fetus and the substantial increase in maternal blood volume. All pregnant patients are advised to take prenatal vitamins that typically contain between 27 and 60 mg of iron. The patient in this question had compliance issues due to nausea caused by her prenatal vitamins. However, even compliant patients can develop iron deficiency anemia, and therefore, all pregnant patients with a hemoglobin $<$11 mg/dL are usually started on iron supplements in addition to their prenatal vitamin.

---

41 A 37-year-old G2P2 comes to see you because she has recently noticed spotting between her periods that is progressively getting worse. The patient now has to wear a panty liner every day because she does not know when the bleeding will occur. The patient does not have any medical problems and takes no medications. The patient denies tobacco, alcohol, or drug use. The patient had two uncomplicated vaginal deliveries 10 and 12 years ago and does not want any more children. The patient is not sexually active and uses no birth control. No abnormalities are noted on physical examination. What is your immediate assessment and plan?

(A) The patient's abnormal uterine bleeding (AUB) necessitates an endometrial biopsy to rule out endometrial hyperplasia and cancer
(B) The patient's AUB is likely due to premature ovarian failure, and chromosomal analysis is indicated to rule out a genetic cause
(C) The patient's AUB should be treated with endometrial ablation since further childbearing is not desired
(D) The patient's AUB is likely due to anovulation necessitating workup for hypothalamic–pituitary–gonadal axis dysfunction.

The answer is A: The patient's abnormal uterine bleeding (AUB) necessitates an endometrial biopsy to rule out endometrial hyperplasia and cancer. The patient in the scenario suffers from intermenstrual bleeding (IMB), an abnormality of menstrual bleeding defined as any bleeding that occurs between normal menstrual periods. All patients older than 35 years with AUB should undergo an endometrial biopsy to rule out endometrial hyperplasia and cancer. While endometrial ablation may be a reasonable treatment option, the first step in the workup of this patient's AUB should be an endometrial biopsy.

42 A 42-year-old, G3P3, complains of a 2-year history of increasingly painful and heavy periods. She says that in her teens and 20s she had relatively painless periods as well as significantly less bleeding. She also complains of pain with bowel movements and sexual intercourse. Her primary care doctor prescribed oral contraceptive pills (OCPs), but she has not had any relief with them. On examination, her uterus is enlarged and globular, and there is no nodularity on rectovaginal examination. β-hCG is negative. Which of the following is the most likely diagnosis?

(A) Primary dysmenorrhea
(B) Adenomyosis
(C) Endometriosis
(D) Pelvic inflammatory disease (PID)
(E) Endometrial cancer

The answer is B: Adenomyosis. Adenomyosis refers to the presence of endometrial tissue within the myometrium (the muscular layers of the uterus). The most common presenting symptoms of adenomyosis are dysmenorrhea and menorrhagia, and physical examination findings include an enlarged, globular uterus. The most common age at diagnosis is between 40 and 50 years; however, this may be due to the fact that definitive diagnosis is only by tissue visualization, and thus, most cases are identified at hysterectomy. This case is not consistent with primary dysmenorrhea as the patient did not develop painful periods until she was approximately 40 years old. Endometriosis is less likely as the patient does not have any relief with OCPs. PID would present more acutely (within days to weeks, not years) and might be seen in conjunction with new vaginal discharge, fevers, and chills. This patient is young and without significant risk factors for endometrial cancer. Furthermore, endometrial cancer usually first presents as painless vaginal bleeding in a postmenopausal woman.

---

43 A 26-year-old G0 reports painful periods for the past 2 years. Her past medical history is unremarkable, she has never had any surgeries, and she does not take any medications on a chronic basis. She experiences severe cramping the entire 4 days of her period, which gradually improves 1 to 2 days afterward. She has tried nonsteroidal anti-inflammatory drugs (NSAIDs) and oral contraceptive pills (OCPs) with little relief. On review of systems, the patient also reports several 2- to 3-week episodes of severe diarrhea and occasional bloody stools over the past couple of years. On bimanual examination, she has diffuse pelvic tenderness, as well as a fixed, retroverted uterus. Which of the following investigations is most likely to reveal the cause of this patient's pain?

(A) Colposcopy
(B) Cystoscopy
(C) Colonoscopy
(D) Endoscopy
(E) Laparoscopy

The answer is C: Colonoscopy. Her history of bloody diarrhea and the examination finding of a fixed retroverted uterus are suspicious for a local inflammatory disease such as Crohn disease. Crohn disease is associated with transmural inflammation of the bowel wall extending out to the serosa, which can lead to the formation of adhesions between the bowel and other abdominal and/or pelvic structures, including the uterus. These adhesions, in turn, can present with dysmenorrhea. The best course of action would be to refer this patient to a gastroenterologist for evaluation of her bowel via colonoscopy. If the colonoscopy is negative, laparoscopy may be considered.

---

44 An 18-year-old G0 presents to her gynecologist complaining of painful periods. She reports that she experiences severe cramping pain beginning 1 week prior to menses, which peaks 1 to 2 days into menses. Her pain is relieved when she gets her period, however, and she reports that she feels normal for the rest of the month. She has had this pattern of pain since she started menstruating at age 15, but it has been getting progressively worse. If initial empiric medical treatment of her condition fails, which of the following will provide definitive diagnosis of this patient's likely condition?

(A) Pap smear with human papillomavirus (HPV) testing
(B) Bimanual examination
(C) Transvaginal ultrasound
(D) Direct visualization via laparoscopy
(E) Serum β-hCG

The answer is D: **Direct visualization via laparoscopy.** This patient has the typical clinical picture of endometriosis: cyclical pain that is worst in the 1 to 2 weeks leading up to menses and during menses. Endometriosis is caused by ectopic endometrial tissue, which is most often in the pelvis but can be located anywhere in the peritoneal cavity. Medical treatment includes suppression of the endometrial tissue via oral contraceptive pills (OCPs), progestins, or gonadotropin antagonists. It is reasonable to try a patient on OCPs if there is a high suspicion for endometriosis and the patient does not wish to become pregnant at the time. Definitive diagnosis, however, is achieved only via direct visualization of endometrial implants via laparoscopy. They may appear as dark brown "powder burns," blue raised "mulberry lesions," or blood-filled "chocolate cysts." Bimanual examination of patients with endometriosis is often normal, although it may reveal uterosacral nodularity or a fixed retroverted uterus in patients with advanced disease. Ultrasound may reveal "ground glass" lesions consistent with ovarian endometriomas, but it is not sensitive for the detection of endometriosis. Serum β-hCG is used to diagnose pregnancy or choriocarcinoma, neither of which is consistent with this patient's presentation of cyclic pelvic pain.

---

45 A 24-year-old G0 complains of headache, irritability, low mood, restlessness, and fatigue that occur mostly in the 2 weeks preceding menstruation. She reports regular 5-day periods every 30 days and says that she feels relatively symptom-free for the week following her period. Which of the following treatments is most likely to be helpful in this patient?

(A) Naproxen
(B) Nortriptyline
(C) Quetiapine
(D) Lorazepam
(E) Fluoxetine

The answer is E: **Fluoxetine.** This patient's presentation is consistent with premenstrual dysphoric disorder, defined by the presence of five or more neurobehavioral symptoms (including sadness, anxiety, mood lability, irritability, decreased interest, difficulty concentrating, fatigue, changes in appetite, changes in sleep, feeling out of control, and a number of physical symptoms including headache and breast tenderness). Symptoms must be present for at least 1 week prior to menstruation and must resolve in the days following. First-line treatment is with selective serotonin reuptake inhibitors (SSRIs) such as fluoxetine.

46 A 17-year-old G0 complains of painful periods. She says that she began menstruating at 14 years of age and has had significant pain and cramping associated with menstruation since then. Her pain is worst on the first and second days of menstruation and is often associated with nausea, vomiting, and headache. Her pain is so severe that she often has to miss school on the first day of her period. She has tried heating pads and baths, which provide some minor relief. Physical examination reveals no abnormalities. Which of the following interventions is considered first-line therapy for this patient's condition?

(A) Acetaminophen
(B) Nonsteroidal anti-infl ammatory drugs (NSAIDs)
(C) Opiate analgesics
(D) Oral contraceptive pills (OCPs)
(E) Gonadotropin antagonists

The answer is B: Nonsteroidal anti-infl ammatory drugs (NSAIDs). This patient likely has primary dysmenorrhea. Primary dysmenorrhea is idiopathic and is thought to be due to increased levels of endometrial prostaglandin production at the onset of menstruation. In support of this hypothesis is the fact that the first-line and most effective treatment for primary dysmenorrhea is NSAIDs, which prevent the formation of prostaglandins via inhibition of the cyclooxygenase enzymes. Second-line treatment for patients who fail NSAIDs is OCPs, which are thought to decrease pain either by suppressing ovulation and/or endometrial proliferation and thus prostaglandin production. Acetaminophen, opiate analgesics, and gonadotropin antagonists are not routinely used in primary dysmenorrhea.

47 A 26-year-old G2P1 at 39 weeks 3 days by last menstrual period (LMP) consistent with a 6-week ultrasound undergoes a scheduled repeat low transverse Cesarean section. Her medical history is complicated by type 1 diabetes mellitus, well controlled on insulin. Visual inspection of the exteriorized uterus reveals two well-circumscribed, firm nodules of approximately 2 to 3 cm in diameter beneath the serosa of the uterus. She has no history of menorrhagia or urinary frequency and was taking oral contraceptive pills (OCPs) prior to pregnancy. What is the most likely diagnosis for these masses?

(A) Fibrous cysts
(B) Leiomyomata
(C) Uterine sarcomas
(D) Endometrial carcinoma

The answer is B: Leiomyomata. Uterine fibroids, also known as leiomyomas, are the most common pelvic tumors in women. They represent the benign proliferation of smooth muscle cells, often thought to originate from a single cell. Most women are asymptomatic, such as this patient. Uterine sarcomas are a rare-type malignant uterine cancer that arises from the smooth muscle of the uterus. It often presents in older women as postmenopausal bleeding and a fungating mass through the external cervical os visible on speculum examination. Endometrial carcinoma also presents as postmenopausal bleeding and would not be likely in this patient. Fibrous cysts are commonly found in breast tissue.

48 Which of the following is the best management in this patient?

(A) Expectant management
(B) Nonhormonal medical therapy
(C) Hormonal therapy
(D) Removal of the masses during the Cesarean section

The answer is A: Expectant management. This patient has asymptomatic leiomyomas found incidentally during a Cesarean section which are likely subserosal given their easy identification on the exterior surface of the uterine corpus. She may have intramural or submucosal fibroids as well. However, since she has no history of symptoms associated with fibroids such as menorrhagia or urinary frequency, she does not need any treatment at this time such as nonhormonal medications, hormonal medications, or surgery for symptom control.

49 A 36-year-old G1P1 presents to her gynecologist with progressively heavier menstrual flow and pelvic pressure. She strongly desires future fertility. Bimanual examination reveals a 16-week-sized uterus, and urine β-hCG testing is negative. Ultrasonography reveals multiple uterine leiomyomas, but cannot comment on the specific location of each fibroid. The patient is considering surgical treatment. What is the next best step in identifying the locations of the uterine fibroids?

(A) Hysterosalpingography (HSG)
(B) Sonohysterography
(C) MRI
(D) CT
(E) Positron emission tomography (PET)

The answer is C: MRI. MRI is the best imaging study for identifying the size and location of leiomyomas, also known as fibroids. It is particularly useful if uterine artery embolization is being considered as a possible treatment option. HSG enables the evaluation of the uterine cavity contour but does not ascertain each fibroid location. Sonohysterography helps identify the location of submucosal fibroids and their distortion of the endometrial cavity. CT and PET are not typically used for the evaluation of leiomyomas.

50 A 32-year-old, G3P0, woman has been referred to an infertility specialist for a history of three consecutive spontaneous abortions at 9, 13, and 18 weeks of gestational ages. She reports menarche at 14, moderate flow menses lasting 6 days with 30-day cycles, and her gynecologic history is negative for abnormal Pap smears. Further workup reveals uterine fibroids. Surgical removal of which fibroid type has been shown to improve fertility outcomes?

(A) Submucous
(B) Intramural
(C) Cervical
(D) Subserosal

The answer is A: Submucous. Submucous and intramural fibroids have been associated with a higher rate of spontaneous abortions and infertility. They are thought to impair implantation, disrupt tubal function, or impede sperm transport. Only the removal of submucous fibroids and not intramural fibroids has been shown to improve fertility outcomes. Subserosal fibroids are not associated with adverse changes to fertility.

---

51 A 19-year-old G1P0 at 10 weeks 1 day of gestational age by her last menstrual period (LMP) presents to the emergency department (ED) with a 3-day history of vaginal bleeding and cramping, which she likens to her menstrual cramps. She had an 8-week ultrasound, which confirmed an intrauterine pregnancy; transvaginal ultrasound in the ED shows a gestational sac in the lower uterine segment. On pelvic examination, the internal cervical os is open and active bleeding is visible. She is diagnosed with an incomplete abortion. What is the next step in the management of this patient?

(A) Discharge home with follow-up in clinic in 1 week
(B) Obtain a β-hCG level
(C) Obtain an abdominal ultrasound
(D) Recommend a dilation and curettage (D&C)

The answer is D: Recommend a dilation and curettage (D&C). As this patient has been diagnosed with an incomplete abortion, the next step in management would be to recommend a D&C to remove any remaining products of conception. While an abdominal ultrasound or β-hCG test could be performed, from the physical examination the patient has an incomplete abortion, in which case these two tests would not change the management. The products of conception are still in the lower uterine segment and will continue to cause bleeding until removed. Therefore, it is not recommended that the patient to go home without intervention.

---

52 A 34-year-old woman presents to her physician with feelings of depression, abdominal bloating, and breast tenderness 5 days prior to her onset of menses last month. She states that symptoms resolved with the onset of her menses and she felt back to herself. She reports that this happened once before, she thinks about 6 months ago. Her periods have always been regular since her onset of menses at the age of 13. What is the next step in the management of this patient?

(A) Instruct her to begin documenting a menstrual diary
(B) Begin treatment with an selective serotonin reuptake inhibitor (SSRI) such as fluoxetine or sertraline
(C) B_6 supplementation
(D) Order follicle-stimulating hormone (FSH) level
(E) Administer depression screen

The answer is A: Instruct her to begin documenting a menstrual diary. In order to make a diagnosis of premenstrual syndrome (PMS), symptoms must occur 5 days before menses in at least two consecutive menstrual cycles, with symptom relief within 4 days of the onset of menses. While this patient has experienced symptoms of PMS, she cannot conclusively say that she experienced them in consecutive months, and it is important for her to document her symptoms in a menstrual diary. This will allow the assessment of a correlation of symptoms with the luteal phase of her cycle, as well as recurrence. SSRIs are second-line treatment for PMS after supportive therapy, but a diagnosis of PMS has not yet been made in this patient. B_6 supplementation is often used as a treatment for PMS, but again we cannot conclude from her history that she has PMS. FSH level can be used to assess for menopause, but as this patient is still menstruating this is unlikely. While a depression screen may be helpful in this patient, her symptoms of depression resolve between cycles making a diagnosis of depression unlikely.

---

53 A 24-year-old woman presents with increased irritability, depressed mood, breast tenderness, and headaches that occur cyclically each month about 5 days before the onset of menses. Symptoms resolve with the onset of menses. She states that this has occurred monthly for the past 2 years. She is subsequently diagnosed with premenstrual syndrome (PMS). What is the first step in the management of this patient?

(A) Selective serotonin reuptake inhibitors (SSRIs) such as fluoxetine and sertraline
(B) Oral contraceptive pills (OCPs)
(C) Spironolactone
(D) Supportive therapy
(E) Gonadotropin-releasing hormone (GnRH) agonists

The answer is D: Supportive therapy. The first step in pharmacologic treatment of PMS is supportive therapy such as nutritional supplements like calcium, magnesium, and vitamin E. Spironolactone can be used as an initial treatment, but is only effective in decreasing bloating, which this patient does not have. SSRIs are second-line treatment after supportive therapy, complex carbohydrate diet, nutritional supplements, or spironolactone has failed. OCPs and GnRH are generally third-line treatments.

---

54 A 34-year-old woman presents to her physician with a 4-day history of fevers, chills, nausea, and vomiting. She also notes pain radiating to her back. A urinalysis detects leukocyte esterase in the urine. What is the next step in the management of this patient?

(A) Obtain a urine culture
(B) Start empiric treatment with trimethoprim/sulfamethoxazole
(C) Give intravenous (IV) fluids and discharge home
(D) Abdominal CT

The answer is A: Obtain a urine culture. This patient presents with signs and symptoms consistent with acute pyelonephritis (the upper urinary tract infection [UTI]). A urine culture should be performed in all cases of upper UTI. Trimethoprim/sulfamethoxazole is reserved for the treatment of uncomplicated UTIs, which this patient does not have. She has a complicated UTI. While patients who present with acute pyelonephritis are often given IV fluids, they must also be started on antibiotics before being discharged home. Abdominal CT to rule out abscess is reserved for those patients with pyelonephritis who fail to defervesce after 72 hours of treatment.

---

55 A 22-year-old sexually active woman presents to her physician with a 3-day history of pain with urination as well as frequent awakening at night with the urge to void. She denies fevers, chills, flank, or suprapubic pain. Upon microscopic examination, 14 leukocytes/mL are noted. What is the next step in the management of this patient?

(A) Reassurance
(B) Obtain urine culture results prior to initiating treatment
(C) Trimethoprim/sulfamethoxazole
(D) Ampicillin and gentamicin

The answer is C: Trimethoprim/sulfamethoxazole. Symptomatic urinary tract infections (UTIs) should always be treated. If pyuria or bacteriuria is present in a patient presenting with symptoms of a lower UTI, a urine culture is not required before starting initial treatment. Of the choices given, for noncomplicated UTIs trimethoprim/sulfamethoxazole is the treatment of choice. Ampicillin and gentamicin are generally reserved for complicated UTIs (upper tract infection in women, any UTI in men or pregnant women, or UTI with underlying structural disease or immunosuppression). This patient's symptoms are most consistent with an uncomplicated, lower UTI.

56 A 16-year-old African-American woman presents to her physician for the fourth time in the last 6 months with signs and symptoms consistent with urinary tract infection (UTI) despite several treatment regimens with antibiotics. Her medical history includes placement of a levonorgestrel intrauterine device (IUD) 1 year ago. She reports that she frequently engages in intercourse with her boyfriend of 2 years. Which of the following is the greatest risk factor for this patient's recurrent UTI?

(A) Levonorgestrel IUD
(B) Young age at first intercourse
(C) African-American race
(D) Frequent sexual intercourse

The answer is D: Frequent sexual intercourse. Risk factors associated with recurrent UTIs include frequent intercourse, long-term spermicide use, diaphragm use, a new sexual partner, young age at first UTI, and maternal history of UTI. IUDs do not increase the risk of UTIs. While young age at first UTI is a risk factor, young age at first intercourse is not. Race is not an independent risk factor for recurrence of UTIs.

57 A 29-year-old woman presents with signs and symptoms consistent with an uncomplicated, lower urinary tract infection (UTI). It is decided to begin treating her with antibiotic therapy. What is the recommended duration of oral antibiotic treatment for an uncomplicated UTI?

(A) 1 day
(B) 3 days
(C) 7 days
(D) 10 to 14 days

The answer is B: 3 days. Single-dose, 1-day treatment is sufficient for some sexually transmitted infections (STIs) including gonorrhea and chlamydia, but is generally not recommended for UTIs. Recent data have shown that 3 days of therapy are equivalent in efficacy to longer durations of therapy. Treatment durations greater than 10 days are generally reserved for complicated UTIs.

58 A 37-year-old G3P2 underwent a tubal reanastomosis subsequent to a bilateral tubal ligation at age 24. Menses is currently 5 days late. A home pregnancy test, confirmed by a serum test at the hospital, is positive. What is the next appropriate step in her management?

(A) Advise pelvic rest until the second trimester
(B) Confirm folic acid intake
(C) Evaluate for a possible ectopic pregnancy
(D) Perform maternal serum screening to evaluate for trisomy 21
(E) Schedule an initial prenatal visit within the next 2 to 3 weeks

The answer is C: Evaluate for a possible ectopic pregnancy. This would include a serum quantitative β-hCG and when appropriate an ultrasound to evaluate the presence of a gestational sac. Because tubal scarring can occur during each tubal surgery, an increased risk of ectopic pregnancy exists. Until certain that this is an intrauterine gestation, any genetic testing should be deferred. The appropriate time to advise patients regarding folic acid intake is prior to conception. There is no evidence that pelvic rest prevents first-trimester miscarriage. Maternal screening for genetic abnormalities is not performed at 5 week's gestation.

---

59 A 24-year-old G1P0010 presents for a preconception consultation. She wishes to conceive in the next year. Three years ago, she has a termination of pregnancy at 10 weeks via suction curettage. Until 18 months ago, she used depot medroxyprogesterone acetate (DMPA) but has used no contraception since. She resumed having very regular menses 5 months after her last DMPA injection, but they are very scant and associated with severe cramping. She regularly checks an ovulation predictor kit that reveals a luteinizing hormone (LH) surge consistently on day 16 of her cycle. She has remained sexually active. Her general medical examination is unremarkable. Her thyroid is of normal size. Gender-specific examination reveals normal internal and external genitalia. Uterus is small and is at mid-position. Ovaries are palpable bilaterally about 2 cm each. Pregnancy test is negative. Which of the following will be the most beneficial in evaluating this patient's differential diagnosis?

(A) Diagnostic laparoscopy
(B) Hysteroscopy
(C) Progesterone challenge
(D) Thyroid function testing
(E) Ultrasound

The answer is B: Hysteroscopy. Hysteroscopy in indicated for this patient with secondary infertility, secondary dysmenorrhea, and scant menses since having a suction curettage. The condition was probably masked due to amenorrhea with DMPA and was only identified after cessation of the contraceptive. Although about 7 months of anovulation is not uncommon subsequent to stopping DMPA, she has a good documentation of regular ovulatory function over the past 13 months. Based on her presentation, Asherman syndrome is the most likely diagnosis. The way to definitively diagnose and treat Asherman syndrome is hysteroscopically.

---

60 A 55-year-old G0P0 presents with a 2-month history of intermittent bright red vaginal bleeding. She went through menopause at the age of 51 and has not had a period since until recently. She presents for a second opinion about the management of postmenopausal bleeding through a hysterectomy. Other than a preoperative complete blood count (CBC), she has had no workup. You recommend an endometrial biopsy but she is concerned that she may have endometrial cancer, and an outpatient endometrial biopsy will not be accurate enough to diagnose endometrial cancer. You explain to her that the diagnostic accuracy of office endometrial sampling techniques is:

(A) 90% to 98%
(B) 80% to 89%
(C) 70% to 79%
(D) 60% to 69%
(E) 50% to 59%

The answer is A: 90% to 98%. A positive test result is highly accurate; however, a negative test result is of limited accuracy and only moderately useful. Given the pretest probability in a postmenopausal patient with new-onset vaginal bleeding, it is reasonable to proceed with endometrial biopsy. When adequate tissue sampling is obtained, the results are highly accurate.

---

61 A 43-year-old woman presents with a 4-month history of abnormal menses. Some months she has periods that last for 12 days; she may then skip 2 weeks and have another really long period. The periods are irregular and heavy. Until 4 months ago, she had been having regular menses with cycles of 28-day length, periods lasting 5 days with moderate bleeding. She has been having occasional hot flashes at night, not sleeping well, and feeling very fatigued. She gives no history of unusual bleeding with procedures. She is currently on no medications, and she denies taking any herbal or over-the-counter remedies.

Physical examination reveals a pleasant, mildly obese woman with a slightly enlarged thyroid gland. Vital signs are BP 146/89 mmHg, P 82 beats/min, T 37°C, and R 20 breaths/min in no acute distress. Her pelvic examination is significant for an enlarged uterus approximately the size of a 3-month pregnancy. She tells you she has had fibroids for 8 years, but they have been asymptomatic. All other pelvic structures appear normal.

Thyroid-stimulating hormone is normal at 4.5. A pregnancy test is negative. A transvaginal ultrasound confirms the presence of three intramural fibroids ranging from 1 to 2 cm in diameter. A saline-infused ultrasound reveals no evidence of endometrial polyps or masses.

You see her back in 3 weeks of follow-up. The endometrial biopsy performed 3 days before her period revealed proliferative endometrium. She had a withdrawal bleed after you gave her progesterone therapy for 10 days. Since that time, she has had no other vaginal bleeding. The most likely diagnosis for this patient is:

(A) Anovulatory bleeding
(B) Hypothyroidism
(C) Polycystic ovary syndrome
(D) Menopause

The answer is A: Anovulatory bleeding. The biopsy reveals changes consistent with estrogen stimulation which responded to progesterone withdrawal so she is not at menopausal. She does not have abnormal thyroid function. The history is not consistent with polycystic ovarian syndrome (PCOS) in general as her periods are more frequent than usual. The intramural uterine fibroids play no role in this patient's symptomatology. The diagnosis of menopause requires no menses for 12 months.

---

62 A 19-year-old G0 college student presents with amenorrhea for the past 6 months. Her menses began at age 12 and were regular until then. She denies sexual activity, and a pregnancy test is negative. Her physical examination is unremarkable except for the milky white discharge she expresses from her nipples. What is the next step?

(A) Transvaginal ultrasound
(B) Measure serum prolactin
(C) Order brain MRI
(D) Get thyroid ultrasound

The answer is B: Measure serum prolactin. Autopsy studies indicate that 6% to 25% of the US population have small pituitary tumors. Forty percent of these pituitary tumors produce prolactin, but most are not considered clinically significant. Clinically significant pituitary tumors affect the health of approximately 14 out of 100,000 people.

---

63 Refer to the patient in Question 62. The prolactin comes back as 175 g/L. What is the next step?

(A) Coned down view of the sella turcica
(B) Cranial radiography
(C) Dual-energy X-ray absorptiometry scanning
(D) Helical CT
(E) MRI

The answer is E: MRI. Although modern high-speed helical CT scanners produce very detailed images, MRI is the imaging study of choice. MRI can detect adenomas that are as small as 3 to 5 mm.

---

64 A 29-year-old G1P0010 woman with regular menses (every 28 days lasting 5 days) is currently trying to conceive. She has not used contraception for 6 months. Her ovulation predictor kit revealed an luteinizing hormone (LH) surge 7 days ago. She presents with acute abdominal/pelvic pain. This clinical picture is most consistent with:

(A) Cystic teratoma
(B) Ectopic pregnancy
(C) Follicular cyst
(D) Hemorrhagic corpus luteum cyst
(E) Serous cystadenoma

The answer is D: **Hemorrhagic corpus luteum cyst.** Cysts are a normal phenomenon in the menstrual cycle. Both follicular and corpus luteum cysts occur monthly. It is not uncommon for cysts to rupture either. Symptoms can range from no symptoms to symptoms that are similar to an acute abdomen. Most patients will be hemodynamically stable, and once pregnancy is ruled out, treatment is largely symptomatic. Duration of pain is probably related to the degree of hemorrhage and can last from several days to several weeks. Ruptured follicular cysts are more common than ruptured corpus luteum cysts that would be anticipated because the mechanism of ovulation requires breaking through the ovarian capsule to release the oocyte.

---

65 A 34-year-old woman, G3P2002, presents to the emergency room (ER) with sudden onset pain that was severe in nature. She rates it as 7/10. The pain has occurred before, and in fact, she has been present to the ER four times in the past 6 months for similar pain. Each time, the pain has resolved within a few hours. The pain does not occur in any pattern with relation to her menstrual cycle. It is always on her left side. Today, the pain is the worst it has ever been and has lasted far longer than on previous occasions. She has been having some anorexia and nausea currently. In physical examination, she is afebrile and normotensive. You note guarding and rebound in the left lower quadrant (LLQ). Bowel sounds are absent. Pelvic examination reveals a normal-sized uterus, extreme tenderness in the left adnexal area when you move the cervix, but no obvious mass in the pelvis. As you review her records, you view an abdominal X-ray from 6 months ago. After reviewing the X-ray, you are able to make the diagnosis of ovarian torsion and prepare the patient for immediate surgery. What finding on the X-ray would support this diagnosis and plan?

(A) Air-fluid levels
(B) Fluid in the pelvic cul-de-sac
(C) Large simple cystic structure
(D) Subdiaphragmatic gas collection
(E) Teeth with roots

The answer is E: Teeth with roots. Typically, a dermoid cyst is not found in the pelvis because of its buoyancy due to sebaceous content. The treatment is to operate on and remove once diagnosed due to the high risk of ovarian torsion. Finding teeth on the X-ray is a strong clue that the mass is a dermoid.

---

66 On a medical mission to rural Honduras, limited facilities for health care are available. A G2P1 at 16 weeks presents for routine prenatal care with a complaint of urinary frequency and dysuria. She is afebrile and does not have costovertebral angle (CVA) tenderness. You would like to perform a urine dipstick to check for a possible urinary tract infection (UTI), but the clinic does not have the supplies. The manager informs you that they do have an old microscope that a previous volunteer physician had donated in case you would like to use it. A clean-catch urine sample is obtained and examined under the microscope. A single drop of her uncentrifuged urine reveals 2 WBC per high power field. What is the likelihood that this patient has cystitis?

(A) 15%
(B) 30%
(C) 50%
(D) 70%
(E) 90%

The answer is E: 90%. Checking a single drop of uncentrifuged urine under the microscope is a very effective way to diagnose a UTI—even if you are not in a Third World country.

---

67 You are called to the emergency room (ER) to evaluate a 25-year-old patient G1P0 with moderate left lower quadrant (LLQ) pain. The pain woke her from sleep and is described as throbbing but constant 4/10. Her last menstrual period (LMP) was 6 weeks ago. She has regular monthly periods and uses condoms inconsistently. She became sexually active at age 16 and has had five lifetime male partners, the present one for almost a year. She has a history of chlamydia treated at age 18. She has not had any regular gynecologic care since then. She appears to be in no distress and her vital signs are as follows: BP 120/72 mmHg, P 88 beats/min, R 18 breaths/min, and BMI 27. Her abdomen is nontender, but her pelvic examination reveals mild tenderness in the left adnexal area. What is your next step?

(A) Qualitative hCG
(B) Quantitative hCG
(C) Vaginal ultrasound
(D) Abdominal ultrasound
(E) Laparoscopy

The answer is B: **Quantitative hCG.** A quantitative hCG above the discriminatory zone (1,500 to 2,000) would be invaluable in the care for this patient. The discriminatory zone is the lowest level of hCG at which an intrauterine pregnancy can be detected.

---

68 Refer to the patient in Question 67. The quantitative hCG is 900 mIU/mL. The patient is stable with an hemoglobin/hematocrit of 12/35. What is your next step?

(A) Admit the patient and repeat quantitative hCG in 48 hours
(B) Admit the patient and schedule laparoscopy
(C) Admit the patient and get a serum progesterone level
(D) Admit the patient and administer methotrexate

The answer is A: **Admit the patient and repeat quantitative hCG in 48 hours.** Traditionally, rise of 53% in quantitative hCG in 48 hours is indicative of an intrauterine pregnancy. However, approximately 15% of normal intrauterine pregnancies are associated with less than a 53% increase in hCG, and 17% of ectopic pregnancies have normal hCG doubling times. There is no indication for surgery or medical management with methotrexate as an ectopic is not yet diagnosed. Serum progesterone level is rarely helpful. Most ectopic pregnancies are associated with a serum progesterone level between 10 and 20 ng/mL. A serum progesterone level less than 5 ng/mL has a specificity of 100% in confirming an abnormal pregnancy. Serum progesterone levels higher than 20 ng/mL usually are associated with normal intrauterine pregnancies. Levels between 5 and 20 ng/mL are considered equivocal.

---

69 Refer to Questions 67 and 68 to answer the question. About 36 hours after admission for observation, the patient complains of worsening left lower quadrant (LLQ) pain that is now 8/10. Her BP is now 100/60 mmHg and pulse is 120 beats/min. Her abdomen is tense and she now has marked LLQ tenderness and rebound. A quick bedside vaginal ultrasound reveals fluid in the cul-de-sac. What is the next step?

(A) Repeat quantitative hCG STAT
(B) Watch patient until 48-hour quantitative hCG can be performed
(C) Call the operating room (OR) to add patient to the OR schedule tomorrow
(D) Take patient to the OR for emergency diagnostic scope
(E) Perform bedside culdocentesis

The answer is D: **Take patient to the OR for emergency diagnostic scope.** The change in pain and physical examination are all indicative of a ruptured ectopic pregnancy, a medical emergency that should be addressed immediately as it still represents 6% of all pregnancy-related deaths.

70 Refer to Questions 67 to 69 to answer the question. During the course of the laparoscopy, you find dense adhesion in the pelvis as well as between the liver and the right diaphragm. A ruptured ectopic is noted in the left distal tube, and a salpingectomy is performed after lysis of adhesions. What do these laparoscopic findings describe?

(A) Normal findings with ectopic
(B) Fitz-Hugh-Curtis syndrome
(C) Asherman syndrome
(D) Kallmann syndrome
(E) Meigs syndrome

The answer is B: Fitz-Hugh and Curtis syndrome. Fitz-Hugh and Curtis syndrome is a complication of pelvic inflammatory disease (PID) with the classic finding of "violin string" adhesion between the liver and the diaphragm. Asherman syndrome is the formation of scarring and dense adhesions within the uterine cavity, especially after pregnancy-related curettage. Kallmann syndrome is a genetic condition resulting in incomplete puberty characterized by hypogonadism. It is associated with anosmia. Meigs syndrome is the triad of ascites, pleural effusion, and benign ovarian tumor.

71 A 17-year-old G0 presents to your office for follow-up 2 weeks after an appendectomy. She was told that in addition to appendicitis the CT scan revealed a left-sided ovarian cyst measuring 4 cm. The radiology report describes a unilocular, homogenous simple cyst with no septations. The operative report does not describe any pelvic findings. She reports menarche at age 13 and has regular periods every 28 to 35 days with mild menstrual cramps. Her last period was 1 week ago. What is the most appropriate next step in managing this patient's ovarian cyst?

(A) Repeat CT scan
(B) Follow-up visit in clinic in 4 to 6 weeks
(C) Abdominal ultrasound
(D) Transvaginal ultrasound
(E) Laparoscopic cystectomy

The answer is B: Follow-up visit in clinic in 4 to 6 weeks. This patient presents to your clinic after an incidental CT finding of what is most likely a functional ovarian cyst. Functional ovarian cysts are a result of normal ovarian function in pubertal women. Usually these are asymptomatic adnexal masses, but they can be symptomatic and require further evaluation and treatment. Since this patient is asymptomatic, the most appropriate next step is to reassure the patient and have her follow-up in clinic in 6 weeks. Abdominal or transvaginal ultrasound is not necessary for the evaluation of an asymptomatic functional ovarian cyst. Repeat CT scan is not necessary at this time, and laparoscopic cystectomy is not indicated as this cyst will likely resolve.

---

72 A 49-year-old woman comes into your office due to concerns of changes in her menses for the past year and a half. Although unpredictable, her cycles have been farther apart and lighter. She had no period the last 7 months but bled for 3 days last month. Her last Pap smear was 9 months ago and was normal. She has no history of abnormal Pap smears or sexually transmitted infection (STI). Her mother had breast cancer at the age of 65. The patient reports taking levothyroxine and hydrochlorothiazide. When should the patient receive an endometrial biopsy?

(A) In the office today, her absence of menses greater than 6 months classifies her bleeding as postmenopausal
(B) In the office today, irregular bleeding at her age indicates the need for endometrial biopsy
(C) If she continues to have irregular bleeding for greater than 5 months, once she passes 12 months of irregular bleeding a biopsy is indicated
(D) She should never have an endometrial biopsy if there is no family history of endometrial cancer
(E) She should not have an endometrial biopsy unless she is amenorrheic for 12 months, and then begins to have irregular bleeding

The answer is E: **She should not have an endometrial biopsy unless she is amenorrheic for 12 months, and then begins to have irregular bleeding.** Postmenopausal bleeding is defined by amenorrhea for a 12-month period followed by vaginal bleeding. If a woman has periods of amenorrhea or irregular bleeding in her late 40s or early 50s, she can be considered perimenopausal.

73 A 55-year-old G3P3 presents to your office for irregular bleeding. She has not had a period in over 3 years and is concerned that she is beginning to have menses again. The patient reports two episodes of vaginal bleeding over the past 2 months, both times with inconsistent flow and length. She has had regular Paps, her last one being 2 years ago. She uses vaginal estrogen cream three times a week for vaginal atrophy and is well controlled on Risperidone for schizoaffective disorder. Which of the following examinations would rule out the most concerning diagnosis of her bleeding?

(A) Pap with HPV cotesting
(B) Endometrial biopsy
(C) CA-125 serum levels
(D) Speculum examination and bimanual examination

The answer is B: Endometrial biopsy. In a woman with postmenopausal bleeding, defined as bleeding after the absence of menses for 12 months or greater, standard of care is to perform an endometrial biopsy to rule out endometrial hyperplasia or malignancy. A pelvic ultrasound can measure the thickness of the endometrium. A smooth endometrial stripe <4 mm is considered benign. A Pap with or without cotesting is not indicated in this woman who had normal cytology in the recent past. CA-125 may be used in the evaluation of adnexal masses in postmenopausal patients. CA-125 can also be used to monitor recurrence of certain cancers. While the components of the physical examination are important for other signs/symptoms associated with her irregular bleeding, they will not definitely rule out endometrial cancer.

---

74 A 28-year-old G0 presents to your office for an infertility workup. She and her partner have been having regular unprotected intercourse for 14 months with no resultant pregnancies. She achieved menarche at the age of 15, with her menses occurring every 2 to 3 months for irregular durations of time. She admits to excessive hair on her face, chest, and lower abdomen. She has no health conditions other than obesity and has never had surgery. Her mother had uterine cancer at the age of 41, and her grandmother had breast cancer at 55 years old. You suspect polycystic ovarian syndrome (PCOS). Which of the following is indicated in her workup for PCOS?

(A) Endometrial biopsy
(B) LH:FSH ratio levels >1
(C) Testosterone levels
(D) Pelvic ultrasound
(E) No further workup is needed

The answer is E: No further workup is needed. The Rotterdam criteria for PCOS require two of the three items below:

1. Irregular menses consistent with anovulation
2. Clinical or laboratory evidence of excess androgen activity
3. Polycystic ovaries by ultrasound

This patient meets criteria 1 and 2.

---

75 A 42-year-old woman G3P3 status posttubal presents to your clinic with a recurrent complaint of intermenstrual bleeding (IMB). She has been having irregular, heavy periods for the past 2 years and has been tried on multiple medical treatments. Her hemoglobin is 8.9 g/dL from labs performed on day 6 of her cycle. Pelvic examination reveals a smooth, mobile 8-week-sized uterus. She wants to pursue a hysterectomy. Which of the following must be performed before she is an eligible candidate for hysterectomy?

(A) Repeat hemoglobin before menses occurs
(B) Endometrial biopsy
(C) Pelvic ultrasound
(D) Follicle-stimulating hormone (FSH) levels

The answer is B: **Endometrial biopsy.** Before a hysterectomy can be performed, there must be an endometrial biopsy done showing no signs of malignancy. Even without a history of irregular menses, an endometrial biopsy with malignant tissue would change the course of treatment for this patient.

---

76 A 48-year-old G2P2 presents to your clinic for irregular bleeding. She states she reached menarche at 13 and has regular monthly menses lasting 6 days each month until 18 months ago when she began having irregular periods that are heavier than usual. The patient also reports a large amount of yellow, foul-smelling discharge for the past 2 weeks. She is sexually active and has had three partners in the last 6 months with whom she usually uses condoms. You perform a pelvic examination and a gonorrhea and chlamydia culture. The results of the culture show that the patient is positive for gonorrhea and negative for chlamydia. What is your next step?

(A) Pelvic ultrasound to evaluate the thickness of her endometrium
(B) Treat her with ceftriaxone and azithromycin, then perform endometrial biopsy
(C) Treat her with ceftriaxone, then perform pelvic ultrasound
(D) Perform endometrial biopsy, then treat with ceftriaxone and azithromycin
(E) Pelvic ultrasound followed by endometrial biopsy

The answer is B: **Treat her with ceftriaxone and azithromycin, then perform endometrial biopsy.** Although this woman has perimenopausal bleeding and should have an endometrial biopsy, sexually transmitted infections (STIs) are a contraindication to the procedure. Any patient with gonorrhea should also be treated for chlamydia due to the high incidence of concurrent infection. Once her infection has been treated, you may proceed with endometrial biopsy. There are no ultrasound criteria to rule out endometrial cancer or hyperplasia in a premenopausal woman.

---

77 While following up on lab reports you had ordered earlier in the week, you come across a report on a new obstetric patient that found an *Escherichia coli* count of 100,000+ colonies on urine culture. You review her chart and no mention is made of her having dysuria. The nurse calls her to find out whether she is having any complaints and reports to you that she is not. Which of the following is the most appropriate next plan of action?

(A) Call in the appropriate antibiotic for her bacteriuria
(B) Reassure the patient that her test was not abnormal since she is asymptomatic
(C) Tell the patient to present for a renal ultrasound
(D) Admit the patient for possible asymptomatic pyelonephritis
(E) Repeat the urine culture

The answer is A: Call in the appropriate antibiotic for her bacteriuria. Asymptomatic bacteriuria is common in pregnancy and can advance to urinary tract infection (UTI) and/or pyelonephritis in 25% to 40% of patients. All patients should have a urine culture performed during pregnancy and treatment of asymptomatic bacteriuria is found.

progesterone withdrawal bleeding
→ anovulatory bleeding
estrogen stimulation responded
to progesterone withdrawal

estrogen withdrawal bleeding
→ sudden ↓ in estrogen
(bilateral oophorectomy,
cessation of exogenous estrogen,
just before ovulation)

progesterone breakthrough bleeding
→ progesterone: estrogen ratio is
high (progesterone only
contraceptive methods)
endometrium becomes
atrophic, ulcerated

CHAPTER

10

Contraception

1 A 25-year-old G0 presents to discuss birth control options. She denies any past medical history and does not smoke tobacco. She is interested in taking a daily birth control pill. You review the risks and benefits with her. You report one of the noncontraceptive benefits to combined oral contraceptive pills (OCPs) is:

(A) Decreased risk of deep vein thrombosis
(B) Decreased risk of ovarian cancer
(C) Decreased incidence of migraine headaches
(D) Decreased risk of high blood pressure
(E) Decreased risk of breast cancer

The answer is B: **Decreased risk of ovarian cancer.** Combined OCPs have many non-contraceptive benefits, including a decreased risk of ovarian cancer, endometrial cancer, ectopic pregnancy, and pelvic inflammatory disease (PID). OCPs increase the risk of deep vein thrombosis, and patients should be screened for a history of migraines with aura and hypertension before starting OCPs.

2 A 21-year-old G0P0 patient calls your office requesting information on emergency contraception. She had unprotected intercourse the previous night and wants to know if Plan B (progesterone only) would still be an efficacious option, as well as any other risks or benefits she should know about before taking the medication. Which of the following statements should be included in her counseling?

(A) Plan B is most effective if taken within 72 hours of unprotected intercourse
(B) Plan B would disrupt a current pregnancy
(C) She can only take it if she is in the last 2 weeks of her cycle
(D) She must take two doses for it to be effective

The answer is A: **Plan B is most effective if taken within 72 hours of unprotected intercourse.** Plan B is a progesterone-only form of emergency contraception. There is an option for a single dose or split dose 12 hours apart. Emergency contraception does not disrupt a current pregnancy and should not be taken if a patient thinks she is already pregnant (although there is no evidence of harm to a patient, the pregnancy, or fetus if taken during pregnancy). Although emergency contraception is available over the counter, details of its availability have been subject to much recent debate.

---

3 A patient who is postpartum day number 1 would like permanent sterilization for birth control.

What can you tell her is one of the benefits of postpartum tubal ligation?

(A) Laparoscopic technology makes the procedure minimally invasive
(B) Greater breastfeeding success
(C) Patients do not need anesthesia
(D) Patients can have the procedure in the first 24 hours postpartum

The answer is D: **Patients can have the procedure in the first 24 hours postpartum.** Postpartum bilateral tubal ligations (BTLs) are typically performed in the first 24 hours after delivery, but can be performed anytime if the patient is in the hospital. There is no link to breastfeeding success. The procedure is performed under general or regional anesthesia with an infraumbilical incision. Direct visualization of the tubes is possible because of the size of the uterus postpartum; therefore, laparoscopy is not used for this procedure. Postpartum BTL has an equal or higher rate of failure when compared with interval procedures.

---

4 A 34-year-old G3P3 patient presents to your clinic for birth control counseling. She has no significant past medical history and has used natural family planning in the past for contraception. She is interested in using the copper intrauterine device (IUD) for birth control since she does not desire children for several years, but is unsure if she would like more children in the future. Due to religious concerns she asks you how the IUD works. Which of the following statements is correct regarding the method in which the copper IUD prevents pregnancy?

(A) By preventing ovulation
(B) By not allowing implantation of a fertilized egg
(C) Blocking the egg from entering the tubes
(D) Causing an inflammatory response that is spermicidal

The answer is D: **Causing an inflammatory response that is spermicidal.** The copper IUD causes a sterile intrauterine inflammatory response that engulfs, immobilizes, and destroys sperm that enter the intrauterine cavity. The decapacitation of the sperm prevents fertilization of an egg. Copper IUDs do not affect ovulation, nor do they act as abortifacients.

---

5 A 34-year-old G0 presents desiring birth control. She states she cannot remember to take a pill every day because she works and travels in different time zones. She has no past medical history but reports smoking 10 cigarettes a day. Her friend has the implantable rod in her arm and she asks you if this could be a possible option for her. After agreeing that this could be a viable option, which disadvantages to this method should she be counseled on?

(A) It only lasts for 3 months
(B) Bleeding patterns may be irregular
(C) It would be unsafe for her to use due to her tobacco use
(D) It is not as effective as other reversible methods

The answer is B: **Bleeding patterns may be irregular.** The implantable rod is a progesterone-only form of birth control, making it safe to use in patients who smoke (although smoking is not an issue for a 26-year-old). It is highly effective (0.4% failure rate) and lasts for 3 years. The main disadvantage is irregular bleeding patterns that may occur in some women throughout its entire use.

---

6 A 17-year-old G1P1 is postpartum and desires contraception. She had failure of birth control pills resulting in her previous pregnancy and does not desire pregnancy for several years. She is breastfeeding and has no other comorbidities. After counseling her on all of the methods of birth control, you encourage her to proceed with the most reliable birth control option for someone with her obstetrical history and future pregnancy plans. Which of the following methods are you most likely to recommend?

(A) Barrier method
(B) Bilateral tubal ligations (BTL)
(C) Intrauterine device (IUD)
(D) Natural family planning
(E) Oral contraceptive

The answer is C: **Intrauterine device (IUD).** Long-acting reversible contraception is the best method for patients who are not planning pregnancy in the near future, but are not of satisfied parity. This patient would be a good candidate for a very effective, reliable, and long-term form of reversible birth control such as an IUD.

7 A 39-year-old G1P1 would like to discuss birth control at her postpartum visit. She is breastfeeding exclusively and plans to attempt pregnancy again in the next year due to her age and desire for at least one more child. She asks about lactational amenorrhea as a form of birth control. Which of the following statements while counseling her on the benefits and risks of this method you should include?

(A) She may ovulate before she has her first period
(B) She may have increased risk of postpartum depression
(C) This method should only be used for the first 12 months postpartum
(D) She should discontinue her prenatal vitamins

The answer is A: She may ovulate before she has her first period. Lactational amenorrhea can be used as a form of birth control for no longer than 6 months postpartum for women who are exclusively breastfeeding. Women may ovulate before their first menses postpartum, so predicting the return of ovulation occurs after the first ovulation has transpired. The failure rate for this method of birth control is 15% to 55%. Prenatal vitamins should be continued given this high failure rate.

8 A 24-year-old G1P1 is being discharged from the hospital after an uncomplicated vaginal delivery. She is breastfeeding and has no comorbidities. She would like a progesterone-only birth control pill for contraception. Upon hospital discharge, which of the following statements should be included in your counseling?

(A) Do not start taking the pill until 3 months postpartum
(B) Use condoms during the first 6 weeks of taking the pill until hormone levels reach full efficacy
(C) Take the pill at the same time every day
(D) Be aware that the pill can decrease the milk supply she produces

The answer is C: Take the pill at the same time every day. The progesterone-only birth control pill will not affect milk supply, can be started within the first 2 weeks postpartum, and does not require backup for more than 2 weeks (depending on when the pill is started). It is very important to be sure to take the pill at the same time each day (within 1 to 2 hours) to ensure that the progesterone levels do not drop enough to allow for ovulation.

9 A 26-year-old G1P1 presents to your office for birth control counseling. She has a friend who uses the hormone-releasing vaginal ring and would like to try this method. After reviewing the risks and benefits with her, she asks you to review the use of the ring with her to ensure she will be using it correctly. Which of the following is most correct regarding the proper usage of the vaginal ring contraceptive?

(A) It should be replaced every week
(B) It should be removed after 3 weeks and replaced 1 week later
(C) It is not safe to use condoms while the ring is in place
(D) She will need to be refitted for the ring annually

The answer is B: **It should be removed after 3 weeks and replaced 1 week later.** The vaginal ring is a highly effective form of birth control that stays in the vagina for 3 weeks and then can be removed for a hormone-free week and menses. The ring should stay in place during intercourse; condoms and spermicide are both permissible with the ring in place. The ring does not need to be fitted as a diaphragm does; the size is the same for all women.

---

10 A 36-year-old G3P3 patient presents for discussion of contraception. She smokes tobacco and has chronic hypertension. She is considering another pregnancy in the next year. You review with her all of the progesterone-only options due to her smoking. She states that she is interested in the depo-provera shot. What are you concerned about for this patient?

(A) An increase in irregular bleeding
(B) Return of regular ovulation after use of depo-provera can be 6 to 18 months
(C) An increased risk of endometrial cancer
(D) A high rate of failure with the depo-provera shot

The answer is B: **Return of regular ovulation after use of depo-provera can be 6 to 18 months.** The depo-provera shot is highly effective and does not increase the risk of thromboembolic events. However, after use of depo-provera there can be a significant delay in the return of ovulation (independent of the number of injections), so this patient who may desire pregnancy in the near future should not start depo-provera.

---

11 A healthy 16-year-old girl presents to the emergency room for the third time this year due to painful ovarian cysts. Examination is significant for a 5-cm mass in the right adnexa. Ultrasonography confirms the presence of a simple ovarian cyst. Which of the following is the most appropriate treatment to prevent further ovarian cyst formation in the future?

(A) Progestin-only oral contraceptives
(B) Continuous low-dose oral estrogen
(C) Combination oral contraceptives
(D) Levonorgestrel intrauterine system (IUS)

The answer is C: **Combination oral contraceptives.** Combination oral contraceptives have many health benefits beyond birth control. The progestin component of combined contraceptives suppresses the secretion of luteinizing hormone, inhibiting ovulation. This prevents ovarian cyst formation and decreases a woman's risk of ovarian cancer. Progestin-only contraceptives ("mini-pills") prevent pregnancy by making the cervical mucus thick and relatively impermeable. Ovulation continues normally in approximately 40% of patients using progestin-only oral formulations. Similarly, continuous low-dose estrogen and the levonorgestrel IUS will not inhibit ovulation and prevent ovarian cyst formation.

---

12 A 33-year-old African-American woman presents to the office requesting the transdermal contraceptive patch for contraception. She has a history of sickle-cell disease, classic migraines, gestational hypertension with her last delivery, and antiphospholipid antibody syndrome with a deep vein thrombosis 3 years ago. On examination, you diagnose a large fibroid uterus. Which of the patient's conditions is an absolute contraindication to the transdermal contraceptive patch?

(A) Sickle-cell disease
(B) Classic migraines
(C) History of gestational hypertension
(D) History of thromboembolic disease
(E) Uterine leiomyoma

The answer is D: **History of thromboembolic disease.** Before considering combined hormonal contraceptives for a patient, careful evaluation is required. Contraceptives containing estrogen are not contraindicated in patients with uterine leiomyomas or sickle-cell disease. Low-dose formulations are not associated with growth of leiomyomas. Reduced menstrual bleeding is often a benefit for both patients with fibroids and sickle cell. A history of gestational hypertension and classic migraines are not absolute contraindications to the use of estrogen-containing medications. A history of a deep vein thrombosis with a known thrombophilia is an absolute contraindication to the use of estrogen-containing contraceptives.

---

13 A 34-year-old, G0, has recently become sexually active with a new partner. She often experiences mittelschmerz (midcycle ovulatory pain) and hopes to find a method of birth control that will decrease this occurrence. Which of the following contraceptive methods would be inappropriate to offer the patient?

(A) Contraceptive vaginal ring
(B) Subdermal contraceptive implant
(C) Depot medroxyprogesterone acetate (DMPA)
(D) Progestin-only oral contraception

The answer is D: Progestin-only oral contraception. Mittelschmerz refers to midcycle ovulatory pain. Birth control methods that inhibit ovulation should decrease the occurrence of mittelschmerz. The contraceptive vaginal ring, subdermal contraceptive implant, and DMPA all inhibit ovulation. Progestin-only oral contraception (the "mini-pill") does not reliably inhibit ovulation, but works primarily by thickening cervical mucus and acting as a barrier, preventing sperm penetration.

---

14 A 19-year-old G0 woman with endometriosis has been on depot medroxyprogesterone acetate (DMPA) for 4 years. She is very satisfied with this method of contraception, her resulting amenorrhea, and with the decrease in her endometriosis associated pain. She wishes to continue using DMPA; however, she is concerned about the U.S. Food and Drug Administration warning that use beyond 2 years should be carefully considered due to the adverse effects on bone mineral density. Which of the following is the most appropriate next step in management?

(A) Advise her that she should immediately change contraceptive methods since she has been on DMPA for over 2 years

(B) Refer her for bone densitometry and recommend that she continue to use DMPA if her results are normal

(C) Place an etonogestrel contraceptive implant because this will have the same side effect profile as DMPA without affecting bone mineral density

(D) Explain that decreases in bone mineral density appear to be substantially reversible after discontinuation of DMPA and weigh her individual risks and benefits

The answer is D: Explain that decreases in bone mineral density appear to be substantially reversible after discontinuation of DMPA and weigh her individual risks and benefits. Special concern has been raised about the adverse effects of DMPA on bone mineral density, resulting from alterations in bone metabolism associated with reduced estrogen levels. Adolescence is a crucial period of bone accretion. However, loss of bone mineral density appears to be substantially reversible after discontinuation of DMPA. Concern about the use of DMPA in adolescents should be weighed against the advantages of compliance, effective contraception, and non-contraceptive benefits. As with all contraceptive options, the balance of overall risk to benefit should be weighted on an individual basis.

---

15 A 25-year-old, G2P2, presents for her routine annual gynecologic examination. She had an Intrauterine device (IUD) placed for contraception 2 years ago and is very satisfied with this method. The patient has no complaints and her physical examination is within normal limits. Routine sexually transmitted infection screening was performed and she was found to be positive for chlamydia. You inform the patient she will be treated with antibiotics. What is the most appropriate next step in management?

(A) Immediately remove the IUD and inform her that she should no longer use IUDs for contraception.
(B) Leave the IUD in place unless treatment fails and infection spreads.
(C) Leave the IUD in place unless she remains with her current sexual partner.
(D) Immediately remove the IUD and consider reinsertion 3 months after successful treatment.

The answer is B: **Leave the IUD in place unless treatment fails and infection spreads.** Asymptomatic IUD users with positive cervical cultures for gonorrhea or chlamydia should be treated promptly. The patient should be counseled to speak to her sexual partner(s) and not to resume intercourse until he has also been successfully treated. The IUD may remain in place unless there is evidence of spread and/or failure of treatment with appropriate antibiotics. Insertion of IUDs with pelvic inflammatory disease (PID) currently or within the past 3 months is contraindicated. However, IUDs should not be withheld due to a remote history of PID.

16 A 30-year-old woman is on medications for seizure disorder, depression, and adult acne. She is taking combined oral contraceptive (COC) for birth control. Which of the following medications will decrease the effectiveness of her COCs?

(A) Carbamazepine
(B) Fluoxetine
(C) Amitriptyline
(D) Tetracycline

The answer is A: **Carbamazepine.** Stimulation of the cytochrome P-450 system will decrease the effectiveness of COCs. Examples of medications that decrease the efficacy of COCs include benzodiazepines, phenytoin, carbamazepine, rifampin, barbiturates, and sulfonamides. Drugs that may have altered biotransformation when contraceptives are used included tricyclic antidepressants, anticoagulants, methyldopa, and phenothiazines. Antibiotics may alter the intestinal flora and interfere with hormone absorption, but this effect is typically not significant enough to decrease the efficacy of COCs. An exception to this is rifampin. This antibiotic has been shown to decrease the efficacy of COCs.

17 A 20-year-old, G1P1, presents to the clinic for contraceptive counseling. She experienced an unintended pregnancy last year and recently delivered. Efficacy is the most important factor to her when choosing a method of contraception. Which method of contraception is this patient most likely to choose?

(A) Subdermal contraceptive implant
(B) Oral contraceptive pills (OCPs)
(C) Condoms
(D) Natural family planning

The answer is A: Subdermal contraceptive implant. Long-acting reversible contraception (including the contraceptive implant and Intrauterine devices [IUDs]) has the highest efficacy. The subdermal contraceptive implant is the most effective method, with 0.05% of women experiencing an unintended pregnancy within the first year of use. IUDs are also highly effective, with a less than a 1% failure rate. OCPs, condoms, and natural family planning methods are less effective and require substantial patient effort.

---

18 A 40-year-old, G4P4, is considering options for contraception. She inquires about the mechanism of action of the levonorgestrel intrauterine system (IUS). Which is the most accurate answer to her question?

(A) It acts primarily as a spermicide
(B) It is an abortifacient
(C) It acts primarily by inhibiting ovulation
(D) It acts by preventing sperm from fertilizing ova

The answer is D: It acts by preventing sperm from fertilizing ova. Intrauterine devices (IUDs) prevent fertilization and thus are true contraceptives; they are not abortifacients. The copper IUD causes an increase in uterine and tubal fluids containing copper ions, enzymes, prostaglandins, and macrophages. This impairs sperm function and prevents fertilization. The levonorgestrel IUS has an array of contraceptive actions: thickened cervical mucus, inhibiting sperm penetration and suppressing the endometrium. Some women do not ovulate as a result of levonorgestrel absorption, but this is not the primary mechanism of action.

---

19 A 40-year-old, G3P3, presents to clinic with a long-standing history of dysmenorrhea and menorrhagia. After pelvic ultrasound, endometrial biopsy, and laboratory evaluation, she has been diagnosed probable adenomyosis. She does not desire pregnancy at this time and states that she is "100% certain that she is finished having children." Which of the following methods of birth control is the most appropriate treatment for her dysmenorrhea and menorrhagia, while having similar efficacy to sterilization?

(A) Etonogestrel contraceptive implant
(B) Copper Intrauterine device (IUD)
(C) Combined oral contraceptives (COCs)
(D) Levonorgestrel-containing intrauterine system (IUS)

The answer is D: Levonorgestrel-containing intrauterine system (IUS). Failure rates of tubal sterilization are comparable to those of intrauterine contraceptives. A clinically significant side effect of the levonorgestrel-containing IUS is a decrease in menstrual blood loss (up to 50%). This IUS is also used to relieve pain related to adenomyosis and endometriosis. Copper IUDs can increase menstrual bleeding and cramping. COCs may successfully treat symptoms of adenomyosis, but are not as effective as sterilization. The contraceptive implant may surpass the efficacy of sterilization; however, the most common side effect is irregular, unpredictable vaginal bleeding that may persist even after several months of use.

---

20 An 18-year-old, G1P1, presents to the emergency room due to a positive pregnancy test with a copper Intrauterine device (IUD) in place. She does not have any pain or bleeding. A pelvic ultrasound shows an intrauterine pregnancy consistent with 6 week's gestation. On examination, the IUD strings are visualized protruding approximately 2 cm from the cervical os. Although unplanned, the patient would like to continue the pregnancy. Which of the following is the most appropriate course of action?

(A) Perform diagnostic laparoscopy to rule out heterotopic pregnancy
(B) Offer termination of pregnancy due to the risk of congenital anomalies
(C) No intervention at this time
(D) Remove the IUD in the emergency room

The answer is D: Remove the IUD in the emergency room. IUDs do not increase the overall risk of ectopic pregnancy. The relative risk of ectopic is greater in women with an IUD than those not using contraception because the IUD offers greater protection against intrauterine pregnancies than extrauterine pregnancies. There is no evidence of increased risk of congenital anomalies with IUDs. Approximately 40% to 50% of women who become pregnant with an IUD in place will experience a spontaneous abortion. Due to this risk, the IUD should be removed if the string is visible. The risk of abortion after removal is 30%. If the IUD is left in place, there is also an approximately two- to fourfold increase in the incidence of preterm labor and delivery.

---

21 A 25-year-old, G2P2, is 4 weeks status post levonorgestrel intrauterine system (IUS) insertion. She returns for routine follow-up. The insertion was uncomplicated, placed during her 6-week postpartum visit. On physical examination, the IUS strings are not visualized. What is the most appropriate next step in localizing the IUS?

(A) Computed tomography (CT) scan
(B) Pelvic ultrasound
(C) X-ray of the abdomen/pelvis
(D) No imaging study needed

The answer is B: Pelvic ultrasound. To determine whether the IUS is in the uterus, a pelvic ultrasound should be performed. If the IUS is correctly placed, but the strings are not visualized, the patient may continue to use the IUS for birth control. When she is ready for IUS removal, this can be accomplished in the office with specific Intrauterine device (IUD) removal devices or in the operating room with hysteroscopy (see *Figure 10-1*).

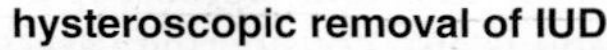
hysteroscopic removal of IUD

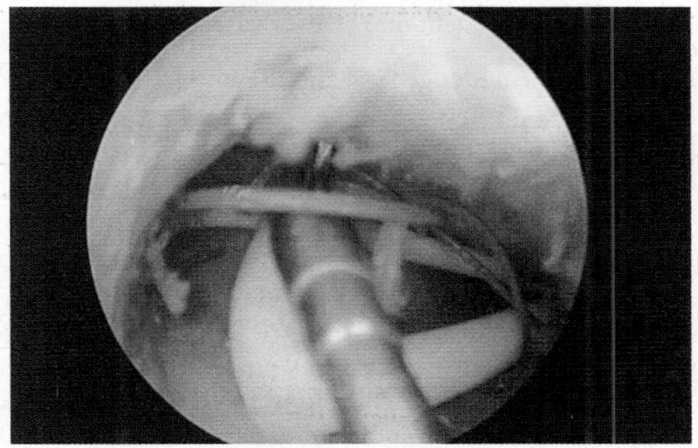

Figure 10-1

If the IUS is not in the uterus, an X-ray of the abdomen/pelvis should be obtained to evaluate for an extrauterine IUS (this would have been a complication of uterine perforation at insertion). *Figure 10-2* shows X-ray presenting IUD (in this case Lippes loop—no longer in use) in right upper quadrant of abdomen.

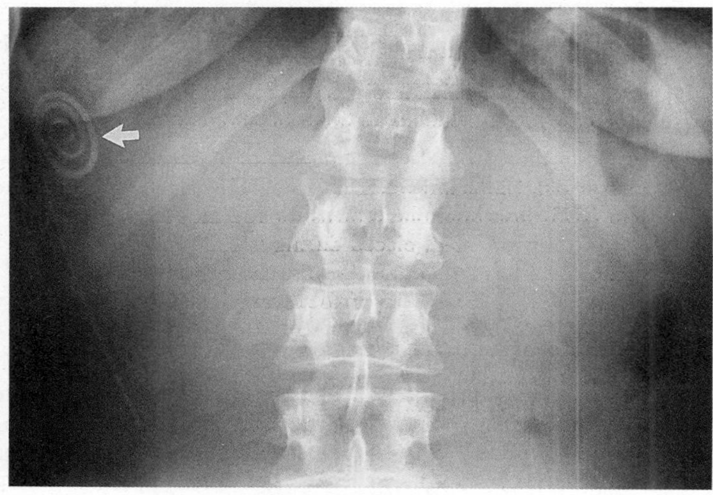

Figure 10-2

A CT scan will also provide this information but at a much higher cost. It is not appropriate to avoid further workup and assume that the IUS was expulsed.

22 A 32-year-old, G3P3, desires a laparoscopic bilateral tubal ligations (BTL). Her husband is also considering vasectomy. Which of the following is the main benefit of BTL over vasectomy?

(A) Usually done under general anesthesia
(B) More easily reversed
(C) Fewer surgical complications
(D) Immediately effective
(E) Less expensive

The answer is D: Immediately effective. The main benefit of BTL over vasectomy is immediate sterility. Couples need to use another method of contraception until male sterility is confirmed by semen analysis (50% achieve azoospermia at 8 weeks, 100% at 10 weeks postprocedure). Risks of laparoscopic BTL include anesthetic complications, infection, bleeding, and injury to surrounding structures. The overall fatality rate is 1 to 4 per 100, 000; this is lower than the fatality rate for childbearing in the United States (approximately 10 per 100,000 births). Minor complications occur in 5% to 10% of vasectomies and include bleeding, hematomas, acute and chronic pain, and local skin infections. Vasectomy is also more easily reversed than most female sterilization; however, patients should consider any sterilization procedure permanent. The cost of laparoscopic BTL in the operating room far exceeds the cost of an outpatient vasectomy.

---

23 A 36-year-old, G4P4, presents to clinic with undesired fertility. She is confident in her desire for permanent sterility. Her deliveries have all been by Cesarean section and her last pregnancy was complicated by gestational diabetes and severe preeclampsia. Her medical history is also significant for obesity and a history of pulmonary embolism during her second pregnancy. Which of the following approaches to sterilization is the most appropriate for this patient?

(A) Minilaparotomy
(B) Hysteroscopy
(C) Laparoscopy
(D) Transvaginal incision

The answer is B: Hysteroscopy. Although minilaparotomy is the most common surgical approach for tubal ligation throughout the world, in the United States it is typically reserved for postpartum tubal ligation. Laparoscopic tubal ligation is immediately effective; however, the patient undergoes general anesthesia and assumes the risk of abdominal surgery. In this patient with obesity and multiple prior surgeries, an approach that avoids abdominal incisions would be optimal. The transvaginal approach offers a convenient port of entry into the peritoneal cavity, but is contraindicated if suspicion of major pelvic adhesions exists. The hysteroscopic approach allows access to the fallopian tubes through the cervix and avoids surgical incisions and general anesthesia.

---

24 A 33-year-old, G4P2022, presents for levonorgestrel intrauterine system (IUS) placement. She is not currently menstruating and strongly desires insertion today. What is the most appropriate course of action?

(A) Schedule the patient for insertion with her next menstrual period
(B) Explain that insertion at a time other than during menstrual bleeding will be more challenging and proceed only if she wishes
(C) Insert the device after obtaining reasonable assurance that she is not pregnant
(D) Refer her to another clinic that may insert the device at a time other than with menstruation

The answer is C: Insert the device after obtaining reasonable assurance that she is not pregnant. There is no scientific reason for the common practice of insertion of intrauterine contraception only during menstrual bleeding. Reasonable assurance that she is not pregnant can be obtained with a sensitive pregnancy test. Allowing insertion at any time during the menstrual cycle gives the patient and her provider more flexibility. Insertion should not be more difficult if she is not currently menstruating.

25 A 27-year-old, G0, and her husband desire to use natural family planning for contraception. They decide to use the calendar method. Based on her regular 28-day cycle, which of the following represents her fertile period?

(A) Days 14 through 21
(B) Days 10 through 17
(C) Days 7 through 14
(D) Days 12 through 19

The answer is B: Days 10 through 17. In most women, ovulation usually occurs near the middle of the cycle. The fertile window of the menstrual cycle lasts only for 6 days, the 5 days preceding ovulation and the day of ovulation (this is related to the life span of the gametes). Additional days are added to the fertile period based on the patient's shortest and longest menstrual intervals. This couple should abstain from intercourse during days 10 through 17 of the patient's menstrual cycle.

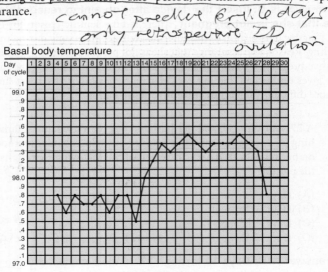

26 A 32-year-old, G1P0, at 39 weeks has decided to use natural family planning following the birth of her first child. After thoroughly researching each method, she has decided to use the basal body temperature method. She takes her basal body temperature method each morning at the same time before getting out of bed. Three days of continuous temperature rises over the baseline indicates which of the following?

(A) The fertile period
(B) Retrospective identification of ovulation
(C) An anovulatory cycle
(D) Absence of cervical mucus

The answer is B: Retrospective identification of ovulation. Couples using the basal body temperature method avoid intercourse until a suitable period after ovulation (see *Figure 10-3*). Three days of continuous temperature rises over baseline indicate that ovulation has occurred and the postovulatory infertile time has begun. This method relies on retrospective identification of ovulation. It is not possible to predict fertile days using basal body temperature. The presence of thin, "stretchy," clear cervical mucus indicates the fertile time. During the postovulatory "safe" period, the mucus is milky or opaque in appearance.

Basal body temperature

Figure 10-3

(Continued)

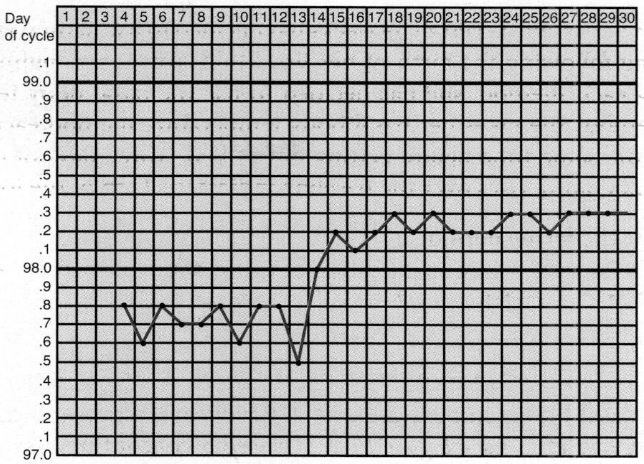
Day
of cycle
1 2 3 4 5 6 7 8 9 10 11 12 13 14 15 16 17 18 19 20 21 22 23 24 25 26 27 28 29 30
.1
99.0
.9
.8
.7
.6
.5
.4
.3
.2
.1
98.0
.9
.8
.7
.6
.5
.4
.3
.2
.1
97.0

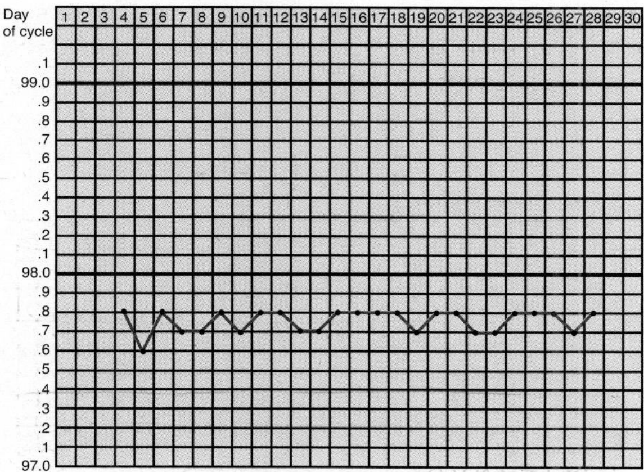
Day
of cycle
1 2 3 4 5 6 7 8 9 10 11 12 13 14 15 16 17 18 19 20 21 22 23 24 25 26 27 28 29 30
.1
99.0
.9
.8
.7
.6
.5
.4
.3
.2
.1
98.0
.9
.8
.7
.6
.5
.4
.3
.2
.1
97.0

Figure 10-3

CHAPTER

11

Family Planning

1 A 22-year-old woman, G2P2, comes to the office 3 days after having unprotected intercourse. She does not desire pregnancy at this time and is requesting the most effective method of emergency contraception.

Which of the following methods of emergency contraception will have the lowest failure rate?

(A) Oral levonorgestrel
(B) Combined oral contraceptive regimens
(C) Oral ulipristal acetate
(D) Insertion of copper intrauterine device (IUD)

The answer is D: Insertion of copper intrauterine device (IUD). The copper IUD has a failure rate of approximately 0.1% if inserted within 5 days of unprotected intercourse. The failure rate for the Yuzpe method (combined oral contraceptive regimens for emergency contraception) is 25% and for Plan B (levonorgestrel) is 11%. An interval greater than 72 hours is associated with an increasing failure rate; however, some evidence of success is seen up to 120 hours after unprotected intercourse. Ulipristal acetate is a selective progesterone receptor modulator and is more effective than the Yuzpe method and Plan B once 72 hours have elapsed.

2 An 18-year-old, G1P0, presents to the office at 6 week's gestation by last menstrual period. Physical examination confirms a 6-week-sized uterus and transvaginal ultrasound reveals an intrauterine pregnancy with a crown–rump length of 6 weeks 2 days. Following counseling, the patient opts to terminate the pregnancy and desires medical abortion.

What laboratory evaluation must be done prior to administering the medications?

(A) Complete blood count
(B) Chlamydia and gonorrhea screening
(C) Beta-human chorionic gonadotropin (β-hCG) level
(D) Rhesus type

The answer is D: Rhesus type. Although the theoretical risk of maternal Rh sensitization during a first-trimester abortion is low, Rh typing and anti-D prophylaxis for Rh-negative patients is recommended. Screening for anemia and sexually transmitted infections (STIs) may be performed, but is not required, prior to medical abortion. With a documented intrauterine pregnancy on ultrasound, β-hCG levels are not clinically useful prior to abortion. These levels may be followed post-procedure to document successful medical abortion; however, typical follow-up after medical abortion consists of a repeat ultrasound to confirm the absence of an intrauterine pregnancy.

---

3 A 25-year-old, G1P0010, presents to the emergency room with 2 days of fever, pelvic pain, and vaginal bleeding. Three days prior to presentation she had an uncomplicated induced abortion at 8-week gestation. She has been taking doxycycline as recommended. Her temperature is 38.2°C (101.2°F), pulse is 96 beats/min, respirations are 16 breaths/min, and blood pressure is 115/75 mmHg. Examination reveals moderate bleeding from an open cervix and a tender, enlarged uterus. On ultrasound, a thickened, heterogeneous endometrial echo is seen, consistent with retained products of conception.

Which of the following is the most appropriate course of action?

(A) Administer antibiotics
(B) Administer an ergot derivative
(C) Administer a prostaglandin analog
(D) Perform a repeat suction curettage
(E) Administer antipyretics

The answer is D: Perform a repeat suction curettage. If the abortion is incomplete, and tissue remains in the uterus, a repeat suction curettage is necessary. All other interventions (administration of antibiotics, ergot derivative, prostaglandin analog, and antipyretics) may be administered concomitantly with suction curettage; however, repeat suction curettage must be performed to clear the uterus of the retained products of conception.

---

4 A 30-year-old, G3P1021, presents to the emergency room 3 days after an induced abortion performed at 9 week's gestation. She has been experiencing severe cramping pain, but minimal vaginal bleeding. She has been taking doxycycline as recommended. In the emergency room she is found to be afebrile, pulse is 80 beats/min, and blood pressure is 120/80 mmHg. On examination, the cervix is closed and the uterus is 12-week size and soft. A collection of blood is seen in the uterus on ultrasound.

Which of the following is the most likely diagnosis?

(A) Normal postabortion findings
(B) Retained products of conception
(C) Septic abortion
(D) Postabortal syndrome

The answer is D: Postabortal syndrome. The enlarged uterus and hematometra on ultrasound are not normal postabortion findings. An infected abortion (complete or incomplete) is a septic abortion. Patients may present with sepsis, shock, hemorrhage, and end-organ failure. Retained products of conception can often be identified on ultrasound, but may be indistinguishable from postabortal syndrome. Postabortal syndrome occurs when the uterus fails to remain contracted after either spontaneous abortions or induced abortions. A collection of blood forms in the uterus (hematometra). Suction curettage is the treatment for both retained products of conception and postabortal syndrome.

5 A 21-year-old, G3P1011, presents with an unintended pregnancy at 6 weeks 5 days. She has a history of one prior delivery by Cesarean section and one ectopic pregnancy successfully treated with methotrexate. Vital signs and a heart, lung, and abdominal examinations are within normal limits. A 7-week-sized retroverted uterus is found on pelvic examination and transvaginal ultrasound reveals an intrauterine pregnancy measuring 6 weeks 6 days by crown–rump length. Following pregnancy options counseling she decides to pursue induced abortion and desires medication abortion if she is eligible.

What procedure is most appropriate for this patient?

(A) Surgical abortion with suction aspiration
(B) Medical abortion with mifepristone alone
(C) Medical abortion with mifepristone and misoprostol
(D) Medical abortion with methotrexate alone
(E) Medical abortion with methotrexate and misoprostol

The answer is C: Medical abortion with mifepristone and misoprostol. At 6 weeks and 5 days, the patient is eligible for a medication abortion. Medication abortion is approved by the Food and Drug Administration for appropriately selected women with pregnancies less than 49 days of gestation. Evidence-based practice supports medical abortion up to 9 week's gestation. History of Cesarean section is not a contraindication to medical abortion and the standard regimen of mifepristone and misoprostol can be used. Mifepristone binds to the progesterone receptor with an affinity greater than progesterone, but does not activate the receptor, therefore, acting as an antiprogestin. This antiprogesterone effect increases the sensitivity of the uterus to exogenous prostaglandin administration. Used alone, mifepristone is not sufficiently effective as an abortifacient. Methotrexate is a dihydrofolate reductase inhibitor that blocks the production of reduced folate needed for DNA synthesis. The use of methotrexate with misoprostol for first-trimester abortion has similar efficacy to the mifepristone/misoprostol regimen; however, approximately 15% to 20% of women using methotrexate regimens may wait up to 4 weeks for complete abortion to occur. Mifepristone and misoprostol regimens are preferable.

---

6 A 22-year-old, G1P0, is transferred to the emergency room after undergoing an induced abortion at 10 weeks by electric vacuum aspiration. She is experiencing brisk, bright red bleeding from the vagina. On arrival, she is afebrile, pulse is 100 beats/min, and blood pressure is 110/65 mmHg. On bimanual examination, the cervix is noted to be 1 cm open and the uterus is small and firm. There is bright red blood on the examining glove. Bedside transabdominal ultrasound is performed and shows an empty uterine cavity, no free pelvic fluid.

What is the most likely etiology of her hemorrhage?

(A) Coagulopathy
(B) Malplacentation
(C) Uterine atony
(D) Uterine perforation
(E) Cervical laceration

The answer is E: Cervical laceration. Hemorrhage is a rare complication of early abortion. It is slightly more common at advanced gestational ages, in multiparous women, and with the use of inhaled anesthetics. Bleeding may be due to cervical injury, incomplete evacuation of the uterus, atony, perforation, placental abnormalities, or coagulopathy. In this case, the most likely cause of brisk, bright red bleeding from the cervix in the presence of good uterine tone and complete uterine evacuation suggests a cervical laceration that occurred with dilation of a nulliparous cervix. This laceration needs to be identified and repaired. Coagulopathy, malplacentation, and uterine perforation are less likely scenarios.

7 A 34-year-old, G3P2, has decided to terminate an unintended pregnancy at 7 weeks. She is contemplating medication abortion and does not have any contraindications to this procedure. During counseling, she is given information on the medication regimen, complications, side effects, and follow-up protocols.

What should the patient expect following administration of mifepristone in clinic?

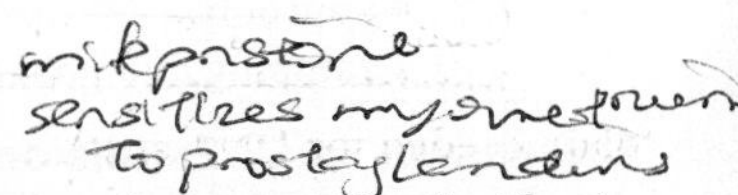

(A) Several hours of heavy bleeding and cramping
(B) Low-grade temperature
(C) Possible diarrhea
(D) No significant symptoms

The answer is D: No significant symptoms. Administration of mifepristone results in sensitization of the myometrium to prostaglandins. Mifepristone is the first step in the medication abortion regimen and usually does not cause significant bleeding. Misoprostol is the second step and is administered by the patient at home. Misoprostol has cervical ripening and strong uterotonic effects. Heavy bleeding and cramping are expected after misoprostol administration. Low-grade temperature and diarrhea are side effects of misoprostol use.

8 A 15-year-old, G1P0010, presents to clinic for contraceptive counseling. She was recently discharged from the hospital, where she was treated for postabortion sepsis. Currently she is completing the recommended antibiotic course. She is afebrile and a pelvic examination does not yield any significant findings. At the time of conception, she was taking combined oral contraceptives. She now desires a long-acting reversible method of birth control.

Which of the following is the most appropriate next step?

(A) Restart combined oral contraceptives
(B) Insert an intrauterine device (IUD)
(C) Administer depot medroxyprogesterone acetate
(D) Place a subdermal contraceptive implant

The answer is D: Place a subdermal contraceptive implant. Long-acting reversible contraceptive methods include copper IUD, levonorgestrel intrauterine system, and the etonogestrel contraceptive implant. IUDs can be used in adolescents and nulliparous patients. However, puerperal or postabortion sepsis within the past 3 months is a contraindication to IUD insertion. Depot medroxyprogesterone acetate is not a reversible method of contraception. Once administered, it maintains a contraceptive level of progestin for at least 14 weeks. While recommending condoms to prevent sexually transmitted infections (STIs) is appropriate, recommending them for contraception when the patient desires a more effective method is not.

9 A 21-year-old, G0, is interested in using a copper intrauterine device (IUD) for contraception. Thorough counseling includes benefits and potential disadvantages of intrauterine contraception.

Which of the following disadvantages is increased by her nulliparity?

(A) Altered bleeding patterns
(B) Infection following insertion
(C) Expulsion
(D) Cramping and pain after insertion

The answer is C: Expulsion. Nulliparity is a risk factor for IUD expulsion; a woman who has expelled one IUD has a 30% chance of subsequent expulsions. Altered bleeding patterns, including menorrhagia and dysmenorrhea, are potential disadvantages for all copper IUD users. Nulliparous patients should not have increased cramping and pain after IUD insertion is completed.

---

10 A 34-year-old woman presents to clinic for her depot medroxyprogesterone acetate injection. It has been 16 weeks since her last injection and she has a positive pregnancy test. She decides to terminate the pregnancy. During her appointment for the surgical abortion, she receives counseling regarding post-procedure contraceptive options. She decides on an intrauterine device (IUD).

When is the optimal time to insert the IUD?

(A) With her first post-procedure menstruation
(B) Six weeks after the abortion
(C) Immediately after the procedure
(D) At a routine gynecologic appointment

The answer is C: Immediately after the procedure. An IUD can be inserted immediately after a surgical abortion. The expulsion rate for IUDs inserted immediately after first-trimester procedures is not significantly different from expulsion rates after delayed insertion. Studies comparing immediate versus delayed insertion of IUD after abortion show a high loss to follow-up rate among the delayed group. Waiting for commencement of menstruation or for a routine gynecologic appointment puts the patient at risk for repeated unintended pregnancy.

---

11 A 27-year-old, G1P0010, is receiving her discharge instructions after an uncomplicated first-trimester surgical abortion. She is told that she will be receiving one prescription medication from the clinic.

What is the most appropriate prescription medication to discharge the patient home with?

(A) Oral contraceptive pills
(B) Uterotonic agents
(C) Antibiotics
(D) Opioid analgesics

The answer is C: Antibiotics. Post-procedure antibiotic prophylaxis is recommended following all surgical abortion procedures. This reduces the incidence of postabortal salpingitis and endometritis. Postoperative pain management after first-trimester surgical abortion often requires little more than ibuprofen. In the absence of hemorrhage, the routine use of uterotonic agents (such as methergine) postoperatively is not necessary. All forms of hormonal contraception and intrauterine devices (IUDs) may be initiated immediately after completing first-trimester surgical abortions; oral contraceptive pills are one of many options.

---

12 A 15-year-old presents to her pediatrician with 2 months of amenorrhea and is diagnosed with an unintended pregnancy at 8 week's gestation. She desires termination of pregnancy. The pediatrician refers her to an obstetrician–gynecologist to obtain the abortion.

What information should she provide to the patient regarding parental involvement requirements for abortion?

(A) Laws regarding parental involvement are consistent between most states
(B) Adolescents can bypass parental involvement requirements by utilizing the judicial bypass system
(C) Adolescents rarely travel out-of-state to obtain abortion care due to parental involvement requirements
(D) Parental involvement requirements involve parental notification, not consent

The answer is B: Adolescents can bypass parental involvement requirements by utilizing the judicial bypass system. Laws regarding parental involvement differ by state and may include parental notification or consent. Adolescents can bypass parental involvement requirement by utilizing the judicial bypass system; however, the courts in certain states may be unprepared to handle judicial bypass requests from adolescents, placing them at risk for delays in obtaining their procedures. The passage of parental notification and consent laws have been shown to increase the frequency with which adolescents travel out-of-state for abortion care.

13 In 1973, Roe v. Wade resulted in the replacement of unsafe, illegal abortions by safer, legal procedures. This legislation also stimulated research into how to perform abortions more safely.

Which of the following procedural changes has resulted from evidence-based medicine?

(A) Performance of most abortions now occurs in a hospital setting
(B) Suction curettage replaced sharp curettage
(C) Performance of abortions at no earlier than 7 week's gestation
(D) Administration of uterotonics after each abortion procedure

The answer is B: Suction curettage replaced sharp curettage. Suction curettage has been shown to be safer and faster than dilation and sharp curettage, which was previously the standard method for performing first-trimester abortion. Since Roe v. Wade, abortions have been moved to the outpatient setting, where the majority of abortions can be performed safely and economically. Abortions are also being performed at earlier gestational ages due to the ability to identify intrauterine pregnancies on transvaginal ultrasound. Uterotonics are not necessary after all abortions; blood loss is minimal in uncomplicated first-trimester procedures.

14 Which of the following statements is most accurate regarding public health and abortion worldwide?

(A) Abortions occur less frequently in countries where it is illegal
(B) The majority of abortion-related deaths occur in developing countries
(C) Approximately 75% of abortions worldwide are safe
(D) Most abortion-related complications occur as a result of anesthesia complications

The answer is B: The majority of abortion-related deaths occur in developing countries. Highly restrictive abortion laws are not associated with lower abortion rates. Nearly half of all abortions worldwide are unsafe and nearly all unsafe abortions occur in developing countries. Almost all abortion-related deaths occur in developing countries. Complications related to anesthesia are relatively rare; the majority of abortion-related complications worldwide are related to hemorrhage, infection, injury to pelvic/abdominal organs, and toxic reactions to substances taken to induce abortion.

CHAPTER

12

Sexually Transmitted Infections

1 An 18-year-old, G0, woman presents to the office with lower abdominal pain during menstruation. She usually has cramping with menstruation, but never as bad as this particular cycle. She has had a dull pain in her lower abdomen bilaterally for approximately 2 weeks before presentation. On examination, her temperature is 100.7 and she is diffusely tender to palpation in her lower abdominal quadrants. On pelvic examination, purulent discharge from her cervical os is noted, and she cries out in pain when her cervix is palpated.

What organism most likely precipitated the patient's presentation?

(A) *Gardnerella vaginalis*
(B) *Chlamydia trachomatis*
(C) Herpes simplex virus (HSV)
(D) *Candida albicans*
(E) *Trichomonas vaginalis*

The answer is B: *Chlamydia trachomatis*. The patient's condition is most consistent with pelvic inflammatory disease (PID), a complication of cervicitis caused by untreated *Chlamydia*, *Neisseria gonorrhea*, or both. Its symptoms can include diffuse mild-to-severe lower abdominal pain, dyspareunia, dysmenorrhea, and/or purulent discharge. On physical examination the patient may have a tender lower abdomen bilaterally, and/or fever, though up to 50% of patients will not present with a fever. Pelvic examination may reveal cervicitis with purulent discharge and cervical motion tenderness. The other organisms can cause vaginal irritation and discharge, but do not cause PID and are not associated with cervical motion tenderness. *Gardnerella* is associated with bacterial vaginosis (BV), HSV causes genital herpes, *C. albicans* causes yeast infections, and *T. vaginalis* causes trichomoniasis.

2 A 28-year-old woman presents to your office complaining of vaginal discharge for the past week. She describes the discharge as grayish white in color. She says that she has been sexually active with a monogamous partner for the past 3 years. Her current medications include only oral contraceptives. On physical examination, a thin, white discharge is present on the vaginal walls. Cervix is not inflamed and there is no cervical discharge. A fishy odor is present. The vaginal pH is 5.0. A wet mount is shown in *Figure 12-1*.

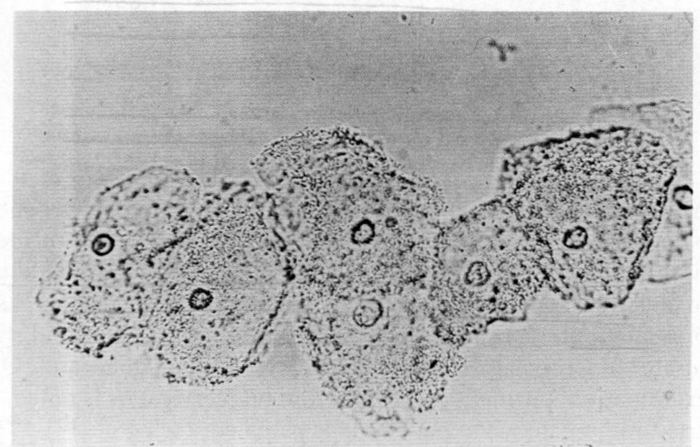

Figure 12-1

Which of the following is the most likely diagnosis?

(A) Trichomoniasis
(B) *Chlamydia*
(C) BV
(D) Candidiasis

facultative anaerobic organisms NOT STI

The answer is C: BV. BV is a polymicrobial infection characterized by an overgrowth of facultative anaerobic organisms. This is not a sexually transmitted infection but rather a sexually associated infection. Women with BV often complain of a "fishy" odor and a thin grayish white discharge. Diagnosis is defined by three out of four of the following criteria:

- Normal gray discharge
- pH > 4.5
- Positive "whiff test"
- Presence of clue cells on wet smear

3 While assisting on a laparoscopic cholecystectomy, you notice localized fibrosis and adhesions that have formed between the liver surface and the diaphragm (see *Figure 12-2*).

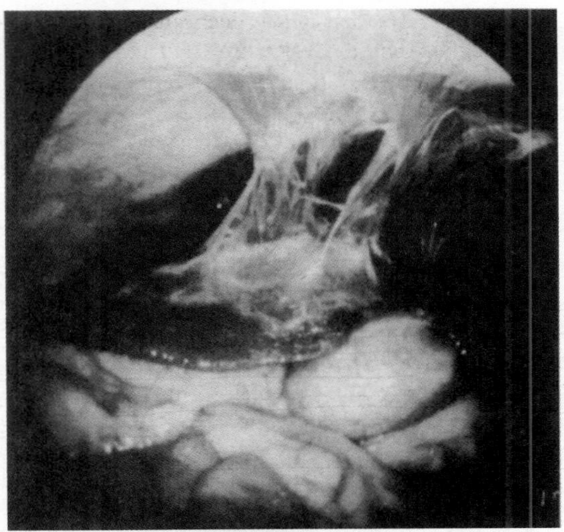

Figure 12-2

Based on these findings, this 28-year-old female patient likely has a history of what condition?

(A) HSV
(B) *Chlamydia*
(C) Syphilis
(D) Lymphogranuloma venereum
(E) Chancroid

The answer is B: *Chlamydia.* Based on the description, this patient has Fitz-Hugh and Curtis syndrome. This is caused by chlamydial infection as well as gonorrhea.

4 A 21-year-old G1P1 who recently emigrated from India presents to your office after she noticed bleeding from a lesion on her labia. She has noticed this bleeding over the past few months but waited to go to the physician since she had no pain. She finally decided to seek medical attention due to the size of the lesion. Her medication list only includes oral contraceptives. On physical examination, a beefy, red ulcer is present on the labia (see *Figure 12-3*). Fresh granulation tissue surrounds the ulcer. The vaginal wall, vaginal vault, and cervix appear to be unaffected.

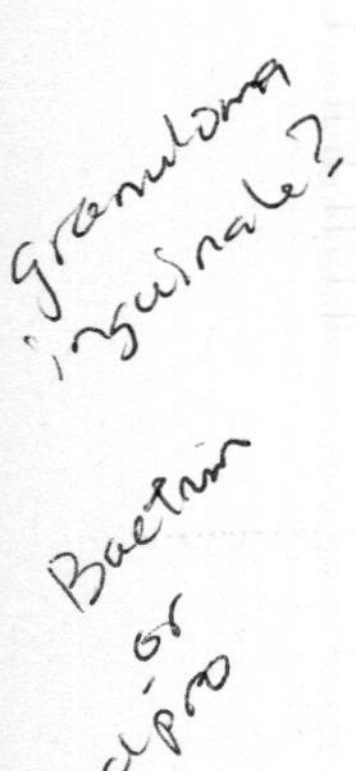

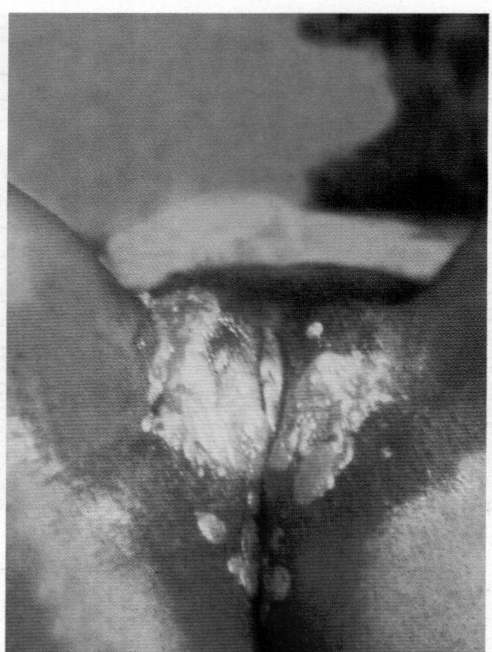

Figure 12-3

The diagnosis can be established by which of the following?

(A) Staining for Donovan bodies
(B) Presence of serum antibodies to *C. trachomatis*
(C) Culturing *Haemophilus ducreyi*
(D) Culturing *Calymmatobacterium granulomatis*

The answer is A: Staining for Donovan bodies. Granuloma inguinale occurs rarely in the United States but is endemic in India, Papua New Guinea, central Australia, and western Africa. Lesions are raised and bleed easily. Diagnosis is made based on high clinical suspicion or based on the presence of dark-staining Donovan bodies on biopsy. Treatment includes either trimethoprim/sulfamethoxazole or ciprofloxacin.

5 A 23-year-old woman presents to your clinic with complaints of vulvar pain. The patient's history is significant for a new sexual partner and a recent history of flu-like symptoms and vaginal burning. On physical examination, extremely painful shallow ulcers with red borders are appreciated on the vulva, vagina, and perineal region (see *Figure 12-4*).

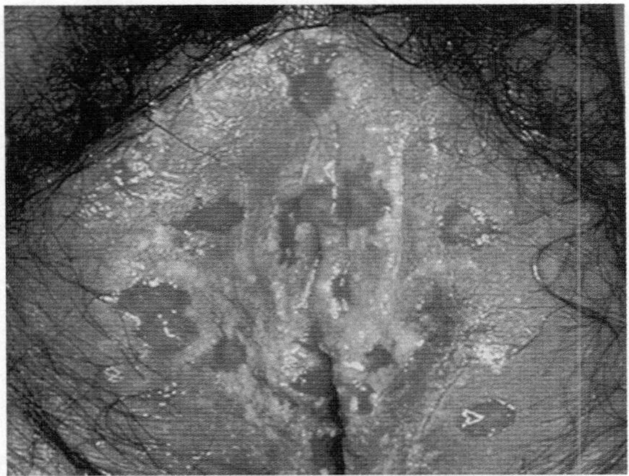

Figure 12-4

Which of the following is the most appropriate course of treatment for this patient?

HSV painful ulcers

(A) Penicillin
(B) Azithromycin
(C) Doxycycline
(D) Acyclovir
(E) Ciprofloxacin

The answer is D: Acyclovir. Based on the prodromal symptoms and painful ulcers, this patient likely has HSV. Appropriate treatment is acyclovir.

---

6 While working in the emergency department, a 15-year-old female patient arrives with severe acute abdominal pain. Before the start of her abdominal pain, the patient recalls having some fever and chills. She reports that her menses is regular and that she is sexually active. She recently started having intercourse with a new partner. Pregnancy test is negative and urinalysis is normal. On physical examination, the patient has muscular guarding and rebound tenderness. On pelvic examination, patient has cervical motion tenderness. Vital signs are significant for tachycardia and fever (102.2).

Which of the following is the most likely diagnosis?

muscular guarding, rebound tenderness

(A) Ovarian torsion
(B) Endometriosis
(C) PID
(D) Kidney stone
(E) Ruptured ovarian cyst

The answer is C: PID. PID is characterized by muscular guarding, cervical motion tenderness, or rebound tenderness. Patient may also have elevated white blood count and fever. PID is considered the most severe form of sexually transmitted infection.

---

7 A patient presents to your office for her annual examination. She admits to having intercourse with multiple sexual partners over the past year. Her only medication is an oral contraceptive pill (OCP) which she takes very regularly. She has no new symptoms or concerns. On physical examination, a painless punched-out ulcer is appreciated on the left labia (see *Figure 12-5*).

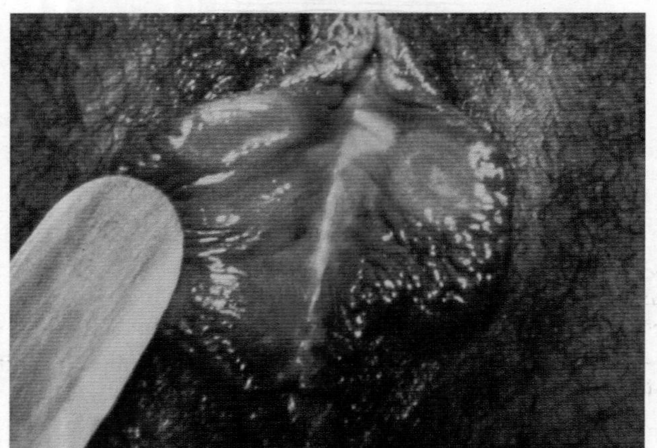

Figure 12-5

After appropriate testing and treatment, you counsel the patient to practice safer sex in the future.

If this patient had not been treated, what would be the next sequelae?

(A) Argyll-Robertson pupil
(B) Gummas on the skin and bones
(C) Tabes dorsalis
(D) Rash involving palms and soles

syphilis
primary stage
→ painless chancre

The answer is D: Rash involving palms and soles. Based on the description of a hard painless chancre, this patient likely has syphilis. The primary stage of syphilis is characterized by painless chancre. Secondary stage includes a red rash involving the palms and soles (see *Figure 12-6*).

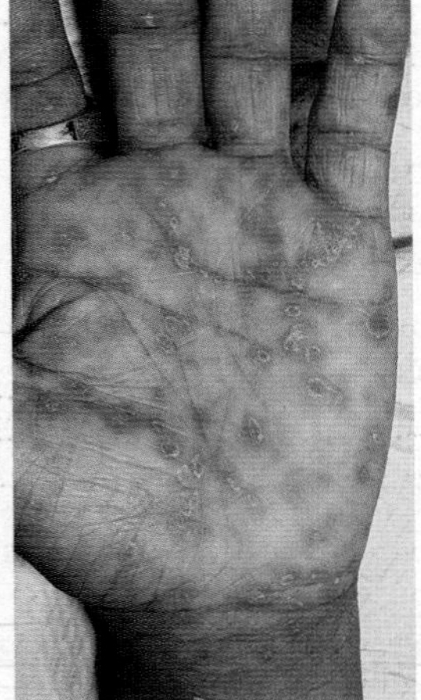

Figure 12-6

Tertiary stage is characterized by Argyll-Robertson pupil, tabes dorsalis, paresis, gummas of skin and bone, and aortic aneurysm.

---

8 A 24-year-old patient presents to your office with complaints of a 1-week history of vulvar itching and vaginal discharge. She endorses that she has had intercourse with two individuals in the past 6 months without the use of a condom. On physical examination, the vulva is edematous. Yellow-green discharge is present on the vaginal walls and at the cervical os. The cervix is strawberry red (see *Figure 12-7*).

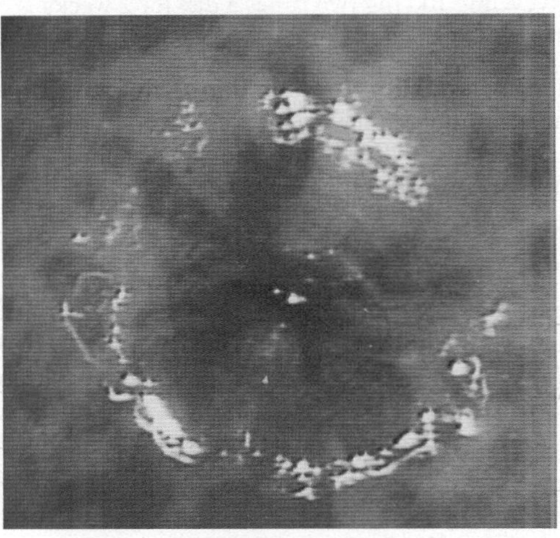

Figure 12-7

Wet smear of vaginal secretions shows epithelial cells, white blood cells (WBCs), and flagellate protozoa. You prescribe an antibiotic.

What warning do you give about this particular treatment?

(A) Avoid sun overexposure
(B) Avoid taking on an empty stomach
(C) Avoid taking with grapefruit juice
(D) Avoid alcohol

The answer is D: Metronidazole. *T. vaginalis* is a flagellate protozoan that is transmitted by sexual contact and causes a yellow-green frothy discharge. In 10% of the population, *T. vaginalis* can cause petechiae or "strawberry patches" on the upper vagina and cervix. Diagnosis is made by wet smear of vaginal discharge. Treatment of trichomoniasis is oral metronidazole—major side effect is antabuse effect—alcohol may cause an upset stomach, vomiting, stomach cramps, headaches, sweating, and flushing (redness of the face).

---

9 A 60-year-old woman presents to your clinic with a painless macule on her right labia. She states that she first noticed the spot 3 weeks ago. You notice on examination that the area has begun to ulcerate and that she has mild, nontender, inguinal lymphadenopathy. Given this history and subsequent physical examination findings, what is the most appropriate antimicrobial treatment?

(A) Penicillin G 2.4 million units IM once
(B) Acyclovir 400 mg orally three times a day for 1 week
(C) Ceftriaxone 250 mg IM once
(D) Doxycycline 100 mg two times a day for 2 weeks
(E) Metronidazole 500 mg orally twice a day for 2 weeks

The answer is A: Penicillin G 2.4 million units IM once. A painless macule or chancre and nontender lymphadenopathy is suggestive of primary infection with *Treponema pallidum*, the infectious agent in syphilis. The preferred treatment for primary syphilis is IM Penicillin G.

---

10 A 26-year-old, G0, woman presents to your clinic. One of her recent sexual partners has been treated for a sexually transmitted disease (STD) but she cannot remember what the specific infection was called. Recently, she has noticed an increase in odorless discharge and some pelvic cramping. Gram stain and wet prep of her cervical mucus show many WBCs and no gram-negative diplococci.

Which of the medications would be the best treatment for this patient?

(A) Penicillin G 2.4 million units IM once
(B) Acyclovir 400 mg orally three times a day for 1 week
(C) Ceftriaxone 250 mg IM once
(D) Doxycycline 100 mg two times a day for 1 week
(E) Metronidazole 500 mg orally twice a day for 2 weeks

The answer is D: Doxycycline 100 mg two times a day for 1 week. The most common cause for non-gonococcal cervicitis/urethritis is *Chlamydia* infection. Because *Chlamydia* bacteria thrive in intracellular environments, they are often not seen on gram stain and are difficult to culture. This patient should be treated with doxycycline for suspected *Chlamydia* infection. Penicillin G is used to treat syphilis, acyclovir is used for the control of genital herpes, ceftriaxone would be appropriate for gonococcal cervicitis, and metronidazole is used to treat both *T. vaginalis* and BV which would have been apparent on wet prep.

---

11 A 45-year-old woman is brought to the operating room for a laparoscopic cholecystectomy. Upon displacing the liver, the surgeon notices fibrous capsular adhesions on the superior aspect of the liver. This condition is most likely to a consequence of which of the following gynecologic issues?

(A) Past *C. trachomatis* infection
(B) Multiple Cesarean deliveries
(C) Untreated endometriosis
(D) Metastatic ovarian carcinoma
(E) Overgrowth of candida vaginallis

The answer is A: Past *C. trachomatis* infection. The vignette is describing Fitz-Hugh and Curtis syndrome, a complication of PID which involves liver capsule inflammation and occasionally presents as pleuritic right upper quadrant (RUQ) pain. The acute presentation can often mimic cholecystitis or pyelonephritis. Even after treatment of the infection, adhesions may remain.

---

12 A 13-year-old girl is brought to see you by her mother who is a patient of yours. The mother recently read that the Food and Drug Administration has approved two vaccines for human papillomavirus (HPV). This virus, which causes genital warts, is also linked to certain types of cervical cancer. The girl's mother is interested in starting the vaccination series for her daughter and would like to know more about how the vaccination works and how well it prevents cervical cancer.

What HPV subtypes account for 70% of the cervical cancers worldwide?

(A) 16, 18
(B) 18, 33
(C) 4, 35
(D) 33, 4
(E) 16, 35

The answer is A: 16, 18. Although the majority of HPV infections are asymptomatic, as many as 15% of HPV cervical infections will progress to cervical intraepithelial neoplasia or carcinoma. The Pap smear is a screen for the presence of HPV-related dysplastic change. The quadrivalent vaccine, Gardasil, protects against HPV subtypes 6, 11, 16, and 18. Of these 16 and 18 are responsible for >70% of cervical cancers worldwide. Of course, with greater access to vaccination this may change in future generations.

---

13 A 19-year-old G0 patient presents to your office after 3 days of general malaise. The patient is currently sexually active with three male partners and admits that she often has unprotected sex. She is now complaining of multiple, painful bumps on her genitals. On physical examination, you see clusters of vesicles on erythematous skin around her vulva and anus. HSV screen is positive for HSV-2. During the dormant phase of this disease, where does the virus typically reside?

(A) The virus is typically cleared with acyclovir treatment; there is no dormant stage
(B) Cell bodies in the dorsal root ganglia of sacral sensory nerves
(C) Cell bodies of squamous epithelial cells of mucous membranes
(D) Incorporated into the DNA of squamous epithelial cells
(E) Axons of cutaneous sensory nerves

The answer is B: Cell bodies in the dorsal root ganglia of sacral sensory nerves. Clustered vesicles on an erythematous base suggests herpes; HSV-2 is the most common virus involved in genital herpes. It is thought that the virus, or potentially the viral capsid, travels retrograde up the axons of sensory nerves and resides in the cell bodies of the dorsal root ganglia of sacral nerves. HPV remains in squamous epithelial cells and can incorporate itself into the cellular DNA.

---

14 A 23-year-old, G0, woman with her last menstrual period (LMP) 1 week ago presents to the emergency department complaining of intense pelvic pain, fever of 103, and uncontrollable vomiting. The patient is currently sexually active and admits to intermittent condom usage. In the emergency room, the patient sits motionless and mentions that the ride over seemed to make the pain much worse.

Urine pregnancy test is negative. She winces with pain and pulls away when the examiner touches her cervix. The examiner notices a purulent discharge coming from the cervical os.

What is the most appropriate next step in patient management?

(A) Prescribe methotrexate and ask her to follow up as an outpatient
(B) Admit the patient to the hospital and treat with cefotetan
(C) Perform a Pap smear with high-risk HPV testing and ask her to follow up as an outpatient
(D) Rush the patient to the operating room for emergent laparoscopic evaluation
(E) Prescribe metronidazole and ask her to follow up as an outpatient

The answer is B: Admit the patient to the hospital and treat with cefotetan. This scenario describes a patient with PID. Although PID may be treated as an outpatient, indications for hospitalization include when the patient does not respond to or cannot tolerate outpatient oral treatment, pregnancy, severe fever, nausea and vomiting, tubo-ovarian abscess (TOA), or when other surgical emergencies cannot be excluded. Intravenous (IV) cefotetan is adequate therapy for most PID hospitalizations.

---

15 A 60-year-old postmenopausal woman comes to your clinic for a wellness visit. She has been divorced for 2 years and sexually active, but has not been to see you for 4 years. She reports three partners for the last 18 months. According to the current U.S. Preventive Services Task Force (USPSTF) guidelines, which of the following services related to the detection of sexually transmitted infections should be offered to your patient?

(A) Pap smear and HIV test
(B) DNA polymerase chain reaction for herpes and wet prep
(C) Wet prep and Venereal Disease Research Laboratory (VDRL)
(D) Hepatitis C test and VDRL
(E) DNA polymerase chain reaction for herpes and HIV test

The answer is A: Pap smear and HIV test. The sexual health components of the USPSTF guidelines for a 60-year-old sexually active woman include testing for HIV, syphilis and gonorrhea, as well as a Pap with HPV testing every 5 years to age 65. A wet prep is a clinical test to assist in the diagnosis of vaginitis and is not appropriate in an asymptomatic woman. VDRL is a serum test, which can suggest syphilis.

---

16 A 45-year-old woman presents to the emergency department with a 1-week history of malaise, headache, and eye pain. Examination shows bilateral, painless, inguinal lymphadenopathy and a scaly, maculopapular rash on the hands and feet. Laboratory studies show a positive VDRL and rapid plasma reagin (RPR).

How long ago did this patient first become infected?

(A) 5 days
(B) 5 weeks
(C) 5 months
(D) 5 years

The answer is C: 5 months. Primary syphilis, a painless genital chancre and nontender inguinal lymphadenopathy, occurs 3 to 12 weeks after initial inoculation. This presentation suggests secondary syphilis that can present 4 to 8 weeks after resolution of the initial chancre of primary syphilis. Thus, a patient with secondary syphilis may have been initially exposed between 2 and 6 months from presentation and it is important to notify all appropriate sexual partners. It is important to remember that many patients never notice the primary chancre, as it is painless, and up to 75% of patients never develop the symptoms of secondary syphilis.

---

17 A 22-year-old G0 presents to the emergency room with RUQ pain and a fever of 102.1 that began suddenly 3 days ago. Patient also reports intermittent nausea and vomiting but denies diarrhea and constipation. Physical examination showed RUQ tenderness with a positive Murphy's sign. Complete blood count was within normal limits with the exception of a WBC count of 13,500 cells/mm^3. Comprehensive metabolic panel was within normal limits.

What is the most likely diagnosis in this patient?

(A) Fitz-Hugh and Curtis syndrome
(B) Hepatitis A
(C) Hepatitis B
(D) Acute cholelithiasis
(E) Gastroesophageal reflux disease
(F) Peptic ulcer disease

The answer is B: Hepatitis A. Fitz-Hugh and Curtis syndrome, or perihepatitis, consists of infection of the liver capsule and peritoneal surfaces of the anterior RUQ, with limited liver stroma involvement; thus, aminotransferases are usually normal.

---

18 A 23-year-old woman presents to the emergency room complaining of lower abdominal pain and subjective fever. On examination she was noted to have mucopurulent cervical discharge and tenderness on bimanual examination. If left untreated, which condition is this patient most at risk for developing?

(A) Chronic pelvic pain (CPP)
(B) Ovarian cancer
(C) Hepatitis B
(D) Urinary incontinence
(E) Ovarian torsion

The answer is A: Chronic pelvic pain (CPP). Patients with gonococcal or chlamydial infection that lead to ascending PID are at increased risk for CPP. It is important to recognize the potential for increased presentation of CPP in areas with high prevalence of STDs. As many as 30% of women with PID will develop CPP, the severity and duration of infection are directly related to the development of CPP.

---

19 A 19-year-old woman presents to the emergency department complaining of cauliflower-like lesions on her vulva (see *Figure 12-8*).

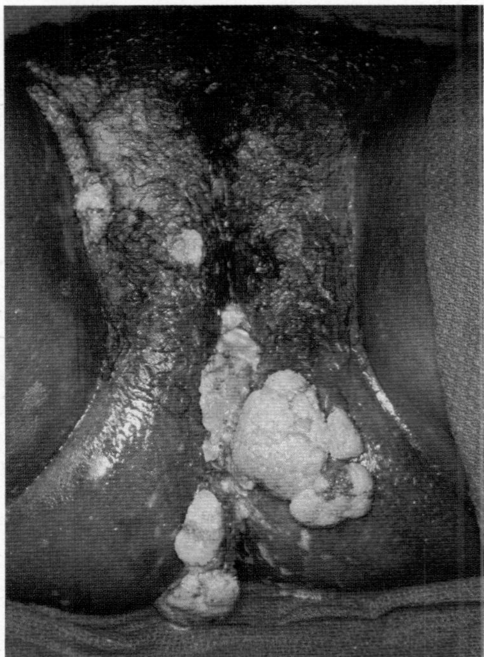

Figure 12-8

They have been present for several months but are now beginning to interfere with intercourse. You diagnose genital warts.

Which viral subtypes are responsible for most cases of this disease?

(A) Types 6 and 11
(B) Types 6 and 18
(C) Types 11 and 16
(D) Types 11 and 31
(E) Types 16 and 18

The answer is A: Types 6 and 11. HPV types 6 and 11 cause genital warts but are associated with low to no risk of developing cancer. Condoms do not prevent the transmission of HPV.

20 A 45-year-old sex worker is seen at the local health department with complaint of a malodorous vaginal discharge for 2 weeks. After thorough examination and wet prep you treat her with metronidazole.

What did the wet prep show?

(A) Rods and buds
(B) Clue cells
(C) Flagellated organisms
(D) Parabasal cells
(E) Fat globules

The answer is C: Flagellated organisms. Trichomonads are unicellular, flagellated, anaerobic organisms. They cause sexually transmitted vaginitis characterized by abnormal vaginal odor and pruritus of the vulva and vagina. The classic sign of *Trichomonas* is a "strawberry cervix," though this finding is only seen in about 10% of cases. Metronidazole is the treatment of choice.

---

21 A 19-year-old G0 presents to her gynecologist for an annual well-woman examination. She is sexually active with multiple male partners, receives depot medroxyprogesterone injections every 3 months for contraception, and says that she "almost always" uses condoms. On examination, the gynecologist notices a single 1 cm round ulcer with a clean-cut margin on the inner surface of the patient's labia majora. The patient reports that she had noticed this lesion a couple days prior but that it is not painful.

Which of the following pathogens is the likely cause of this patient's lesion?

(A) *T. pallidum*
(B) *H. ducreyi*
(C) Herpes simplex
(D) Varicella zoster
(E) *C. trachomatis*

The answer is A: *T. pallidum*. Syphilis is caused by the spirochete *T. pallidum*, and primary syphilis is characterized by a painless ulcer at the site of inoculation known as a chancre. *H. ducreyi* is the causative organism of a chancroid. A chancroid can look like a chancre, but it is a painful lesion. Herpes simplex causes painful vesicular lesions in a random pattern. Varicella zoster causes chicken pox upon initial infection (diffuse vesicles on an erythematous base that itch) and shingles upon latent reactivation (exquisitely painful vesicular lesions that follow a dermatomal pattern). Symptoms of *C. trachomatis* infection can include abnormal vaginal discharge and dysuria, as well as severe lower abdominal pain, fever, and possible sepsis if the infection progress into PID.

---

22 You are in the Student Run Free Clinic and see a 20-year-old G0 LMP 2 weeks ago on OCPs who complains of painful bumps near her vagina. She is currently sexually active with a new male partner of 3 to 4 months and rarely uses condoms. She became sexually active at age 16 and has had six lifetime partners. She denies any history of sexually transmitted infections. Her past medical history and surgical history are unremarkable. On physical examination she is anxious but in no distress. Her vital signs are stable and she is afebrile. Her examination is remarkable for left inguinal lymphadenopathy and a cluster of tender vesicles on her left labia majora. The most appropriate evaluation of this patient is:

(A) GC/*Chlamydia* DNA, HSV I and II IgM and IgG; Pap
(B) GC/*Chlamydia* DNA, HSV I and II IgA and IgG
(C) GC/*Chlamydia* DNA, HIV, RPR
(D) GC/*Chlamydia* DNA, HSV I and II IgM and IgG, lipid profile

The answer is C: GC/*Chlamydia* DNA, HIV, RPR. A Pap is not indicated in a 20-year-old and neither is a lipid profile. Antibody screening is not used for screening of genital HSV since such a large percentage of the population has had prior exposure to HSV. Finally, any patient who presents with an STD should be screened for other STDs.

---

23 Mary G presents to clinic for evaluation of a 3-day history of vaginal irritation with itching and redness. She describes a white odorless discharge. She is a 25-year-old married school teacher, G0, LMP 3 weeks ago on OCPs. Her past medical and surgical histories are unremarkable. Her medications include her OCPs as well as ampicillin she is taking for strep throat that she caught from her class. Pulmonary embolism (PE) reveals an erythematous vulva as well as a thick white odorless discharge. Wet mount is shown in *Figure 12-9*.

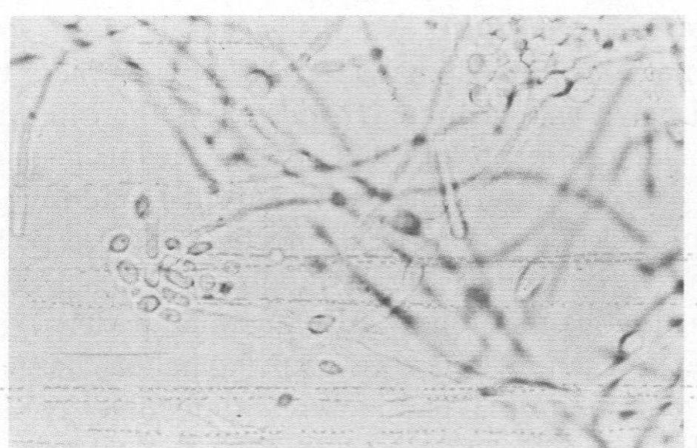

Figure 12-9

The best treatment option for this patient is:

(A) Metronidazole gel
(B) Oral metronidazole
(C) Fluconazole
(D) Azithromycin
(E) Doxycycline

The answer is C: Fluconazole. The patient is noted to have budding yeast on her wet mount consistent with the diagnosis of candidiasis. The pH would be normal. We should also expect a negative Whiff test, the amine or "fishy" odor produced by adding a few drops of KOH to the secretions.

24 You are in the Student Free Clinic seeing a 29-year-old G3P3003 LMP last week on OCPs who complains of vaginal irritation and odor. The patient is married but concerned about infidelity. She was diagnosed with Herpes 3 years ago after her husband cheated on her so she is very suspicious.

PE reveals a thin foamy discharge with odor that worsens when the specimen is collected for wet mount that is shown in *Figure 12-10*.

What is the treatment of choice?

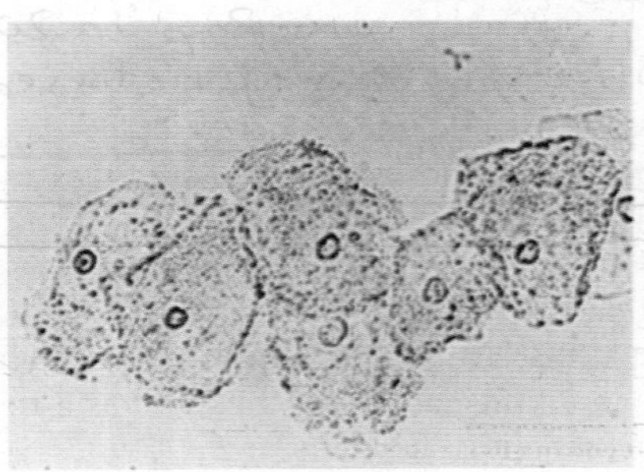

Figure 12-10

(A) Azithromycin for patient and her husband
(B) Azithromycin for patient only
(C) Tetracycline for patient and her husband
(D) Tetracycline for patient
(E) Metronidazole for the patient only

The answer is E: **Metronidazole for the patient only.** BV is not considered an STD and as such the partner does not need treatment.

25 A 21-year-old G0 presents to the emergency room with right-sided abdominal pain, nausea, fever, and vaginal discharge. Her LMP was 2 weeks ago. She denies any medical problems and has not had any surgical procedures. She has several sexual partners and reports inconsistent condom use. Physical examination findings include right lower quadrant rebound tenderness (see *Figure 12-11*). There is yellow discharge at the cervical os and a palpable right adnexal mass. WBC count is 19,000. β-Human chorionic gonadotropin is negative.

What is the most appropriate next step?

(A) Admit to hospital for IV antibiotics
(B) Admit to hospital for surgical intervention
(C) Discharge home with oral antibiotics
(D) Further imaging with computed tomography (CT) is required

The answer is A: **Admit to hospital for IV antibiotics.** This patient most likely has PID with a TOA.

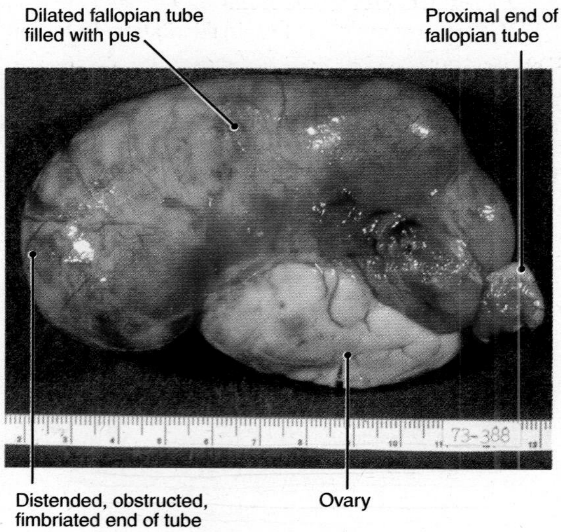

Figure 12-11

She is acutely ill with fever and physical examination suggests a TOA. She requires immediate hospitalization and treatment with IV antibiotics. This clinical picture is often associated with *N. gonorrhea* and *C. trachomatis* but many cases are polymicrobial. Patients should be hospitalized when other causes of an acute abdomen cannot be ruled out, if they are pregnant, if they have failed to respond to previous treatment with oral antibiotics, if they have severe illness, including nausea, vomiting, and fever, or if they have a TOA. IV treatment is for severe PID and the Centers for Disease Control and Prevention guidelines recommend cefotetan 2 g IV q12 or cefoxitin 2 g IV q6h + doxycycline 100 mg PO or IV q12h. CT scan is not required as the history and physical examination have provided enough information to illicit a diagnosis. Oral antibiotics are not sufficient to address the TOA or her severe clinical presentation. Surgical intervention is not appropriate at this time.

CHAPTER

13

Neoplasia

1 A 37-year-old woman with a history of kidney transplant for lupus nephritis presents to the gynecologist for her annual examination. Her last Pap smear and human papillomavirus (HPV) testing were done 1 year ago and were negative. She reports no change in her transplant rejection medications. On examination, her blood pressure is 116/72 mmHg, and her breast examination reveals fibrocystic changes. When is the patient due for her next combined cervical cytology and HPV DNA testing?

(A) Today
(B) In 1 year
(C) In 2 years
(D) In 3 years
(E) In 4 years
(F) In 5 years

The answer is A: Today. According to the American College of Obstetricians and Gynecologists (ACOG) recommendations, patients on immunosuppressants such as this patient should have annual Pap smears. Since she is between 30 and 65 years old, she could have co-testing for HPV. Otherwise, indications for screening in the general population are to start Pap smears at age 21 regardless of the age of onset of intercourse and for Pap smears to be done every 3 years for women aged 21 to 65 years. Women aged 30 to 65 years can extend that period to every 5 years with co-testing for HPV. However, women under 30 years old should not have HPV co-testing.

2 A 17-year-old presents to the local teen clinic concerned about several days of new frothy, yellowish-green discharge with a foul odor. She endorses sexual intercourse with one male partner in her lifetime. Her last encounter was 1 week ago. She uses combined oral contraceptives for pregnancy prevention. She reports no history of cervical cytology screening. Testing today includes a pregnancy test, wet prep, and nucleic

acid amplification tests of cervical samples. What should the clinic recommend for this patient regarding cervical cytology screening?

(A) Immediate cervical cytology
(B) Cervical cytology in 1 year
(C) Cervical cytology in 2 years
(D) Cervical cytology in 3 years
(E) Cervical cytology in 4 years

The answer is E: **Cervical cytology in 4 years.** The recommendation for cervical cytology screening in the general population is to start cervical cytology screening with Pap smears at age 21 regardless of the age of onset of intercourse. Pap smears should be done every 3 years for women 21 to 65 years old. Women aged 30 to 65 years can extend that period to every 5 years with co-testing for human papillomavirus (HPV). However, women under 30 years old should not have HPV testing because younger women often clear abnormal cytology results consistent with HPV infections within 2 years.

---

3 A 47-year-old, G0, with a 30-pack-year smoking history presents for follow-up regarding a new diagnosis of squamous cell carcinoma based on a satisfactory loop electrical excision procedure (LEEP). She reports intercourse onset at age 22 and a history of 20 to 30 male partners in her lifetime. She has a copper intrauterine device (IUD) for pregnancy prevention; she uses condoms infrequently for sexually transmitted infection (STI) prevention. She denies any history of STIs, including negative HIV testing done 1 month ago. Which of the following is the most significant risk factor for cervical squamous cell carcinoma in this patient?

(A) History of cigarette smoking
(B) Age of first intercourse
(C) Use of an IUD
(D) Number of sexual partners in her lifetime
(E) History of STIs

The answer is D: **Number of sexual partners in her lifetime.** Most risk factors for cervical squamous carcinoma are related to the risk of acquiring human papillomavirus (HPV), an STI. The patient's greatest risk factor is having multiple sexual partners. Women with six or more partners have a threefold increased risk. IUD use is not a risk factor for cancer. The other options are risk factors, but they do not increase her risk as much as her history of multiple sexual partners. Tobacco use is a dose-dependent risk factor.

---

4 A 67-year-old woman with a new diagnosis of cervical squamous cell carcinoma based on cold-knife cone biopsy is undergoing an examination under anesthesia for clinical staging of her cervical cancer. She does not have any urinary symptoms. In the operating room, a soft mass is palpable in the posterior and lateral vaginal fornices extending into the surrounding tissues, but it does not extend into the lower vagina. On rectovaginal examination, the mass does not extend into the pelvic wall. What is the clinical staging for this patient based on International Federation of Gynecology and Obstetrics (FIGO) criteria?

(A) Stage I
(B) Stage II
(C) Stage III
(D) Stage IV

The answer is B: Stage II. Cervical squamous cell carcinoma spreads primarily through direct extension into the surrounding tissue. Stage I is limited to the cervix. Stage II includes extension into the parametrial tissues and/or upper two-thirds of the vagina. Stage III signifies involvement of the lower one-third of the vagina and/or pelvic wall. Stage IV reflects bladder or bowel involvement resulting in signs and symptoms of hydronephrosis or bowel obstruction, respectively.

---

5 A 31-year-old G1P0 at 24 weeks 2 days by last menstrual period (LMP) dating with no prenatal care presents to the emergency department for vaginal bleeding after intercourse. She denies any loss of fluid and reports normal fetal movements. On examination, fundal height is 25 cm, and fetal heart tones by Doppler are 140 bpm. Sterile speculum examination reveals scant dark blood in the posterior vaginal vault and a friable appearing cervix. Combined cervical cytology with human papillomavirus (HPV) DNA is done, and the results show high-grade squamous intraepithelial lesion (HGSIL). What is the next step in the management for this patient?

(A) Repeat combined cervical cytology in 4 to 6 months
(B) Repeat combined cervical cytology in 12 months
(C) Immediate colposcopic examination
(D) Colposcopic examination at 6-week postpartum visit
(E) Immediate endocervical curettage
(F) Endometrial biopsy at 6-week postpartum visit

The answer is C: Immediate colposcopic examination. Except for a cervical cytology result of atypical squamous cells of undetermined significance (ASCUS), all other results should be followed up with colposcopy. Endocervical curettage and endometrial biopsies are typically avoided during pregnancy due to the risk of causing preterm labor, premature rupture of membranes, or hemorrhage cases of placenta previa.

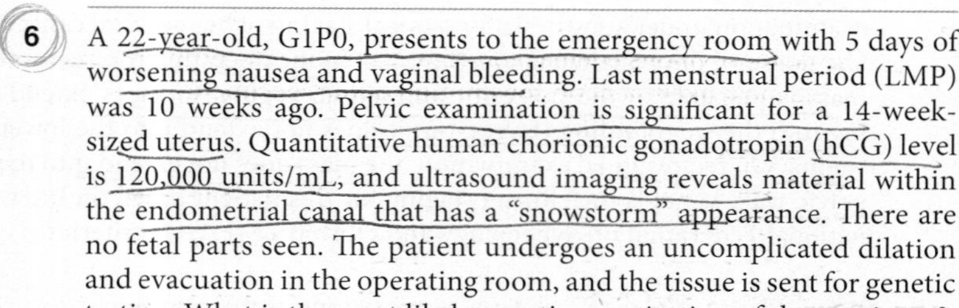

6 A 22-year-old, G1P0, presents to the emergency room with 5 days of worsening nausea and vaginal bleeding. Last menstrual period (LMP) was 10 weeks ago. Pelvic examination is significant for a 14-week-sized uterus. Quantitative human chorionic gonadotropin (hCG) level is 120,000 units/mL, and ultrasound imaging reveals material within the endometrial canal that has a "snowstorm" appearance. There are no fetal parts seen. The patient undergoes an uncomplicated dilation and evacuation in the operating room, and the tissue is sent for genetic testing. What is the most likely genetic constitution of the specimen?

(A) 69, XXX
(B) 69, XXY
(C) 46, XX
(D) 46, XY

The answer is C: 46, XX. Complete moles have chromosomes entirely of paternal origin as a result of fertilization of a blighted ovum by a haploid sperm that replicates. Rarely fertilization of a blighted ovum by two sperm occurs. The karyotype of a complete mole is usually 46, XX and rarely 46, XY. Partial hydatidiform moles result from double fertilization of a normal haploid egg or from fertilization by a diploid sperm. The karyotype is 69, XXX or 69, XXY. Complete moles are more common than partial moles and are more likely to undergo malignant transformation. *Figure 13-1* shows typical snowstorm pattern seen with molar pregnancy.

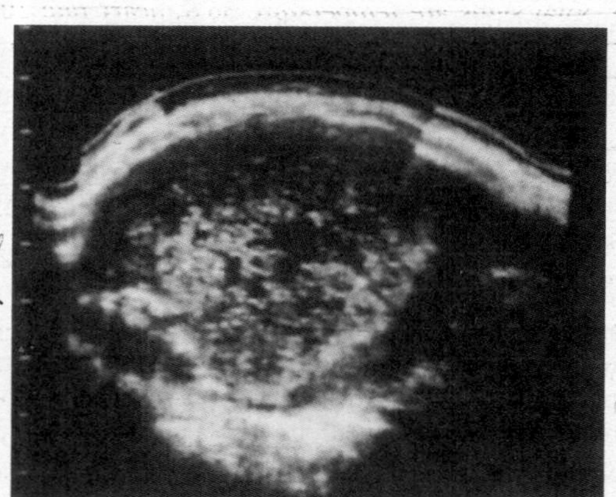

Figure 13-1

7 A 28-year-old, G3P2, presents to clinic for routine obstetric care. Last menstrual period (LMP) was 12 weeks ago. A 10-week-sized uterus is found on pelvic examination, and a subsequent ultrasound reveals a grossly abnormal fetus without cardiac activity. The patient opts for

uterine evacuation. Pathology inspection notes the presence of fetal parts, focal villous edema, and focal trophoblastic proliferation. What is the most likely genetic constitution of the specimen?

(A) 46, XX
(B) 46, XY
(C) Triploidy
(D) Aneuploidy

The answer is C: Triploidy. In cases of partial mole, the ultrasound reveals an abnormally formed fetus. The fetus of a partial mole is usually a triploid and results from dispermic fertilization of a normal ovum. This consists of one haploid set of maternal chromosomes and two haploid sets of paternal chromosomes. Pathology inspection of partial moles typically shows focal villous edema and focal trophoblastic proliferation. Diffuse villous edema and trophoblastic proliferation are usually found with complete moles.

---

8 An otherwise healthy 24-year-old G0 presents to her gynecologist because of irregular, heavy vaginal bleeding for the past few days. She also complains of worsening nausea, vomiting, headache, and dizziness over the past few weeks. She reports that her last regular menstrual period before her current bleeding started was 6 weeks ago. On examination, she has a slight tremor in both hands, an enlarged 10-week-sized uterus, and blood coming from the cervical os. Urine β-hCG is positive. Vital signs are temperature 36.8, heart rate 100 beats/min, blood pressure 160/100 mmHg, and respiratory rate 16 breaths/min. What is the most likely diagnosis?

(A) Missed abortion
(B) Incomplete abortion
(C) Gestational hypertension
(D) Molar pregnancy
(E) Ectopic pregnancy

The answer is D: Molar pregnancy. This patient has numerous findings that are consistent with a molar pregnancy. The most common presenting symptom for a molar pregnancy is heavy or irregular bleeding early in pregnancy, and physical examination reveals size greater than dates in about half of the patients. A molar pregnancy also produces high levels of hCG, which can lead to nausea and vomiting. The α-subunit of hCG is structurally identical to that found in thyroid-stimulating hormone (TSH), luteinizing hormone (LH), and follicle-stimulating hormone (FSH). Therefore, patients with molar pregnancies may also have signs of hyperthyroidism, like nervousness, anorexia, or tremor, as well as large theca lutein cysts on the ovaries from stimulation by an LH/FSH analog. In a patient without baseline hypertension (such as this patient), preeclampsia before 20 week's gestation is highly suggestive of a molar pregnancy. A missed abortion, an incomplete abortion, pure gestational hypertension, or an ectopic pregnancy would not have this constellation of symptoms.

---

9 A 48-year-old perimenopausal woman presents with a chief complaint of perineal and perianal burning. Vulvar colposcopy reveals multiple acetowhite lesions; biopsy of these lesions reveals vulvar intraepithelial neoplasia (VIN). What is the expected course of this patient's condition?

(A) Spontaneous regression without treatment is very common in this age group
(B) Progression of untreated disease in this patient's age group may be as high as 100%
(C) Treatment with topical 5-fluorouracil (5-FU) and Imiquimod is as effective as surgical resection
(D) Post-treatment recurrence rates are as high as 60%

The answer is B: **Progression of untreated disease in this patient's age group may be as high as 100%.** Though spontaneous regression of VIN may occur in women younger than 40, in the 40+ age group the risk of progression of untreated disease to invasive vulvar cancer is as high as 100%. Conservative treatment with 5-FU and Imiquimod may be used to preserve vulvar anatomy; however, effectiveness is much lower than with surgical resection (40% to 75%). The risk of recurrence of disease following treatment is around 30%.

---

10 A 26-year-old G0P0 with a history of vulvar condylomata presents to your office complaining of "a yeast infection that won't go away" despite treatment with topical antifungals. She is obese (body mass index [BMI] 31), smokes half a pack of cigarettes daily, and takes lisinopril/hydrochlorothiazide for moderate hypertension. On examination, she is found to have multifocal vulvar lesions; biopsy reveals vulvar intraepithelial neoplasia (VIN) with moderate dysplasia (VIN II). Which of the following is a risk factor for VIN?

(A) Nulliparity
(B) History of vulvar condylomata
(C) Obesity
(D) Cigarette smoking
(E) Hypertension

The answer is D: **Cigarette smoking.** Any patient with vulvar pruritus that does not respond to topical antifungals should be carefully examined for potential malignant lesions. This young woman's vulvar neoplasia is almost certainly correlated with human papillomavirus (HPV) infection. However, while vulvar condylomata (genital warts) are caused by HPV, they are usually associated with the low-risk serotypes 6 and 11, whereas VIN is most commonly associated with types 16 and 18. Cigarette smoking is an independent risk factor for VIN; this is thought to be due to an enhancing effect of chemicals contained in cigarette smoke upon HPV serotypes 16 and 18. Nulliparity, obesity, and hypertension have not been shown to be associated with increased risk of vulvar neoplasias.

---

11 A 43-year-old otherwise healthy patient undergoes wide local excision of a vulvar intraepithelial neoplasia (VIN). What follow-up surveillance is necessary for this patient?

- **(A)** Pap smears every 6 months for 2 years and then annually after that
- **(B)** Examination by a gynecologist every 6 months for 2 years and then annually after that
- **(C)** Biopsy of excisional margins every 6 months for 2 years and then annually after that
- **(D)** Colposcopy of the entire genital tract every 6 months for 2 years and then annually after that
- **(E)** Human papillomavirus (HPV) testing every 6 months for 2 years and then annually after that

The answer is D: Colposcopy of the entire genital tract every 6 months for 2 years and then annually after that. At least one-third of women who undergo wide local excision for VIN will have recurrence of their disease somewhere along the genital tract, so aggressive follow-up surveillance with colposcopy of the entire genital tract (not just around the previous site) is imperative.

---

12 A 54-year-old G3P2102 presents to your office for the first time with a chief complaint of "feminine itching." She has not had a gynecologic examination since the birth of her last child 25 years ago and underwent menopause 3 years ago. She says that she has had significant pruritus "for years," occasionally accompanied by cracking and bleeding of the affected area. She is clearly nervous, saying she has not sought treatment for this issue sooner because she is afraid that something is "really wrong." On examination, a single 3-cm lobular mass is noted on the right labia majora. Careful examination also reveals an enlarged, painless right inguinal lymph node. The patient denies any recent weight loss, pain, or changes in bowel or bladder habits. Surgical staging confirms that this mass is squamous cell carcinoma with unilateral nodal involvement. What is the recommended course of treatment?

(A) Wide radical local excision with ipsilateral inguinal lymph node dissection
(B) Modified radical vulvectomy with bilateral inguinal lymph node dissection
(C) Radical vulvectomy, bilateral inguinal lymph node dissection, and pelvic exenteration

The answer is C: Radical vulvectomy, bilateral inguinal lymph node dissection, and pelvic exenteration. A 3-cm vulvar lesion with ipsilateral inguinal lymph node involvement and no evidence of metastasis is consistent with stage III disease. Recommended treatment for stage III and stage IV squamous cell carcinoma of the vulva is radical vulvectomy, bilateral inguinal–femoral lymph node dissection, and pelvic exenteration. Modified radical vulvectomy with bilateral inguinal lymph node dissection is the recommended treatment for stage II disease, and wide radical local excision with ipsilateral inguinal node dissection is the treatment for stage I. Neither of these options would be appropriate in this case given the presence of nodal metastasis.

---

13 A 28-year-old, G1P0, presents to the emergency department with hemoptysis. She reports that she has had increasing cough and shortness of breath over the past 8 weeks and that she coughed up a dime-sized blood clot this morning. On review of systems, the patient endorses heavy and irregular vaginal bleeding. She says that she had a spontaneous abortion 6 months ago and that she started having increasingly irregular and heavy periods about 4 months ago. On examination, her uterus is enlarged to 12-week size. Serum β-hCG is elevated, hemoglobin is 10 mg/dL, and chest X-ray reveals two dense areas in her lungs, one in the right upper lobe and one in the left lower lobe. Which of the following is the most likely diagnosis?

(A) Missed abortion
(B) Incomplete abortion
(C) Choriocarcinoma
(D) Molar pregnancy
(E) Ectopic pregnancy

The answer is C: Choriocarcinoma. This woman's presentation is concerning for choriocarcinoma metastatic to the lungs. Choriocarcinoma is a malignant tumor that can arise in the uterus after any pregnancy. Approximately half of the choriocarcinomas occur after molar pregnancies, one-quarter after normal term pregnancies and one-quarter after abortion (spontaneous or therapeutic) and ectopic pregnancies. The most common presentation is heavy and irregular vaginal bleeding, and many patients present with the signs of metastatic disease. The most common metastatic locations include the lung and the central nervous system, but choriocarcinoma is notorious for metastasizing anywhere.

14 A 69-year-old woman presents to her gynecologist complaining of vulvar itching for the past 3 months. She was prescribed a topical antifungal cream by her primary care provider 1 month ago, but did not experience any relief. Examination reveals a 6-cm red, raised lesion with sharp borders and small pale eczematous islands over the vulva and inner thigh. What is the next step in the management of this patient?

(A) Prescribe single-dose oral fluconazole
(B) Prescribe oral valacyclovir
(C) Prescribe oral doxycycline and administer intramuscular ceftriaxone
(D) Prescribe hydrocortisone cream
(E) Perform a biopsy of the lesion

The answer is E: Perform a biopsy of the lesion. This patient has a classic presentation of extramammary Paget disease, a rare intraepithelial adenocarcinoma of the vulva. The most common presentation is prolonged vulvar itching in a woman over the age of 60, and lesions are often described as "velvety red." Furthermore, any pruritic vulvar lesion that does not respond to antifungal treatment (especially in a postmenopausal woman) is suspicious for malignancy and should be biopsied. Twenty percent of patients with biopsy-confirmed Paget disease will have coexistent invasive adenocarcinoma. In the absence of invasive disease, wide local excision is the appropriate management.

15 A 46-year-old asymptomatic patient with known human papillomavirus (HPV) 18 infection has had three Pap smears in the past year that revealed high-grade squamous intraepithelial lesions (HGSILs). However, multiple cervical biopsies have failed to show any evidence of neoplasia. Which of the following conditions is most likely to account for these findings?

(A) Ovarian neoplasm
(B) Endometrial neoplasm
(C) Vaginal neoplasm
(D) Occult cervical neoplasm
(E) Chronic HPV infection

The answer is C: Vaginal neoplasm. A patient with multiple abnormal Pap smears and multiple negative cervical biopsies should raise suspicion for vaginal neoplasm. Endometrial neoplasm would be suggested if there were abnormal glandular cells on Pap smear, and ovarian neoplasm is unlikely to be detected at all on Pap smear. Chronic high-risk HPV infection puts this patient at risk for cervical, vaginal, and vulvar neoplasia. This patient should have thorough examination and colposcopy of the vagina with biopsies of any suspicious lesions.

16 A 58-year-old woman with the history of polycystic ovary syndrome presents to her family physician for heavy postmenopausal bleeding for the last week. Speculum examination reveals dark blood in the vaginal vault with a normal-appearing cervix. Bimanual examination reveals a 9-week-sized uterus with no adnexal masses. Rectovaginal examination reveals no masses in the rectovaginal cul-de-sac. An in-office endometrial biopsy is performed and sent for pathology. After histologic grade, what is the second most important prognostic factor for endometrial carcinoma?

(A) Extent of uterine tube involvement
(B) Depth of myometrial invasion
(C) Location of lymph node metastases
(D) Involvement of bladder or bowel

The answer is B: Depth of myometrial invasion. Prognosis for endometrial carcinoma is based first on histologic grade and then on depth of myometrial involvement. Grade 1 is well differentiated, grade 2 is moderately differentiated, and grade 3 is poorly differentiated. Most patients have grade 1 or 2 lesions at the time of diagnosis. Thus, a patient with a grade 1 lesion limited to the endometrium has a significantly better prognosis than a patient with a grade 3 lesion with myometrial involvement.

17 A 67-year-old P0, obese woman with a 40-pack-year history presents to her gynecologist for daily postmenopausal bleeding for the last 5 months. She reports menses onset at age 11 and menopause at age 54. She has had no abnormal Pap smears and reports negative human papillomavirus (HPV) testing. Which of the following is thought to be protective against endometrial cancer?

(A) Nulliparity
(B) Obesity
(C) Smoking
(D) Early menarche
(E) Late menopause
(F) Negative Pap/HPV history

The answer is C: Smoking. Smoking is thought to be protective against endometrial cancer by purportedly increasing the rate of estrogen metabolism in the liver through the cytochrome P450 system. All of the other options are risk factors for the development of endometrial hyperplasia and endometrial cancer, due to their effects of prolonged estrogen exposure or increased levels of estrogen exposure.

18 A 54-year-old P0 woman presents to her internist for a checkup for her type 2 diabetes mellitus. Her blood glucose has been well controlled on metformin alone. However, she reports new onset of light irregular vaginal bleeding for the last several weeks. She denies dysmenorrhea or dyspareunia. She reports menarche at age 15, menopause at age 49, and no history of using hormone replacement therapy. She has been widowed since age 50 and recently met a man with whom she has become sexually active for the last month. What is the most likely cause of her postmenopausal bleeding?

(A) Endometrial atrophy
(B) Endometrial cancer
(C) Endometrial polyps
(D) Endometrial hyperplasia

The answer is A: Endometrial atrophy. The most common cause of postmenopausal bleeding is atrophy, the natural progression of the endometrial lining thinning after menopause. However, patients who present with postmenopausal bleeding must be evaluated for other causes.

19 A 59-year-old G4P1102 woman with a BMI of 32 and a history of irritable bowel syndrome presents to her internist with complaints of dull, nonradiating pain in her right lower quadrant that has been occurring intermittently and irregularly over the last few weeks. She reports frequent bloating with flatus and diarrhea alternating with constipation, which are lifelong symptoms. She also reports decreased appetite the past several months and unintentional weight loss. She denies fevers, chills, nausea, or vomiting. Which of the following symptoms is not typically associated with ovarian cancer?

(A) Early satiety
(B) Urinary frequency
(C) Pelvic pain
(D) Dyspareunia

The answer is C: Pelvic pain. Pelvic pain is not strongly associated with ovarian cancer. Symptoms associated with ovarian cancer are nonspecific and include bloating, early satiety, anorexia, unintentional weight loss, fatigue, constipation, urinary frequency, dyspareunia, and irregular menstrual bleeding. Since symptoms are usually nonspecific, most patients diagnosed with ovarian cancer are found to have stage III or stage IV ovarian cancer at the time of diagnosis.

20 A 57-year-old woman presents to her internist for her annual examination and reports persistent spotting for the past 3 months. She reports menopause at age 51 with no history of hormone replacement therapy. She had a cold-knife cone biopsy for an abnormal Pap several years ago, with normal Pap smears since that time. An in-office endometrial biopsy is unsuccessful due to cervical stenosis, and the patient is subsequently consented for a dilation and curettage in the operating room. What serum tumor marker may help predict this patient's response to future treatment if endometrial carcinoma is diagnosed?

(A) CA 19-9
(B) CEA
(C) CA-125
(D) HE4

The answer is C: CA-125. All of the options are tumor markers associated with ovarian cancer. However, of these tumor markers, only CA-125 is known to be frequently elevated in women with advanced-stage uterine cancer.

21 A 37-year-old G1P0 Chinese exchange student presents 9 weeks after her last normal menstrual period to the emergency room. Her blood pressure on arrival was 205/115 mmHg, and she is in a postictal state. A pregnancy test is positive with a qualitative β-hCG of 1,500,000 mIU. Her uterus is of 15-week size, and a snowstorm pattern without evidence of gestational sac is noted on pelvic ultrasound. Such a presentation will most frequently be associated with:

(A) Abruption placenta
(B) Aneurysm
(C) Chronic glomerulonephritis
(D) Molar pregnancy
(E) Pregnancy-induced hypertension

The answer is D: Molar pregnancy. Based on her age and ethnicity, this patient is at an increased risk of a molar pregnancy. She most likely had an eclamptic seizure. The treatment for her condition after control of the blood pressure and seizure prophylaxis is a dilation and curettage to remove the products of conception. She is at high risk for hemorrhage during the procedure. Blood products and uterotonics should be readily available. In addition, due to the high hCG levels, this patient with gestational trophoblastic disease (GTD) is at risk for invasive mole, choriocarcinoma, and placental site trophoblastic tumor and should be followed by a center that monitors and treats GTD. She is also at risk for persistent GTD and should be followed until the hCG reaches zero.

Her sonogram is consistent with a complete molar pregnancy, of which about 5% of women progress to preeclampsia or eclampsia. It is recommended that suction curettage be used rather than sharp curettage in order to limit the risk of vascular spread.

---

22 A 25-year-old G3P2103 who underwent a postpartum tubal ligation 6 weeks ago has a Pap smear reported as an high-grade squamous intraepithelial lesion (HGSIL). At the time of her postpartum examination, no visible lesions were noted on the cervix. The next step in her management should be

(A) Cold-knife cone biopsy
(B) Colposcopically directed biopsies
(C) Hysterectomy
(D) Laser therapy
(E) Local chemotherapy

The answer is B: Colposcopically directed biopsies. In addition, an endocervical curettage should be considered. A cold-knife cone and loop electrical excision procedure (LEEP) or laser cone are performed when there is a mismatch between the Pap smear and colposcopically directed biopsies. In extreme cases, a 25-year-old patient might require a hysterectomy for treatment, but this patient's workup and prognosis are far removed from such extreme interventions. Just because she has had a BTL does not make a hysterectomy a more acceptable procedure.

---

23 A 35-year-old G2P1 presents with scant first-trimester bleeding. An ultrasound report describes an empty gestational sac. Which of the following statements is correct regarding this presentation?

(A) It is caused by an abnormality of the placenta
(B) It is the result of a genetic error
(C) The quantitative β-hCG is likely to be unusually low
(D) It is most often due to paternal causes
(E) The risk of severe hemorrhage is increased

The answer is B: It is the result of a genetic error. The quantitative β-hCG is likely to be unusually low. The remainder of the responses refer to molar pregnancy, which typically presents with sonographic findings of a snowstorm pattern. In cases of molar pregnancy, the β-hCG is typically very elevated above what would be expected for the same gestation of a normal pregnancy, there is an increased risk of hemorrhage, and the culprits for this placental condition are paternal X chromosomes.

24 A 24-year-old G0 presents to the resident clinic as a referral from the Student Health Service with an atypical squamous cells of undetermined significance (ASCUS) Pap. She had a Pap about 2 to 3 years ago, and it

was normal. She became sexually active at age 17 and has had five lifetime partners. She and her male partner have been together for over a year. She started having periods at age 13 and has regular cycles on her own. Her last period was 1 week ago on oral contraceptives. She has a history of herpes simplex virus well controlled with daily acyclovir. Her physical examination is normal. What is the next step?

(A) Repeat the Pap
(B) Get high-risk human papillomavirus (HPV) typing
(C) Get low-risk HPV typing
(D) Perform colposcopy
(E) Perform a conization

The answer is B: **Get high-risk human papillomavirus (HPV) typing.** ASCUS Pap is best followed up with high-risk HPV typing. If it is negative, then the Pap is handled as normal and screening repeated in 3 years. If high-risk HPV typing is positive, one would proceed to colposcopy. There is no indication for low-risk HPV typing.

---

25 You are seeing a 21-year-old white woman in the Student Health Clinic for follow-up of an abnormal Pap. She became sexually active at age 17 and has had four lifetime partners, but has been with her current partner for over a year. They initially used condoms with the oral contraceptive pills (OCPs), but they were both tested for sexually transmitted diseases (STDs) at the Student Health Clinic and all was negative almost a year ago. She returned last month for her first Pap and was told it was abnormal. She has never had an STD but has not received the Gardasil vaccine. Her cytology report reveals atypical squamous cells of undetermined significance (ASCUS). What is the next step?

(A) Repeat the Pap in 1 month
(B) Proceed with colposcopy
(C) Obtain high-risk human papillomavirus (HPV) typing
(D) Perform a loop electrical excision procedure (LEEP)
(E) Counsel on hysterectomy

The answer is C: **Obtain high-risk human papillomavirus (HPV) typing.** If high-risk HPV typing is negative, we can repeat the Pap in 3 years. If it is positive, we can proceed with colposcopy. Colposcopy is not recommended for ASCUS without + high-risk HPV testing. A LEEP and hysterectomy would be overly aggressive and not indicated.

---

26 You are seeing a patient with your community preceptor who is a 24-year-old black woman G1P1001 on Depo-Provera. Your preceptor is about to call her with the results of her Pap. It showed low-grade squamous intraepithelial lesion (LGSIL). Your preceptor wants to know what you would recommend as follow-up. You review her history. The patient had a normal Pap 2 years ago when she was pregnant and has never had an STD. She became sexually active at age 16 and has had four lifetime partners but has been married for about 2 years. She has not had Gardasil. She smoked a pack of cigarettes per day until her pregnancy but has not smoked since. What would you recommend?

(A) Repeat Pap immediately
(B) Gardasil and repeat Pap in 1 year
(C) Repeat Pap in 1 year
(D) Gardasil and repeat Pap in 6 weeks
(E) Colposcopy immediately

The answer is B: Gardasil and repeat Pap in 1 year. Gardasil is beneficial even after exposure to human papillomavirus (HPV). An LGSIL Pap is generally repeated in 1 year. If it is still LGSIL or higher, one would proceed with colposcopy.

---

27 You are in the resident clinic seeing a patient for follow-up of an abnormal Pap showing high-grade squamous intraepithelial lesion (HGSIL). The patient is a 25-year-old white woman G3P0212 last menstrual period (LMP) 2 week's ago on oral contraceptive pills (OCPs). She became sexually active at 16 and has had eight partners including two in the past year. She has a history of chlamydia around age 18. She has recurrent genital herpes that she controls with acyclovir. What is the next step in the evaluation of this patient?

(A) Repeat Pap now
(B) Repeat Pap in 1 year
(C) Colposcopy and biopsies
(D) High-risk human papillomavirus (HPV) typing
(E) Hysterectomy

The answer is C: Colposcopy and biopsies. An HGSIL Pap does not need repeating—it warrants immediate further investigation into colposcopy. HPV typing adds no value and would not change your plan.

---

28 You are assisting in the Resident Colposcopy Clinic. The resident asks you to establish a plan for a 25-year-old Latin woman G0 with regular menses on NuvaRing. She became sexually active at age 16 and has had four lifetime partners. She has been with her present partner about 6 months. She has used oral contraceptive pills (OCPs) and NuvaRing but has not used condoms since her teens. She had all normal Paps until a month ago when her Pap was high-grade squamous intraepithelial lesion (HGSIL). You look in the colposcope and see the view in *Figure 13-2*. Where should biopsies be performed?

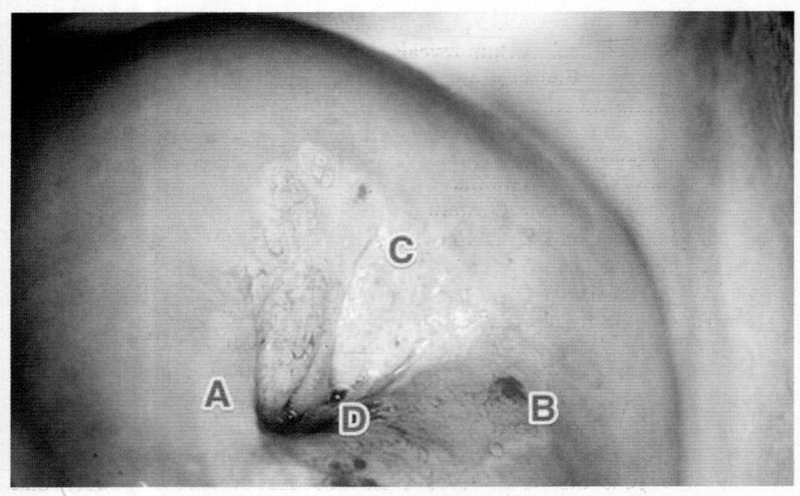

Figure 13-2

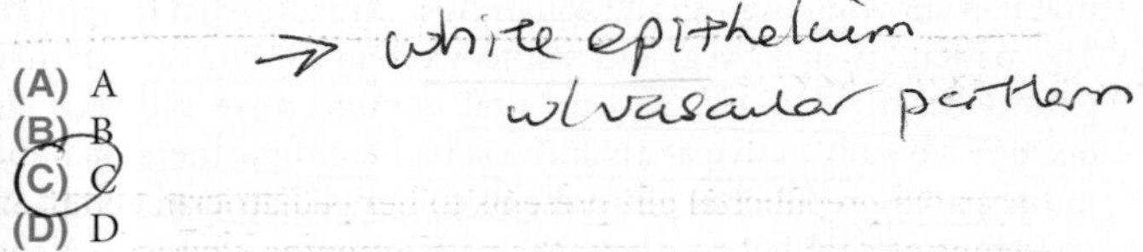

(A) A
(B) B
(C) C
(D) D

The answer is C: C. The white epithelium with vascular pattern is the most ominous looking area on this cervix.

29 You see the patient in Question 28 for the results of her colposcopic biopsies. They reveal cervical intraepithelial neoplasia II–III (moderate-to-severe dysplasia). What is the next step?

(A) Repeat Paps every 6 months
(B) Loop electrical excision procedure (LEEP)
(C) Hysterectomy
(D) Endometrial biopsy
(E) Endometrial ablation

The answer is B: Loop electrical excision procedure (LEEP). The LEEP offers the best chance for cure while maintaining fertility. Endometrial biopsy and ablation do not address the problem. The former would not add to the diagnostic decision making, and the latter would not improve treatment.

30 A 7-year-old girl presents to her pediatrician with her parents who are concerned about her early sexual development. She is developing breasts, axillary hair, and pubic hair, and they are noticing body odor. A thorough clinical workup reveals the child has an irregular, echogenic, thickly septated ovarian mass on her left ovary. What type of tumor is responsible for this child's clinical presentation?

(A) Dysgerminoma
(B) Embryonal carcinoma
(C) Sertoli-Leydig cell tumor
(D) Endodermal sinus tumor
(E) Granulosa-theca cell tumor

The answer is E: Granulosa-theca cell tumor. Granulosa cell tumors are the most common type of ovarian gonadal stromal cell tumor. These are functional tumors that produce estrogen and inhibin. Clinically, these tumors are associated with symptoms that result from hyperestrogenism. In a prepubertal girl, excess estrogen will cause isosexual precocious puberty resulting in early development of secondary sexual characteristics. Sertoli-Leydig cell tumors produce androgens and would result in heterosexual precocious puberty and cause this child to have clinical signs of virilization. Dysgerminomas are germ cell tumors that may produce lactate dehydrogenase (LDH) or hCG. Endodermal sinus tumors may produce α-fetoprotein (AFP). Embryonal carcinoma may produce AFP or hCG.

---

31 A 9-year-old prepubertal girl presents to her pediatrician complaining of worsening abdominal pain over the past 3 months. Physical examination demonstrates Tanner stage I development and right lower quadrant tenderness. CT scan demonstrates a complex right-sided ovarian mass, and she undergoes an exploratory laparoscopy to remove the mass. The resulting pathology reveals chaotically arranged cartilaginous, dermal, and neural tissue. This is consistent with which of the following tumor types?

(A) Dysgerminoma
(B) Mature teratoma
(C) Immature teratoma
(D) Embryonal carcinoma
(E) Endodermal sinus tumor

The answer is C: Immature teratoma. All of the tumors listed represent the types of ovarian germ cell tumors. Teratomas are the most common type of ovarian germ cell tumor, and they are classified as benign or malignant based on their histologic components. Immature teratomas are malignant tumors composed of endoderm, mesoderm, and ectoderm. The presence of neural tissue makes this an immature teratoma. Mature teratomas contain tissue from all three germ layers; however, they are benign and do not have neural components. Dysgerminomas, embryonal carcinomas, and endodermal sinus tumors do not contain the variety of tissue types seen in teratomas.

---

32 A 67-year-old woman presents with abdominal discomfort and bloating, 30-lb weight loss, decreased appetite, and fatigue. Vital signs are stable. Physical examination demonstrates a menopausal woman with a large left adnexal mass detected on bimanual examination. You perform a transvaginal ultrasound that shows an 8-cm complex mass with solid and cystic components, thick irregular septations, and an irregular surface. Based on your clinical assumptions, what is the most likely course of management for this patient?

(A) Chemotherapy
(B) Abdominal exploration with surgical resection
(C) Neoadjuvant chemotherapy, abdominal exploration, and surgical resection
(D) Abdominal exploration with surgical resection followed by chemotherapy
(E) Abdominal exploration with surgical resection followed by radiation

The answer is D: Abdominal exploration with surgical resection followed by chemotherapy. This patient presents with symptoms and clinical findings suspicious for advanced-stage ovarian cancer. Prior to surgery, this patient would likely undergo further radiologic studies to assess the extent of disease. Surgery should be the initial step to establish a histologic diagnosis and determine appropriate staging. Since this patient is menopausal, it is recommended to undergo a total hysterectomy with bilateral salpingo-oophorectomy along with removal of the suspicious mass. Chemotherapy following surgical debulking of the tumor is recommended for nearly all ovarian cancer patients. Neoadjuvant therapy is only used in those with very advanced-stage cancer or those who may not be able to tolerate surgical intervention. Radiation is not nearly as effective as chemotherapy and is rarely used in the treatment of ovarian cancer.

---

33 A 77-year-old woman with a history of cancer 10 years ago presents to your clinic complaining of abdominal discomfort, bloating, and weight loss. Symptoms have been increasing in severity for about 3 months. On physical examination, her abdomen is soft with mild lower abdominal tenderness. On pelvic examination, you palpate masses bilaterally. Assuming the masses are cancer, what is the most likely primary source of the tumors?

(A) Bone
(B) Liver
(C) Breast
(D) Gastrointestinal tract
(E) Lymph nodes

The answer is D: Gastrointestinal tract. Metastatic cancer to the ovary is responsible for 5% to 10% of all ovarian cancers. Krukenberg tumor is the name given to an ovarian tumor that is metastatic from another site. These tumors are usually infiltrative, mucinous, and bilateral. Out of the potential sources, cancer of the gastrointestinal tract is responsible for 30% to 40% of metastatic cancer to the ovary. Breast is the second most common source. Gynecologic cancers can also metastasize to the ovary.

---

34 A 26-year-old G2P2 presents for her annual gynecologic examination and would like to discuss her risk of ovarian cancer. Menarche occurred at age 14. She used oral contraceptive pills (OCPs) for 3 years prior to the birth of her first child when she was 23. She breastfed both of her children for 1 year each. Her mother is 46 and currently is undergoing chemotherapy for ovarian cancer, and she had a maternal aunt who passed away in her 80s from breast cancer. What is this woman's greatest potential risk factor for developing ovarian cancer?

(A) BRCA (breast cancer gene) mutation
(B) Hereditary nonpolyposis colorectal cancer (HNPCC) mutation
(C) Family history
(D) Early menarche
(E) Late childbearing

The answer is A: BRCA mutation. This woman has a significant family history with a first-degree relative with ovarian cancer and a second-degree relative with breast cancer. This family history may indicate a need for BRCA genetic testing which, if positive, is associated with up to a 60% lifetime risk for developing breast cancer. An HNPCC mutation is associated with various types of cancer, including ovarian but the associated risk is much less than with the BRCA mutation. A positive family history in a first-degree relative is associated with a 5% lifetime risk of developing cancer. Nulliparity is associated with increased risk of ovarian cancer, but late childbearing is not. Early menarche is associated with an increased risk of ovarian cancer, but this patient did not start menarche at an early age.

---

35 A 58-year-old white woman recently completed surgery and chemotherapy for stage III ovarian cancer. She presents to your office today to discuss how she will be monitored for a recurrence. In addition to a complete physical examination, you recommend which of the following laboratory or radiographic studies to check for recurrence?

(A) CT scan
(B) Positron emission tomography (PET) scan
(C) Pelvic ultrasound
(D) CEA testing
(E) CA-125 testing

The answer is E: CA-125 testing. CA-125 testing every 3 months along with a complete physical examination is the best way to monitor for a recurrence. CA-125 is most useful for post-treatment surveillance when it was elevated preoperatively. The combination of physical examination and CA-125 testing has been shown to detect recurrent disease in 90% of patients. CT scans, PET scans, and pelvic ultrasounds may be useful for detecting recurrences in certain patients, but these are not standard follow-up tests for all ovarian cancer patients.

---

36 A 36-year-old G0 presents to your clinic complaining of abnormal periods, acne, thinning hair on her scalp, and increased coarse hair on her face, abdomen, and thighs. She has no significant past medical history. She denies any history of abnormal pelvic examinations or Pap smears. She has taken oral contraceptive pills (OCPs) for 10 years. In addition to her complaints, on physical examination, you note vaginal atrophy and you palpate a mass in the right adnexa. What is the most likely cause of her complaints?

(A) Adrenal tumor
(B) Dysgerminoma
(C) Granulosa cell tumor
(D) Serous cystadenocarcinoma
(E) Sertoli-Leydig cell tumor

The answer is E: Sertoli-Leydig cell tumor. Sertoli-Leydig cell tumors are functional gonadal stromal tumors that account for less than 1% of ovarian cancers. These tumors produce hormones such as testosterone and androstenedione. Clinically, the androgens produced by these tumors result in female masculinization and in severe cases virilization. Granulosa cell tumors are also hormone-producing ovarian cancers; however, they produce estrogen that can cause precocious puberty in a prepubertal girl. Dysgerminomas are germ cell tumors that may produce lactate dehydrogenase (LDH) and estradiol, but not androgens. An adrenal tumor can produce androgens; however, an ovarian tumor is more consistent with this woman's physical examination finding of an adnexal mass. Serous cystadenocarcinoma is the most common type of ovarian cancer but would not result in these clinical findings as these tumors do not produce hormones.

---

37 A 28-year-old G2P1001 at 15 week's gestation returns to your clinic to discuss her lab results from her new obstetric visit. You inform her that all of her laboratory results were within normal limits with the exception that her Pap smear cytology was reported at low-grade squamous intraepithelial lesion (LGSIL). After further discussion, she tells you she has had previous abnormal Pap smears in the past but has never had further workup done. According to the current standard of care, what is the preferred approach in monitoring her cervical dysplasia?

(A) No further workup until postpartum period
(B) Repeat Pap smear at 32 week's gestation
(C) Monitor for changes in pelvic examination or symptoms of irregular spotting at monthly obstetric exams
(D) Colposcopy during this pregnancy

The answer is D: Colposcopy during this pregnancy. While it is acceptable to wait until the postpartum period for further workup of a woman with LGSIL, in the non-adolescent woman it is preferred to do a colposcopy during the pregnancy. Repeating a Pap smear later in the pregnancy would not change the guideline recommendations, and cytology changes are not monitored by physical examination findings. Note that the goal of colposcopy during pregnancy is to rule out cancer; therefore, endocervical curettage and aggressive biopsies are avoided unless truly suspicious lesions are identified.

---

38 A 27-year-old G4P3013 returns to your clinic to follow up on the results of her annual Pap smear. She has had a full annual examination including Pap smear since the age of 21 and has never had abnormal cervical cytology. Her STD screening at her last examination was normal. The cytology of her Pap smear showed high-grade squamous intraepithelial lesion (HGSIL). You discuss the management options to the patient, and she decides to have a colposcopy. The biopsy results of the colposcopy you perform are insufficient to give a histology report. Which of the following options is the next best step in management for this patient?

(A) Repeat Pap smear at 6-month intervals for a year
(B) Repeat colposcopy to obtain better sample
(C) Perform diagnostic excisional procedure such as Loop electrical excision procedure (LEEP)
(D) Request that the lab repeats their tests on the biopsy samples given

The answer is C: Perform diagnostic excisional procedure such as Loop electrical excision procedure (LEEP). When a colposcopy following HGSIL is unsatisfactory, current guidelines recommend going to an excisional procedure. The other options are not recommended without a satisfactory colposcopy.

39 A 26-year-old G0 presents to your clinic for follow-up on her Pap smear results. Her menses occur at 34-day intervals and last approximately 4 days. She denies any irregular spotting or dyspareunia. The patient reports coitarche at age 15. The cytology results from the Pap smear show low-grade squamous intraepithelial lesion (LGSIL). She previously had not had any abnormal Pap smears and has no history of STDs. What is the next best step in management?

(A) Repeat Pap smear in 6 months, biopsy if abnormal at that time
(B) Repeat Pap in 12 months
(C) Colposcopy with biopsy
(D) Loop electrical excision procedure (LEEP)
(E) Cold-knife cone

The answer is B: Repeat Pap in 12 months. Repeat Pap in 1 year is recommended. If repeat Pap is normal, return to routine screening, otherwise proceed with colposcopy.

---

40 A 27-year-old G4P3013 returns to your clinic to follow up on the results of her annual Pap smear. She has had a regular annual examinations including Pap smear since the age of 19 and has never had abnormal cervical cytology. The patient reports having had chlamydia twice in her life and was treated both times. Her STD screening at her last examination was normal. The cytology of her Pap smear showed atypical squamous cells of undetermined significance (ASCUS). What are the treatment options for this patient?

(A) Repeat Pap smear at 6 months, if negative return to annual screening
(B) Repeat Pap smear at 6 and 12 months, if both negatives return to annual screening
(C) Proceed with colposcopy
(D) High-risk human papillomavirus (HPV) testing

The answer is D: High-risk human papillomavirus (HPV) testing. HPV testing or repeat Pap in 1 year is recommended. If HPV testing or repeat Pap is normal, return to routine screening, otherwise proceed with colposcopy.

CHAPTER

14

Menopause

1 A 52-year-old, G4P4004, presents for an annual gynecologic examination. She had four vaginal deliveries, each one greater than 4,000 g. Her last delivery was 18 years ago. She had a third-degree laceration that was repaired without incident. Currently she denies fecal incontinence. She also denies the loss of urine with coughing. Her last menstrual period was 11 months ago.

While asking about exercise, she mentions that she has recently decreased her athletic activity despite being an avid tennis player in the past. Her activity has been limited due to a sensation like there is a soft ball between her legs after exercising for more than an hour.

While performing a speculum examination that retracts the posterior vaginal wall, the patient bears down and a bulge is noted in the anterior vaginal wall. What is the diagnosis?

(A) Cystocele
(B) Enterocele
(C) Rectocele
(D) Urethrocele urethra
(E) Vaginal vault prolapse after hysterectomy

The answer is A: Cystocele. A cystocele occurs when the supportive tissue between the bladder and the vagina weakens and the bladder herniates into the vagina. Symptoms determine the need for treatment of this condition. An enterocele is a herniation of intestines into the vagina. A rectocele is the herniation of the rectum into the vagina. An urethrocele occurs when the tissue surrounding the urethra sags downward into the vagina. Vaginal vault prolapse occurs after a hysterectomy. It is defined by the International Continence Society as descent of the vaginal cuff and occurs when the upper vagina bulges into or outside the vagina.

2 A 73-year-old woman presents with severe vaginal dryness and burning. She had taken estrogen orally until 3 years ago when her physician made her stop because of worries about increasing her risk of heart attacks. Initially she tolerated the change well but began progressively having more and more vaginal irritation, especially with intercourse. You note the thinned tissue around the urethra and at the introitus. No discharge is noted externally. There is no evidence of leukoplakia.

Upon speculum examination, you note atrophic vaginal epithelium with scant thin clear vaginal secretion. Measurement of pH is 6.0. Whiff test is negative. KOH prep is negative.

What will you find on her wet mount?

(A) Columnar cells
(B) Parabasal cells
(C) Ciliated cells
(D) Clue cells
(E) Pseudohyphae

The answer is B: Parabasal cells. These cells are prevalent in women with decreased estrogen such as postmenopausal women who are not on estrogen therapy. They are also shown to be present in the postpartum period and in lactating women. Columnar cells are found most commonly in the endocervix and in areas of metaplasia. Ciliated cells are more common in the fallopian tubes. Clue cells are found in bacterial vaginosis. While the pH of the menopausal vagina is elevated to greater than 5, the negative whiff test and gradual onset of symptoms after stopping estrogen therapy make hypoestrogenism the most likely source of this patient's complaint. The discharge is not characteristic of candidiasis and the pH is too high in addition to a negative KOH prep.

3 A 43-year-old woman whose last menstrual period (LMP) was 2 weeks ago complains of decreased libido over the past 6 months. During that time, she has noticed no increase in vaginal dryness except when her husband tries to initiate sex. It has gotten so bad that her husband of 16 years complains constantly. She is concerned that he may have an affair if things do not change.

The trouble began about 8 months ago when he did not make tenure and has been unable to find a new position as a philosophy professor. She was promoted a year ago and her job requires long hours. She typically rises at 5 am each weekday to put in 12-hour days. Since her husband is very "traditional," she is expected to cook dinner and wash the dishes and clothes in the evenings. She resents having to perform these functions since she is the primary breadwinner and her unemployed spouse refuses to help out. Her husband typically attempts to initiate sex when she finally gets to bed after 10 pm. But they only have sex one to two times a month and she has stopped having orgasms with him but has no problem attaining orgasm with masturbation.

What is the most likely explanation for this patient's decreased libido?

(A) The contextual nature of female sexual response
(B) Premature menopause with atrophy
(C) The linear nature of female sexual response
(D) An underlying metabolic condition such as diabetes
(E) A stress reaction culminating in anorgasmia

The answer is A: **The contextual nature of the female sexual response.** The nonlinear model of female sexual response acknowledges that female sexual functioning proceeds in a more complex and circuitous manner than male sexual functioning as described by Masters and Johnson. Furthermore, female functioning is dramatically and significantly affected by numerous psychosocial issues. This is in contradistinction to a more linear biologic model that presumes men and women respond in the same manner. There is no evidence she has experienced menopause; her vaginal dryness is more likely related to lack of arousal. She is capable of having orgasms as indicated by successful masturbation.

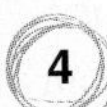

4 A 42-year-old woman, G7P5207, presents for a routine annual examination. Until 4 months ago, her menses were normal. Over the past 3 months she has not had a period and has noticed symptoms associated with "the change of life." These include moodiness, vaginal dryness, difficulty sleeping through the night, occasional hot flashes, and excessive fatigue during the day. As a result, she has stopped exercising which she feels contributed to her recent 7 lb weight gain.

Past medical history reveals hypothyroidism diagnosed 5 years ago for which she takes 0.125 μg of levothyroxine. Her last thyroid-stimulating hormone (TSH) level 6 months ago was 4.7. She is otherwise healthy and reports no other remarkable history. Her general physical examination is unremarkable, as are her vital signs. On pelvic examination, you note an irregular, mildly enlarged uterus.

Which of the following tests is the most appropriate?

(A) Follicle-stimulating hormone (FSH)
(B) Luteinizing hormone (LH)
(C) Pregnancy test
(D) Sonogram
(E) TSH

The answer is C: **Pregnancy test.** A qualitative β-human chorionic gonadotropin such as a urine pregnancy test should be considered in this woman who belongs to the age group of women who are most likely to have an unintended pregnancy. FSH would be appropriate to determine if the patient is entering the climacteric/menopause. A sonogram would be indicated if the pregnancy test is positive to help date the pregnancy. A sonogram would be indicated if the pregnancy test is negative to determine the cause of uterine enlargement. A TSH could be considered after determining whether or not the patient is pregnant since it has been 6 months since the level was checked and if she is pregnant, her thyroid medication may need to be titrated. There is no compelling reason to order an LH at any point in this particular patient.

---

5 A 54-year-old, G3P2012, woman with an last menstrual period (LMP) 2 years ago presents with episodes of increased sweating, palpitations, emotional lability, and a 20-lb weight loss over the past 6 months. She complains of debilitating anxiety. Vital signs are as follows: P 116 beats/min, respiration 18 breaths/min, blood pressure (BP) 138/92 mmHg. General physical examination reveals an anxious, thin middle-aged woman in no acute distress. Pelvic examination reveals a grade 1 cystocele, decreased rugae in the vagina, a 10-week irregular uterus, and a 4-cm right adnexal mass. Transvaginal ultrasound reveals the presence of hyperechoic lines and dots, regional diffuse bright echoes, and a "hair/fluid level" in the right adnexa. The most likely diagnosis leading to this patient's symptoms is:

(A) Dysgerminomas
(B) Mucinous cystadenoma
(C) Placental site tumor
(D) Serous cystadenoma
(E) Struma ovarii

The answer is E: Struma ovarii. A struma ovarii can be part of a benign cystic teratoma (dermoid). Patients present with symptoms of hyperthyroidism and an adnexal mass.

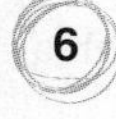

A 55-year-old white woman, G3P2103, presents to you 4 years post menopause with history of vaginal bleeding for 3 to 4 days last month. She is diabetic managed with Metformin and has well-controlled hypertension. She went through menopause without incident and was never on hormones. Her last Pap was 5 years ago and was normal. Her history is otherwise unremarkable. On examination she is in no apparent distress. She is afebrile with BP 138/82 mmHg, P 88 beats/min, body mass index (BMI) 35. Her pelvic is remarkable for moderate vaginal atrophy. Her cervix is noted to be stenotic while performing a Pap and barely allows a cytobrush. She is not bleeding and her uterus is 8-week size. Her ovaries are not palpable.

What is your next step?

(A) Perform in office endometrial biopsy
(B) Perform vaginal ultrasound
(C) Schedule dilation and curettage in hospital
(D) Schedule office hysteroscopy
(E) Schedule hysterectomy

The answer is B: Perform vaginal ultrasound. Since you have already encountered cervical stenosis while obtaining a Pap, an endometrial biopsy may prove difficult. Because transvaginal ultrasonography in postmenopausal patients with bleeding has an extremely high negative predictive value, it is a reasonable first approach. Endometrial thickness ≤4 mm requires no further workup. If the lining is >4 mm, then further evaluation is indicated in the form of endometrial biopsy or hysteroscopy.

7 Your patient is a 64-year-old, G2P2, who went through menopause around age 52 and complains of vaginal bleeding. She has a history of hypertension controlled with medication as well as diet-controlled diabetes. Her surgical history is negative. She is taking estradiol 1 mg per day.

Her vital signs are stable with a BMI of 24 and her pelvic examination is notable only for a pink, elastic vaginal mucosa, normal-appearing cervix, 6- to 8-week-sized uterus, and nonpalpable ovaries. She has no hemorrhoids.

What is this patient's greatest risk factor for endometrial hyperplasia or cancer?

(A) Hypertension
(B) Diet-controlled diabetes
(C) BMI of 24
(D) Taking estradiol
(E) Her age of 64

The answer is D: Taking estradiol. Unopposed estrogen increases the risk of endometrial hyperplasia and cancer. The addition of a progestin, either continuous or cyclic, would decrease her risk of endometrial cancer. Although obesity contributes to one's risk of endometrial cancer through peripheral conversion of androgens to estrogens in fatty tissue but her BMI of 24 does not fall into the obese category.

8 Refer to the vignette in Question 7 to answer the question. The patient admits that she was prescribed a second medication to take with her estrogen when she went through menopause. She took it only 10 days or so of each month but it made her have periods and she felt bloated so she stopped taking it about 10 years ago but has not told her doctor. She has felt great.

What medication was the patient prescribed?

(A) Tamoxifen
(B) Medroxyprogesterone
(C) Levothyroxine
(D) Methotrexate
(E) Doxycycline

The answer is B: Medroxyprogesterone. Unopposed estrogen is indicated for menopausal symptoms in a woman who has had a hysterectomy, but increases the risk of endometrial hyperplasia and cancer in a woman with intact uterus. In the latter, a progesterone or progestin is added to decrease the risk of malignancy. Medroxyprogesterone is probably the most common progestin prescribed for hormone therapy. It can be given continuously or cyclically, usually for 10 days and in the latter case, it triggers a withdrawal period.

---

9 Refer to Question 8 to answer the question. You perform an endometrial biopsy and it is benign. You contact the patient and relate the diagnosis. What is your recommendation?

(A) Continue with unopposed estrogen since the patient has proven she is not at high risk
(B) Continue estradiol but add continuous or cyclic medroxyprogesterone to decrease the risk of endometrial changes
(C) Consider stopping hormones since she is 13 years postmenopausal
(D) Consider an endometrial ablation and resuming cyclic estrogen/progesterone therapy
(E) Continue estradiol alone but perform an endometrial biopsy on a yearly basis

The answer is C: Consider stopping hormones since she is 13 years postmenopausal. Hormone replacement is indicated for menopausal symptoms and should be administered for the shortest time possible. The patient should consider stopping hormones, either by tapering or all at once. You should counsel her that she may experience menopausal symptoms but that they usually resolve in a few months. Continuing unopposed estrogen would not be recommended since it would still increase her risk of endometrial hyperplasia or cancer. Continuing hormones but adding progesterone, cyclic or continuous, would not be indicated without first discussing the effects of long-term therapy and at least discussing the discontinuation of hormones. An ablation would not be indicated prior to resumption of hormones as it would mask early changes. Yearly biopsies with continuation of unopposed estrogen would not be a next step although it may be a negotiable plan in a patient whose quality of life suffered significantly off estrogen and could not tolerate the side effects of progesterone.

CHAPTER

15

Sexuality

1 A 36-year-old, G3P3, woman presents to the office with sexual concerns. The patient is currently married and is in a monogamous relationship with her husband of 13 years. The patient has three children living at home with her husband. The patient reports that she no longer has as much sexual desire as she did when she was younger and that this has become a source of stress within her marriage. The patient states that when she does have sex she does not experience any pain but does seems to reach orgasm less often these days. The patient's current medical problems include asthma, depression, acne, and a torn meniscus for which she underwent recent knee surgery.

First-line treatment for which of the patient's medical issues is most likely to be the cause of her current sexual complaints?

(A) Asthma
(B) Depression
(C) Acne
(D) Knee surgery

SSRIs

The answer is B: Depression. A common side effect of selective serotonin reuptake inhibitor is sexual concerns. This can range from decreased libido to difficulty having orgasm. Treatments such as albuterol for asthma, antibiotics for acne, and anti-inflammatories are not likely to cause sexual dysfunction.

2 A 54-year-old, G0, woman comes to your office to discuss sexual dysfunction. The patient reports that sex is becoming progressively uncomfortable and would like to know if there is anything she can do to improve this aspect of her relationship with her husband. The patient's medical issues include fibromyalgia and difficulties with fertility. The patient's last menstrual period was 2 years ago and she now reports that she does not experience any spotting or pelvic cramping. The patient takes a daily multivitamin and denies any alcohol or tobacco use.

The patient read that testosterone can be used to treat sexual function and would like to know if it would be helpful in her case.

What group of women is most likely to benefit from testosterone?

(A) Women with polycystic ovarian syndrome
(B) Women with fibromyalgia
(C) Women who have undergone menopause
(D) Women who are postpartum

The answer is C: Women who have undergone menopause. Testosterone has been shown to be beneficial for sexual dysfunction in women who have undergone menopause either surgically or "naturally."

3 A 32-year-old, G0, woman presents to your clinic with the complaint of sexual dysfunction. The woman has recently entered her first sexual relationship and is very hesitant to discuss her problems with you today. The patient says that she has pain during intercourse and is unsure if she has ever had an orgasm. After a complete history and physical examination you find no causative underlying conditions evident.

What is the first step in addressing this patient's sexual dysfunction?

(A) Referral to a sex therapist
(B) Reassurance and giving the patient permission for sexual thoughts and attitudes
(C) Writing a prescription for the patient's partner to obtain Viagra
(D) Initiating transdermal testosterone therapy

The answer is B: Reassurance and giving the patient permission for sexual thoughts and attitudes. The initial step in the treatment of sexual dysfunction is offering permission that sexual thoughts are normal, as well as sexual practices. The next step is offering limited information regarding many aspects of sexual function, then offering specific suggestions and advice, and ultimately referral to intensive therapy.

4 A 21-year-old presents to discuss a dramatic decrease in sexual desire that she has been experiencing for many months. The patient is in a 4-year monogamous relationship with her boyfriend and this is very unusual for their relationship. The patient says the problem is causing her a great deal of distress and would like to know if there is anything that she can do to improve her issue. She is a healthy nonsmoker, and has no current or past sexually transmitted infections. She is home from college during her Christmas break for her appointment in the office.

What is the most important factor in obtaining a complete sexual history?

(A) The use of language that the patient understands
(B) The provider feeling comfortable with obtaining all aspects of the sexual history
(C) The patient feeling secure that the encounter is confidential
(D) The provider being nonjudgmental regarding sexual orientation and premarital sex

The answer is D: The provider being nonjudgmental regarding sexual orientation and premarital sex. A complete sexual history is imperative to being able to diagnose sexual dysfunction. Providers must be nonjudgmental in the context of the interview, be able to assure the confidentiality of the interview, use language that patients understand and is professional, and be comfortable with the interview.

---

5 A 33-year-old, G1P1, comes to your office to discuss a concerning sexual issue. The patient reports that she has been having worsening pain during intercourse with her husband for the last year. The patient says that it is not painful during initial insertion of the penis but during deep penetration the patient experiences excruciating sharp pain deep within her pelvis. They use condoms but she denies any sensitivity to latex. The patient says that she now is anxious about having sex because she fears having the pain and would like to know if there is something that can be done to relieve her symptoms. Pelvic examination is remarkable for tenderness and nodularity behind the cervix.

What is your next step?

(A) Course of azithromycin
(B) Trial of oral contraceptives
(C) Diagnostic laparoscopy
(D) Hysterectomy

The answer is B: Trial of oral contraceptives. Patients with painful intercourse with deep penetration may have endometriosis as the etiology of the pain. Uterosacral tenderness and nodularity would increase the probability of the diagnosis. Although diagnostic laparoscopy offers the definitive diagnosis and hysterectomy the definitive treatment, a trial of oral contraceptives, is an excellent first choice of treatment. Tenderness and nodularity should not be confused with cervical motion tenderness, the hallmark of pelvic inflammatory disease.

6 A 27-year-old, G1P1, woman comes to see you to discuss a recent decrease in sexual desire. The patient is in a 7-year monogamous sexual relationship with her husband and states that otherwise they have a great relationship. You start by discussing the four phases of the female sexual response: desire, arousal, orgasm, and resolution.

What is the most likely problem noted in evaluating sexual dysfunction?

(A) The sequence stated above is out of order
(B) There is a missing step in the sequence
(C) There is a lack of satisfaction with the sexual encounter
(D) The patient reports pain with intercourse

The answer is C: There is a lack of satisfaction with the encounter. The diagnosis of sexual dysfunction is when a patient lacks pleasure or satisfaction from the encounter. The sexual response cycle can be normal but not in the above-stated order (for example, arousal may be the first step with desire following), and even may lack one of the aspects of the cycle. Painful intercourse is a different diagnosis than sexual dysfunction, but may contribute to dysfunction given that the encounter is not likely to be satisfactory.

7 A 25-year-old, G0, patient presents to discuss pain with intercourse. The patient is currently sexually active with two male partners. The patient takes birth control regularly but does not use condoms. The patient was recently tested for common sexually transmitted diseases and was found to be negative. The patient tells you that she has had problems with painful intercourse for many years and does not recall a time that she was able to have sex without pain.

Which of the following should be included in your evaluation?

(A) Sexual abuse
(B) Hypothyroidism
(C) Cardiac disease
(D) History of stroke

The answer is A: Sexual abuse. The list of possible etiology for painful intercourse is long and includes evaluation for urinary and bladder issues, bowel problems, hypertension, vulvar skin disorders, endometriosis, and others. A complete history should be performed and sexual abuse must be considered and reviewed with each patient in an open, nonjudgmental, and caring way.

8 A 17-year-old, G0, woman comes to see you to discuss an issue with sexual intercourse. The patient reports that she first became sexually active 1 month ago but that she has experienced pain with each encounter. The patient reports that she had her first period at age 12 and that her periods have been regular ever since. The patient last saw you 6 months ago to obtain oral contraceptive pills (OCPs) because she thought that she may have sex soon. The patient has been with the same boyfriend for 2 years and is taking her OCPs as prescribed.

What is the next step in the workup of this patient's sexual dysfunction?

(A) Description of the pelvic examination and asking for permission to perform the examination
(B) Obtaining a pregnancy test and ensuring the patient is not currently pregnant
(C) Obtaining and evaluating blood work
(D) Obtaining contact information for the patient's sexual partner
(E) Obtaining consent from the patient's parent or legal guardian to perform a pelvic examination

The answer is A: Description of the pelvic examination and asking for permission to perform the examination. Patients with painful intercourse often have significant anxiety regarding examination. Patients must be informed and give permission to proceed with each part of the examination. If at any point they are uncomfortable the examination should be discontinued.

9 A 49-year-old, G0, woman comes to your office with complaints of painful intercourse. The patient recently married for the first time and is finding it difficult to have sexual intercourse with her husband. The patient tells you that she desires sex but feels very anxious and avoids intercourse because she fears the pain.

What is the innervation of the vulva and vestibule?

(A) Femoral nerve
(B) Pudendal nerve
(C) Superior hypogastric plexus
(D) Superior rectal nerve

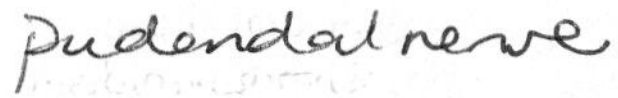

The answer is B: Pudendal nerve. The pudendal nerve innervates the vulva and the vestibule. Needs more clinical information and the direction of the question may need to be changed to a more clinical next step type question rather than a fact question.

10 A 45-year-old patient presents to your office to discuss about decreased libido and would like to know what is causing her current sexual dysfunction. The patient's medical problems include hypothyroidism that is well controlled by synthroid and infrequent migraine headaches. The patient takes birth control pills and a daily multivitamin. The patient denies tobacco use but does report that she drinks two glasses of wine 3 to 4 days per week. She reports that she and her husband are considering separation but they are trying to "work things out" because their two children are still in high school. Based on the patient's history, what is the most likely cause of her dysfunction?

(A) Hypothyroidism
(B) Birth control pills
(C) Alcohol intake
(D) Relationship issues

The answer is D: Relationship issues. Relationship with a patient's partner plays the primary determinant of a patient's sexual satisfaction. The role of birth control pills is controversial, and while alcohol use and untreated or undertreated hypothyroidism could contribute, the primary determinant of sexual satisfaction is still the relationship with the partner.

CHAPTER

16

Reproductive Issues

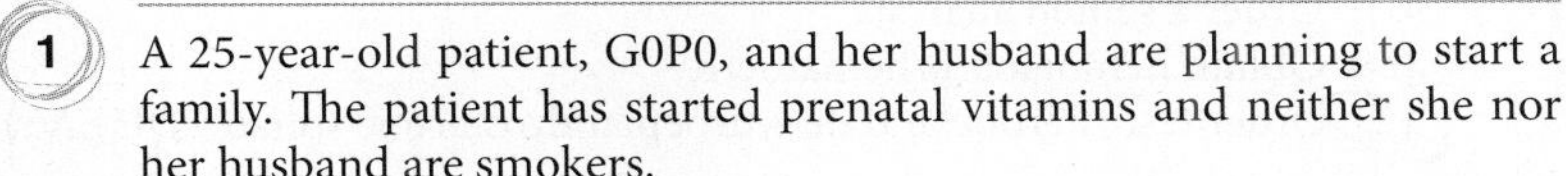

1 A 25-year-old patient, G0P0, and her husband are planning to start a family. The patient has started prenatal vitamins and neither she nor her husband are smokers.

What are the chances that she will become pregnant in the first 3 months?

(A) 10% to 15%
(B) 20% to 25%
(C) 35% to 45%
(D) 45% to 55%

The answer is B: 20% to 25%. The fecundity rate for a normal couple is 20% to 25% in the first 3 months; 80% to 90% of couples are able to conceive within 12 months. Infertility is defined as the failure to conceive after 12 months of unprotected intercourse. Smoking decreases fertility rates.

2 A 26-year-old woman, G0P0, presents to the office with the inability to conceive after 12 months of unprotected intercourse. She has regular periods and her husband has one child from a previous relationship. Her medical history is positive for asthma and history of *Chlamydia* when she was 19. Surgical history is positive for tonsillectomy.

What is the most likely cause of her infertility?

(A) Male factor
(B) Premature ovarian failure
(C) Tubal factor
(D) Polycystic ovarian syndrome (PCOS)
(E) Diethylstilbestrol (DES) exposure in utero

The answer is C: Tubal factor. History of *Chlamydia* is a risk of pelvic inflammatory disease (PID), which is the most common cause of tubal factor infertility. The patient's partner has had a child in the past making male factor unlikely and normal menses makes PCOS as well as premature ovarian failure unlikely. This patient's age makes it very unlikely that she would have been exposed to DES in utero.

---

3 A 24-year-old, G0P0 with a body mass index (BMI) of 34, presents to the office. She has had only three periods in the last year, and she complains of moderate facial hair that she has had treated with laser. She has no recent weight gain or fatigue. She desires pregnancy in the next year.

What is the next step in her workup?

(A) Refer her for assisted reproductive technology
(B) Order transvaginal ultrasound to assess ovaries
(C) Order a semen analysis
(D) Obtain hemoglobin/hematocrit
(E) Order testosterone and dehydroepiandrosterone sulfate (DHEAS)

The answer is E: **Order testosterone and dehydroepiandrosterone sulfate (DHEAS).** The Rotterdam criteria for Polycystic ovarian syndrome (PCOS) only requires two of the following three findings: chronic oligo-ovulation; clinical or laboratory findings of androgen excess; and polycystic-appearing ovaries on ultrasound. This patient has probable anovulatory cycles and hirsutism which leads most likely to a diagnosis of PCOS. She does not need an ultrasound. Testosterone and DHEAS levels would exclude other sources for her hirsutism.

---

4 A 38-year-old, G2P2, presents with her new husband and is interested in trying to conceive. She is in good health, has no history of sexually transmitted infections (STIs), and does not smoke. Her husband has fathered a child in the past.

What single test will assess her chances of getting pregnant?

(A) Thyroid-stimulating hormone (TSH)
(B) Prolactin
(C) Hemoglobin
(D) Follicle-stimulating hormone (FSH)
(E) Progesterone level

The answer is D: **Follicle-stimulating hormone (FSH).** The FSH level on day 3 of the cycle is the best indicator of the reserve the ovary has left. This patient is over the age of 37, which is the time that the rate of fertility declines rapidly.

---

5 Your patient is a 30-year-old G0 with a long history of irregular cycles, hirsutism, and an ultrasound appearance consistent with Polycystic ovarian syndrome (PCOS) who presents for preconception counseling. She is a nonsmoker and is already taking prenatal vitamins. Her husband has fathered a child with a previous partner. She understands the pathophysiology of PCOS and her ovaries. You discuss the use of medication to help her conceive.

What is mechanism of action of this medication?

(A) It is an antiestrogen that results in increased production of Follicle-stimulating hormone (FSH) and luteinizing hormone (LH)
(B) It decreases the conversion of androgens into estrogens which reduces the negative feedback loop on the hypothalamus which increases FSH
(C) It inhibits gluconeogenesis and therefore allows the ovary to respond to normal gonadotropin signals
(D) It interferes with the pulsatile release of FSH and LH from the anterior pituitary

The answer is A: It is an antiestrogen that results in increased production of Follicle-stimulating hormone (FSH) and luteinizing hormone (LH). Clomiphene is an antiestrogen that competitively binds to estrogen receptors in the hypothalamus. This increases the pulsatile gonadotropin-releasing hormone and leads to increased production of FSH and LH. This leads to follicular growth and ovulation. It is an oral medication that is given starting on cycle day 3 or 5 for 5 days.

6 A 29-year-old, G1P0010, presents to your clinic desiring pregnancy. She had one ectopic pregnancy in the past treated with methotrexate. She has not been able to become pregnant despite 2 years of unprotected intercourse. Her husband has a normal semen analysis. She is otherwise healthy and has normal menstrual cycles.

What is the next step in her workup?

(A) Magnetic resonance imaging
(B) Clomid citrate challenge
(C) Hysterosalpingogram
(D) In vitro fertilization

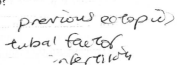

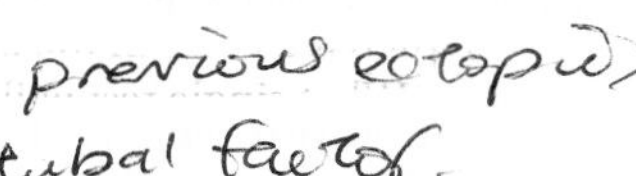

The answer is C: Hysterosalpingogram. This patient's history of a previous ectopic puts her at risk for having tubal factor infertility. A hysterosalpingogram would be used to assess the contour of the uterus as well as the patency of the fallopian tubes.

7 A 24-year-old, G0, and her husband presents to your office for preconception counseling. She has not attempted pregnancy to date because she is concerned about her future pregnancies and wants to know about preimplantation genetic diagnosis. From her statement you ask her about her other medical history.

Which of the following diagnoses is she likely to have?

(A) Polycystic ovarian syndrome (PCOS)
(B) Sickle cell anemia
(C) Hyperstimulation syndrome
(D) Hyperprolactinemia

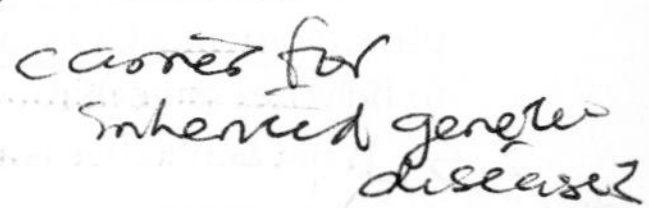

The answer is B: **Sickle cell anemia.** Preimplantation genetic diagnosis is a technique that determines the genetics of an embryo prior to transfer during an in vitro fertilization cycle. Patients use this technique when they have (or are a carrier for) a known inherited genetic disease such as sickle cell anemia, Tay-Sachs disease, cystic fibrosis, hemophilia, fragile X disease, or others.

---

8 A 31-year-old, G0, with a long history of endometriosis presents to discuss future childbearing. She has no genetic family history complicating her prenatal counseling. Her husband is a nonsmoker with no medical problems. She has used birth control pills in the past to control her menses and pain. She would like to proceed with the best option for her to obtain pregnancy quickly.

What would you recommend for this patient?

(A) Use depot leuprolide for 6 months and then attempt pregnancy
(B) Restart birth control pills for 3 months and then attempt pregnancy
(C) Perform laparoscopy with fulguration of endometrial implants and then attempt pregnancy
(D) Start clomiphene therapy cycle with next cycle on days 5 to 9

The answer is C: **Perform laparoscopy with fulguration of endometrial implants and then attempt pregnancy.** Surgical treatment for endometriosis has been shown to improve fertility rates. Medical treatment has been shown to improve symptoms but not to improve fertility rates.

---

9 A 30-year-old, G1P1, presents to clinic with intermittent thin milky discharge from both nipples. The symptoms have been present for the past 6 months. The discharge is non-bloody and is not associated with increased breast tenderness. The patient has also had irregular menses lately. The patient says that up until recently her periods were always very regular. The patient is currently not taking any medications. The pregnancy test in the office is negative. The patient says the discharge occurs spontaneously without manual stimulation and denies any recent changes in bras. In the office, the patient's blood pressure (BP) is 120/75 mmHg, heart rate (HR) 82 beats/min, temperature (T) 98.5, height 5′5″, and weight 179 lb which is 18 lb heavier than when you saw her last year. On physical examination, the breasts are symmetric and no breast lesions or masses are appreciated. A thin white discharge can be manually expressed bilaterally.

What is the most likely mechanism leading to these findings?

(A) Microadenoma of the pituitary gland leading to hyperprolactinemia
(B) Excessive stimulation of the nipple
(C) Renal failure leading to a decreased clearance of prolactin
(D) Hypothyroidism leading to an increased thyrotropin-releasing hormone (TRH) which causes increased prolactin release
(E) Cushing disease leading to increased growth hormone causing hyperprolactinemia

The answer is D: **Hypothyroidism leading to an increased thyrotropin-releasing hormone (TRH) which causes increased prolactin release.** Galactorrhea typically presents with bilateral painless nipple discharge. The discharge is usually thin and milky. Painful, unilateral discharge that is bloody is more concerning for malignancy. The differential diagnosis of galactorrhea is broad. This patient has galactorrhea, irregular menses, and a recent increase in weight. This constellation of symptoms makes hypothyroidism the most likely diagnosis. Primary hypothyroidism results in increased Thyroid-stimulating hormone (TSH) and TRH. The increased TRH can cause increased release of prolactin and resultant hyperprolactinemia and galactorrhea.

10 A 32-year-old, G0, comes for her annual examination. The patient states that she has been under a great deal of stress lately due to work. The patient also reports hair loss, weight gain, and unusually light periods for the past 4 months. The patient attributes most of these symptoms to stress and wonders if there is anything you can do to help. The patient's only current medication is an oral contraceptive pill. The patient is currently not sexually active and her last period ended 2 days ago. The pelvic and breast examinations are normal.

What is the next best step in the care of this patient?

(A) Refer the patient to a psychiatrist
(B) Prescribe alprazolam 0.25 mg PO TID with follow-up in 1 month
(C) Perform a pregnancy test
(D) Tell the patient to keep a daily basal body temperature log and return in 1 month
(E) Obtain a Thyroid-stimulating hormone (TSH) test

The answer is E: **Obtain a Thyroid-stimulating hormone (TSH) test.** The patient in the vignette presents with hair loss, weight gain, and amenorrhea. These symptoms are most likely due to hypothyroidism and the patient's TSH and free T4 should be checked for dysfunction. The primary cause of hypothyroidism in the United States is Hashimoto thyroiditis. Hashimoto thyroiditis is an autoimmune disorder in which the body produces antibodies to the thyroid gland. In hypothyroidism, TSH levels will be elevated and free T4 levels will be low or normal. Treatment of hypothyroidism is hormone replacement for life.

check ↑TSH / free T4

11 A 19-year-old, G0P0, presents to clinic with concern about amenorrhea for 2 months. She is sexually active with one partner and uses the levonorgestrel intrauterine system for contraception. Past history is relevant for a broken humerus when she was 7 and *Chlamydia* found on routine sexually transmitted infection (STI) screening 1 year ago which was treated as an outpatient. She subsequently had a negative test of cure. She has recently started training for a half marathon and has lost 12 lb over the past 3 months; she is 5′6″ and currently weighs 147 lb (BMI 23.7).

What is the appropriate next step?

(A) Serum Follicle-stimulating hormone (FSH)/luteinizing hormone (LH) to evaluate for hypothalamic anovulation secondary to weight loss

(B) Beta-human chorionic gonadotropin (β-hCG) to rule out pregnancy as a result of levonorgestrel intrauterine system failure

(C) Inform the patient that her amenorrhea is due to tubal scarring from pelvic inflammatory disease (PID)

(D) No action required because anovulatory cycles are common in young women. Tell the patient to return if she misses two more periods.

The answer is B: **Beta-human chorionic gonadotropin (β-hCG) to rule out pregnancy as a result of levonorgestrel intrauterine system failure.** β-hCG is the first test in any woman of reproductive years presenting with amenorrhea, regardless of contraceptive method used or reported sexual history. The levonorgestrel intrauterine system (Mirena IUS) has a failure rate of only 0.2% and a very high rate of amenorrhea; however, pregnancy remains a possibility. This patient's weight loss has been less than 10% of her total body mass, and she is currently at a normal BMI; hypothalamic anovulation due to weight loss would not be expected in this case. A past history of *Chlamydia* is relevant for women who are experiencing difficulty in conceiving, as untreated PID can lead to fallopian tube scarring and infertility; this would not be expected to cause sudden amenorrhea in a woman with previously normal menses. Finally, though anovulatory cycles and irregular menses are common in the first few years of menstruation, not only is this expected to have ceased by 19 years of age, it would also be inappropriate to ignore the possibility of pregnancy in any sexually active woman of reproductive age.

12 A 16-year-old is brought in by her mother, who is concerned that her daughter has not yet started to menstruate. The patient's medical history is significant only for well-controlled asthma. She is in her third year of high school, plays on the soccer team, and enjoys spending time with friends. When interviewed without her mother's presence, she denies ever having been sexually active. A urinary pregnancy test is negative. On examination, she is 5′7″ tall and weighs 138 lb

(BMI 21.6). She has Tanner stage V breast development with minimal pubic or axillary hair. Pelvic examination reveals a shortened vagina ending in a blind pouch.

What can you tell the mother?

(A) "With surgery and hormone replacement therapy, your daughter can have a functional female reproductive system."

(B) "This is a genetic condition associated with early menopause and osteoporosis."

(C) "Unfortunately there are no options to give your daughter an opportunity for normal sexual function."

(D) "This condition is associated with an increased risk of gonadal cancer; surgical castration may be indicated."

The answer is D: "This condition is associated with an increased risk of gonadal cancer; surgical castration may be indicated." Androgen insensitivity syndrome (AIS), also known as testicular feminization, occurs when a genetically male individual is born with insensitivity to male sex hormones. This causes a lack of stimulation of the Wolffian system during embryogenesis, which ultimately results in a phenotypically female individual. This condition may not be recognized until the individual does not undergo menarche within the expected time frame. Germ cell malignancy risk is increased and prophylactic gonadectomy is generally performed, though there is controversy over the age by which this should ideally occur. As a genetic male without internal female reproductive organs, there are no surgical or hormonal means of establishing functional female reproductive function, though vaginal reconstruction or dilatation may be employed to allow more normal sexual function. Early menopause and osteoporosis are associated with Turner syndrome (gonadal dysgenesis, or 45X), though individuals with AIS may be prone to decreased bone mineral density, particularly if gonadectomy is performed at a very young age.

---

13 A 24-year-old, G0P0, presents to her obstetrician/gynecologist complaining of amenorrhea. She states that her menses have always been irregular, but have become increasingly rare over the past year and have now been entirely absent for 3 months. She is sexually active with her husband for 2 years; they used to use condoms for contraception, but since she has not been menstruating they have ceased using them. A urinary pregnancy test in the office is negative. She has no history of sexually transmitted infections (STIs). She is 5′6″ and weighs 193 lb (BMI 31.1). Terminal hairs are evident on her jaw and upper lip, she has moderate acne, and the skin of her axillae and the nape of her neck are darkly pigmented. Aside from infertility, what is the major morbidity associated with the condition this woman likely has?

(A) Diabetes mellitus type 2 (DM type 2)
(B) Ovarian carcinoma
(C) Congenital adrenal hyperplasia
(D) Coronary artery disease

The answer is A: Diabetes mellitus type 2 (DM type 2). This patient's symptoms—virilization, obesity, and amenorrhea likely secondary to anovulation—are consistent with a diagnosis of Polycystic ovarian syndrome (PCOS). PCOS consists of a cycle of increased LH:FSH ratio with subsequent failure of follicles to mature, leading to anovulation and polycystic ovaries. Though the initial trigger of this disorder is unclear, it is thought that insulin resistance likely plays a role and DM type 2 is highly increased in these women. Ovarian carcinoma is less likely in anovulatory women, though endometrial cancer risk is increased due to unopposed endometrial proliferation. Congenital adrenal hyperplasia is not known to be associated with PCOS; the virilization commonly seen in these patients is due to excess androgen production in the cystic ovaries. Though individuals with obesity are at increased risk for coronary artery disease overall, it is not specifically linked to the pathophysiology of PCOS.

---

14 A 22-year-old, G0, comes to see you for her annual examination. The patient expresses frustration at not being able to lose weight despite regular exercise and a balanced diet. The patient reports increased feelings of depression and thinks that the extra weight is causing her to have acne. The patient has also noticed stiff dark hairs on her upper lip and chin which is further decreasing her self-esteem. On examination, the patient's BP is 112/85 mmHg, HR 69 beats/min, height 5′3″, and weight 155 lb. The thyroid, cardiac, pulmonary, breast, and pelvic examinations are all normal.

What is the most likely cause of this patient's symptoms?

(A) Steroid abuse
(B) Idiopathic hirsutism
(C) Stein-Leventhal syndrome
(D) 21-α-Hydroxylase deficiency
(E) von Hipple-Lindau disease

The answer is C: Stein-Leventhal syndrome. Stein-Leventhal syndrome, also known as Polycystic ovarian syndrome (PCOS), is one of the most common endocrine disorders in women. In PCOS, chronic anovulation leads to increased levels of androgens and estrogen. Obesity and insulin resistance frequently occur in PCOS. The increased androgens can result in acne and hirsutism as seen in the patient in this question. While the other answer choices can explain some of the symptoms and physical examination findings, PCOS is the most likely disorder to cause these findings in this 22-year-old patient.

15 A 29-year-old, G0, comes to see you for an infertility evaluation. The patient has been trying to conceive for the past 2½ years. The patient's husband recently had a semen analysis, and sperm count and motility were normal. Today, the patient's BP is 122/79 mmHg, pulse (P) 76 beats/min, and T 98.6. The patient's current BMI is 33. Initial labs show an luteinizing hormone (LH) of 36 mIU/mL, Follicle-stimulating hormone (FSH) of 8 mIU/mL, Thyroid-stimulating hormone (TSH) of 1.6, normal dehydroepiandrosterone (DHEA), and mildly elevated androstenedione and testosterone.

What is the best next step in addressing the patient's infertility?

(A) Hysterosalpingography
(B) Combined estrogen and progesterone challenge
(C) Magnetic resonance imaging of the brain
(D) Ovulation induction with clomid
(E) Pelvic ultrasound

The answer is D: Ovulation induction with clomid. The patient likely has Polycystic ovarian syndrome (PCOS). PCOS is one of the most common female endocrine disorders. It is characterized by anovulation, resulting in menstruation irregularities and excess androgens. Other features include obesity, polycystic ovaries, and insulin resistance. The patient in the vignette has failed to conceive for 2.5 years, making anovulation a potential cause of her infertility. In PCOS, chronic anovulation leads to increased estrogen and androgen levels. The high estrogen levels in turn lead to an increased LH:FSH ratio, which is normally approximately 1:1. Although the ratio is not used diagnostically, an increased ratio can often be measured which is exemplified in this question. DHEA is a marker of adrenal androgen production, and normal values exclude adrenal sources of increased androgens. Finally, the TSH is normal in this patient, which indicates thyroid dysfunction is not the cause of her infertility. In patients with PCOS, clomid is used to induce ovulation.

16 A 36-year-old, G3P2012, presents to her primary care physician complaining of several months' poor sleep, heat intolerance, newly irregular menses, and decreased libido. She denies recent changes in weight, diet, or activity, and does not use alcohol or illicit drugs. Her obstetric history includes two uncomplicated, full-term vaginal deliveries and one first-trimester spontaneous abortion. On examination, she is thin and tired-appearing, without exophthalmos or thyromegaly. Vital signs show the following: T 36.8°C, respiratory rate of 17 breaths/min, P 77 beats/min, and BP 142/88 mmHg. Her breasts are nontender, without masses or nipple discharge. Pelvic examination reveals moderately well-estrogenized vaginal mucosa and a small, nontender uterus with regular contours and no palpable adnexal masses. A urinary pregnancy test is negative.

What laboratory values are appropriate to check at this time?

(A) Follicle-stimulating hormone (FSH)/luteinizing hormone (LH), prolactin, Thyroid-stimulating hormone (TSH), complete blood count (CBC), basic metabolic panel (BMP)
(B) CBC, BMP, serum ferritin/total iron-binding capacity (TIBC)
(C) Endometrial biopsy and CT abdomen/pelvis
(D) Adrenocorticotropic hormone (ACTH), dehydroepiandrosterone (DHEA), 24-hour cortisol, and memantine challenge

The answer is A: Follicle-stimulating hormone (FSH)/luteinizing hormone (LH), prolactin, Thyroid-stimulating hormone (TSH), complete blood count (CBC), basic metabolic panel (BMP). Premature ovarian failure is defined as the loss or decline of normal ovarian function prior to age 40. Women may present with irregular menses or amenorrhea, fatigue or poor concentration, hot flashes, vaginal dryness, and other signs/symptoms of menopause. Many of these symptoms may, however, be caused by other conditions, most commonly endocrine conditions such as thyroid dysfunction. In cases of premature ovarian failure, serum FSH will be increased while LH is decreased, whereas TSH, prolactin, and CBC/BMP give a good overview of basic hematologic and endocrine function, helping to distinguish true ovarian failure from another common underlying process. CBC and serum ferritin/TIBC tests for anemia; while anemia could cause some of her symptoms, such as fatigue and pallor, it would not on its own explain her menstrual irregularity. Endometrial biopsy and CT abdomen/pelvis may be indicated if preliminary testing suggests a malignant or other intrauterine process; however, these are invasive and expensive tests and should not be performed as part of an initial evaluation unless there is high suspicion for malignancy or other relevant disease process. ACTH, DHEA, and cortisol levels test for adrenal/hypothalamic/pituitary axis function; a primary disease process in this system would be unusual in this patient's age bracket, and in any case these would rarely be initial tests ordered in the absence of high clinical likelihood for a specific pathology.

---

17 A 37-year-old, G1P1, presents to clinic with 3 months of amenorrhea. Her history is significant for obesity (BMI 30.6), occasional headaches, and moderate hypertension well controlled with lisinopril/hydrochlorothiazide. Her one pregnancy was uncomplicated, and the infant was born at term by normal spontaneous vaginal delivery. She and her husband are sexually active and use condoms for contraception. A urinary pregnancy test is negative. Serum Follicle-stimulating hormone (FSH)/luteinizing hormone (LH) are both low.

What is the most likely diagnosis?

(A) Polycystic ovarian syndrome (PCOS)
(B) Early menopause
(C) Prolactinoma
(D) Missed abortion

The answer is C: Prolactinoma. Though the trademark sign of prolactinoma is galactorrhea due to elevated prolactin levels, in some women the nipple discharge may be missed or entirely absent. Prolactin is a competitive inhibitor of both FSH and LH, leading to amenorrhea; early menopause would present with high FSH and low LH. PCOS, though more common in obese women, is generally accompanied by signs of virilization (hirsutism, acne, etc.). Missed abortion would not cause the gonadotropin depression seen in this woman, and (if recent enough) would still present with elevated β-hCG.

---

18 A 16-year-old is brought into her primary care physician's office because her mother is concerned that her daughter has not starting menstruating yet. In conversation with the teenager, her doctor learns that she has been having low pelvic pain for the past few months. On speculum examination, a dark bulging mass is identified 5 cm from the vaginal introitus, and the hymenal ring is identified distal to the bulging mass.

What is the most likely etiology of this patient's condition?

(A) Failure of fusion of the paramesonephric duct and the urogenital sinus
(B) Failure of fusion of the mesonephric duct and the urogenital sinus
(C) Failure of fusion of the paramesonephric duct and the vitelline duct
(D) Failure of fusion of the mesonephric duct and the vitelline duct
(E) Failure of fusion of the urogenital sinus and the vitelline duct

The answer is A: Failure of fusion of the paramesonephric duct and the urogenital sinus. This patient has primary amenorrhea from a congenital abnormality known as a transverse vaginal septum, in which the upper vagina (derived from the paramesonephric or Müllerian duct) fails to fuse with the lower vagina (derived from the urogenital sinus). In addition to primary amenorrhea, patients can present with pelvic pain and pressure from blood building up in the uterus and upper portion of the vagina (known as hematocolpos). An imperforate hymen may have a similar presentation, but on examination this patient had a visible hymenal ring, which excludes this diagnosis. The mesonephric or Wolffian duct develops into the epididymis, the vas deferens, and the seminal vesicle in men. The vitelline duct joins the yolk sac to the midgut in the early embryo.

---

19 A 19-year-old sexually active college student presents requesting oral contraception to help clear up acne. Gender-specific history reveals she uses condoms inconsistently and has had no menstrual period for 7 months. Three pregnancy tests at home have been negative.

Menarche began at 14. Periods occurred irregularly three to four times a year, never heavy. Coitarche was at 17. Vital signs are as follows: P 88 beats/min, R 18 breaths/min, BP 110/68 mmHg, BMI 25, and height 4′10″.

General physical examination reveals a short-statured, well-proportioned woman with a moderate case of acne. Gender-specific examination reveals the presence of both axillary and pubic hairs in the appropriate distribution. Breast examination is Tanner stage 2. External genitalia appear normal as does a speculum examination that reveals a normal vagina with a single cervix. After Gonococcal/*Chlamydia trachomatis* specimens are obtained, a bimanual examination reveals a normal-sized uterus. Adnexa were nonpalpable bilaterally. Both estrogen and testosterone levels are low. Follicle-stimulating hormone (FSH) is 35. Pregnancy test is negative. Gonococcal/*Chlamydia trachomatis* is negative.

What is the most likely diagnosis for this patient?

(A) Androgen insensitivity syndrome (AIS)
(B) Congenital adrenal hyperplasia
(C) Hypothalamic hypogonadism
(D) Swyer syndrome
(E) Turner syndrome

The answer is E: Turner syndrome. Short stature, which becomes evident by age 5, is the most common presentation of Turner syndrome. An early loss of ovarian function is also very common. Initially, the ovaries develop normally, but by birth most ovarian tissue degenerates leaving what are referred to as gonadal streaks. Many affected girls present with primary amenorrhea but a small percentage of girls with Turner syndrome retain normal ovarian function through young adulthood. Additional signs of Turner syndrome include webbed neck, lymphedema, skeletal abnormalities, heart defects, and kidney problems. They typically have normal intellectual development.

---

20 A 15-year-old sexually active adolescent girl presents with primary amenorrhea. Vital signs are as follows: BP 110/68 mmHg, P 88 beats/min, R 16 breaths/min, BMI 24, and height 5′0″. An examination reveals normal external genitalia. A three-dimensional (3D) ultrasound reveals the presence of uterus, tubes, and ovaries bilaterally. On speculum examination, she has an unobstructed vagina and a patent cervical os. Breasts are Tanner stage 2. She has scant axillary hair, Tanner stage 2, which has developed over the past 6 months. Follicle-stimulating hormone (FSH) and luteinizing hormone (LH) are low; Thyroid-stimulating hormone (TSH), estrogen, and testosterone levels are all within normal limits. She relates that she has grown 2″ in the last 3 months.

What is the most likely diagnosis?

(A) Androgen insensitivity syndrome (AIS)
(B) Anorexia nervosa
(C) Constitutional delay
(D) Turner syndrome
(E) Congenital adrenal hyperplasia

The answer is C: Constitutional delay. This patient has constitutional delay. The most common cause of hypogonadotropic hypogonadism (low FSH and LH levels) in primary amenorrhea is constitutional delay of growth and puberty. The condition is commonly familial. Using Tanner staging as a guide, watchful waiting is appropriate for constitutional delay of puberty.

---

21 A 14-year-old adolescent presents with a history of primary amenorrhea. Her past medical history is unremarkable as is her family history. Her vital signs are as follow: P 90 betas/min, respiratory rate 14 breaths/min, BP 124/76 mmHg, and BMI 21. General physical examination reveals no evidence of acne. She has no axillary or pubic hair. External genitalia are of normal female. Breasts are Tanner stage 4. She is not sexually active so a three-dimensional (3D) pelvic ultrasound was performed revealing no evidence of a uterus.

What is the next step in evaluation?

(A) Chromosomal analysis
(B) Estrogen level
(C) Follicle-stimulating hormone (FSH) level
(D) Speculum and bimanual examination
(E) Testosterone level

The answer is A: Chromosomal analysis. The patient does not have a uterus. This suggests a congenital explanation for her amenorrhea. In this case, the next appropriate step is to determine the chromosomal complement. Since the patient has abnormal uterine development, Müllerian agenesis is the most likely cause but there are syndromes such as Swyer and Androgen insensitivity syndromes (AISs) that occur in genetically male individuals. A karyotype analysis should confirm that the patient is 46, XX in cases of Müllerian agenesis.

22 Refer to the vignette in Question 21 to answer the question. In this case, the chromosomal analysis reveals XY.

What hormone is implicated in this case of amenorrhea?

(A) Estrogen
(B) Testosterone
(C) dehydroepiandrosterone/sulfate (DHEA/S)
(D) Follicle-stimulating hormone (FSH)
(E) Thyrotropin-releasing hormone (TRH)

The answer is B: Testosterone. Androgen insensitivity syndrome (AIS) is a genetic condition, occurring in approximately 1 in 20,000 individuals. The genotype is 46 XY. AIS is a condition that affects sexual development before birth and during puberty. Fetal testes produce Müllerian-inhibiting hormone (MIH) and testosterone. MIH causes the fetal Müllerian ducts to regress so uterus, fallopian tubes, cervix, and upper vagina do not develop. Testosterone is implicated in the development of normal male external genitalia and the genitalia differentiate into female. At puberty, the testes are stimulated to produce testosterone at high levels and some is aromatized to estrogen which produces breast growth, though it may be late. Women with AIS are amenorrheic and infertile. Since pubic and axillary hair depends on testosterone and its effect on receptors, these patients have sparse to no pubic or axillary hair. Affected individuals have undescended testes that are at risk for cancer in later life so they are removed after puberty and sexual differentiation.

---

23 A 15-year-old adolescent presents with a complaint of a vaginal discharge. Further history reveals she had attempted to have intercourse with her 16-year-old boyfriend for the first time a week earlier. The attempt was painful and her boyfriend commented that he could not "enter" her. They presumed it was due to her hymen. A second attempt was equally uncomfortable and the boyfriend became frustrated because he still could not enter her vagina.

Past medical history is positive for asthma that does not require medication. Gender-specific history reveals she has never had a menstrual period, but her family medicine doctor had told her 9 months ago that everything seemed normal and she should just wait a bit longer since she had normal breast and axillary hair development.

General physical examination reveals vital signs as follows: P 78 beats/min, R 16 breaths/min, BP 126/82 mmHg, and BMI 28. Lungs clear to auscultation. A 10-cm solid, nontender mid-abdominal mass is noted on deep palpation. No skeletal or hearing abnormalities noted.

Gender-specific examination: Tanner stage 4, breasts and external genitalia normal. Patient could not tolerate a speculum examination and it was impossible to perform a satisfactory bimanual examination partly due to the patient experiencing vaginismus.

What is the most likely diagnosis?

(A) Androgen insensitivity syndrome (AIS)
(B) Imperforate hymen
(C) Swyer syndrome
(D) Turner syndrome
(E) Vaginal agenesis

The answer is E: Vaginal agenesis. Sometimes called Mayer-Rokitansky-Küster-Hauser syndrome, patients with vaginal (Müllerian) agenesis may be missing some or all of the vagina and/or the uterus. Patients with Müllerian agenesis present in adolescence with primary amenorrhea, cyclic pain, and normal growth and development. After gonadal dysgenesis, Müllerian agenesis is the second most common cause of primary amenorrhea.

24 A 14-year-old girl presents to the resident clinic with complaint of no periods for the past 6 months. Menarche was at age 11 with regular periods for the last 2 years. Five months ago she noted facial hair that has increased to the point of requiring shaving almost daily. She is very embarrassed about this situation since it is impacting her social life.

On physical examination, breasts are Tanner stage 3. Hirsutism is not noted due to the patient shaving. Examination of the external genitalia reveals an enlarged clitoris, approximately 1 cm in diameter.

What is the most likely cause of her symptoms?

(A) Exogenous testosterone administration
(B) Brenner tumor
(C) Hyperthyroidism
(D) Polycystic ovarian disorder
(E) Sertoli-Leydig tumor

The answer is E: Sertoli-Leydig tumor. Sertoli-Leydig cell tumors are also called arrhenoblastomas and are remarkable for the androgenic manifestations from hirsutism to outright virilization. Brenner tumors account for 1% to 2% of ovarian neoplasms and typically present in the fifth decade.

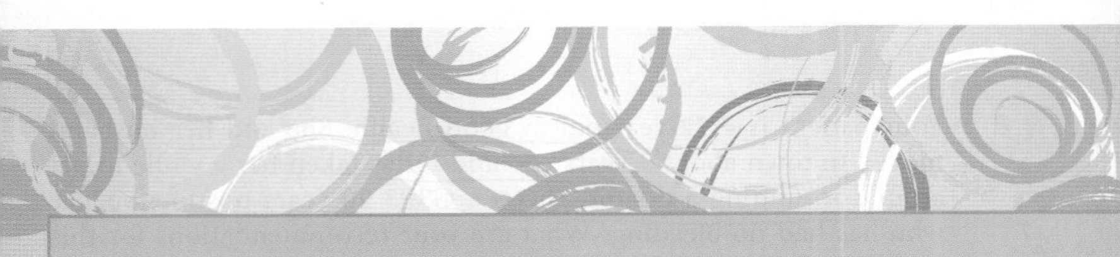

Practice Exam

1 A 17-year-old G0 last menstrual period (LMP) about a month ago on birth control pills presents to the resident clinic concerned about several days of a yellow discharge with unpleasant odor. She became sexually active at age 15 and has had three male partners, the present one for about a month. Her last encounter was 1 week ago. She has never had a Pap. Testing today includes a pregnancy test, wet prep, and nucleic acid amplification tests of cervical samples. What should the clinic recommend for this patient regarding cervical cytology screening?

(A) Immediate cervical cytology
(B) Cervical cytology in 1 year
(C) Cervical cytology in 2 years
(D) Cervical cytology in 3 years
(E) Cervical cytology in 4 years

21y/o start Papsmear

2 A 29-year-old G1P1 comes to see you concerned about recent changes in her menses. Menarche was at age 13 and her periods became regular by age 14. They are normally monthly and predictable and last 4 to 5 days with moderate flow and minimal cramping. She started oral contraceptive pill (OCP) at age 19 and stopped them in her mid-20s to have a baby and does not recall anything unusual. She resumed the pill after breastfeeding a year and stopped them again to get pregnant about 6 months ago. Her periods are still regular and last 4 days but she is now noting bleeding about 10 days before her period. It is dark but requires a pad and lasts 2 days. What term best describes this bleeding pattern?

(A) Menorrhagia
(B) Dysfunctional uterine bleeding
(C) Oligomenorrhea
(D) Intermenstrual bleeding

3 Your patient is a 72-year-old in good health. She and her husband moved to town about 5 years ago and it has taken her a while to get around to finding a doctor. She is a G3P3 20 years postmenopause who has had no bleeding. What are your recommendations for this patient?

(A) Colonoscopy, pneumococcal vaccine, lipid screen, Pap
(B) Mammogram, bone densitometry, pneumococcal vaccine, lipid screen, Pap
(C) Mammogram, bone densitometry, colonoscopy, lipid screen, Pap
(D) Mammogram, bone densitometry, colonoscopy, pneumococcal vaccine, Pap
(E) Mammogram, bone densitometry, colonoscopy, pneumococcal vaccine, lipid screen

4 A 20-year-old, G0, woman presents to the office with a 2-week history of lower abdominal pain that worsened during menstruation 3 days ago. She usually has cramping with menstruation, but never as bad as this particular cycle. She admits to pain with intercourse for the last few days. She became sexually active at age 16 and has had four partners. She has been with her current partner about 2 months. On examination, her temperature is 100.7 and she is diffusely tender to palpation in both lower abdominal quadrants with guarding. On pelvic examination, purulent discharge is noted from her cervical os, and she cries out in pain when her cervix is palpated. What will probably be your treatment of choice?

(A) Metronidazole
(B) Azithromycin
(C) Acyclovir
(D) Ampicillin and gentamicin
(E) Leuprolide

5 A 24-year-old woman, G2P2002 last menstrual period (LMP) 2 weeks ago, presents to your office complaining of vaginal discharge for the past week. She describes the discharge as grayish white in color. She says that she has been sexually active with a monogamous partner for the past 3 years. Her current medications include only oral contraceptives. On physical examination, a thin, white discharge is present on the vaginal walls. Cervix is not inflamed and there is no cervical discharge. A fishy odor is present. The vaginal pH is 5.0.

A wet mount is shown in *Figure 1*:

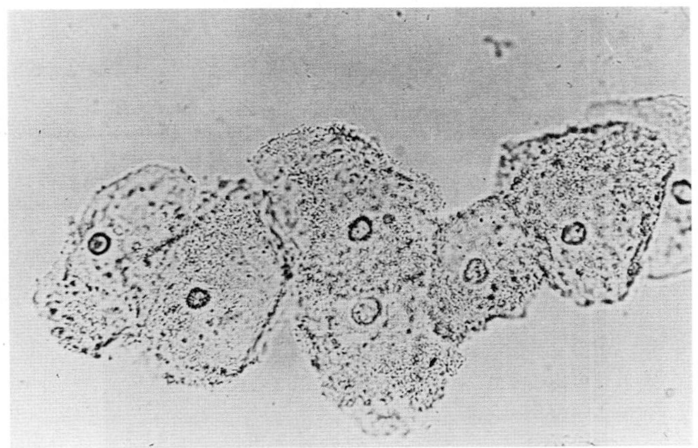

Figure 1

Which of the following is the most likely diagnosis?

(A) *Trichomonas*
(B) *Chlamydia*
(C) Candidiasis
(D) Bacterial vaginosis

BV

6 While on your gynecology rotation you scrub into a diagnostic scope for ruptured ectopic pregnancy. The patient is a 23-year-old black woman, G3P1011, with a history of ectopic pregnancy treated with methotrexate in the past who presented with right lower quadrant pain, vaginal bleeding, and quantitative human chorionic gonadotropin (hCG) of 1,500. Vaginal ultrasound revealed an empty uterus and blood within the cul-de-sac. Although there were dense pelvic adhesions, the right fallopian tube and ectopic are successfully removed. At the completion of the surgery, the attending physician takes a look at the rest of the pelvis and points out filmy adhesions between the liver and the right hemidiaphragm (see *Figure 2*). Based on these findings, this 23-year-old female patient likely has a history of what condition?

Fitz Hugh Curtis

(A) Herpes simplex virus (HSV)
(B) Chlamydia
(C) Endometriosis
(D) Ruptured appendicitis

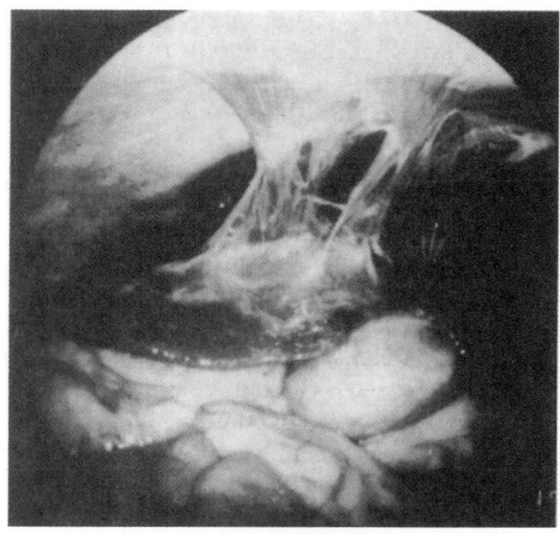

Figure 2

7 A 31-year-old G3P0202 presents at 28 weeks with possible rupture of membranes more than 2 days ago. She denies contractions and has had no bleeding. She says the baby has had decreased movements. The patient's vital signs are as follows: temperature (T) 100.2, heart rate (HR) 103 beats/min, blood pressure (BP) 122/76 mmHg, and O_2 saturation 98% on room air. Fetal heart tone (FHT) are 180s. The fundal height is 26 cm and the uterus is moderately tender. Sterile speculum examination reveals minimal pooling but positive ferning. What is the most likely diagnosis?

tachycardia?

(A) Chorioamnionitis
(B) Pelvic inflammatory disease
(C) Placental abruption
(D) Placental insufficiency

8 You are on the labor and delivery service watching a G2P1001 who is undergoing a trial of labor after Cesarean section (TOLAC). Her first Cesarean was for footling breech and she is felt to be a good candidate. She has been 5/100/0 for a few hours but her contractions are now picking up and she complains of increased pain with contractions and expresses a desire for epidural. While awaiting anesthesia you notice a change in the fetal monitor with new-onset variables and now late decelerations. The patient complains of severe abdominal pain and you check her cervix and note the head is now at −4 station. What is the next step?

(A) Antibiotics
(B) Amnioinfusion
(C) Pitocin
(D) Stat Cesarean
(E) Epidural

umbilical cord?

9 A 23-year-old white woman, G1P1 last period 1 week ago on oral contraceptives, presents to your clinic with complaints of left groin pain. The patient became sexually active at 8 years ago and admits to five lifetime partners. She has been with her current partner for 2 months. Review of systems is remarkable for malaise and some dysuria. On physical examination, she has tender lymph nodes in the left groin area and painful shallow ulcers with red borders on the right labia (see *Figure 3*). Which of the following is the most appropriate course of treatment for this patient?

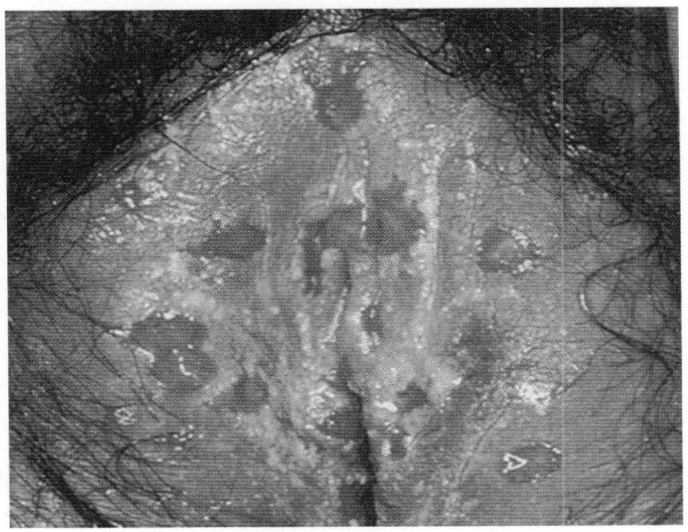

Figure 3

(A) Penicillin
(B) Azithromycin
(C) Doxycycline
(D) Acyclovir
(E) Ciprofloxacin

10 A 24-year-old G0 on oral contraceptive pills (OCPs) presents to your office with complaints of a 1-week history of vulvar irritation and vaginal discharge. She has had two partners in the past 6 months without the use of condoms. On physical examination, the vulva is edematous. Yellow-green discharge is present on the vaginal walls and at the cervical os. The cervix is strawberry red (see *Figure 4*). Wet smear of vaginal secretions shows epithelial cells, white blood cells (WBCs), and flagellate protozoa. You prescribe an antibiotic. What warning do you give about this particular treatment?

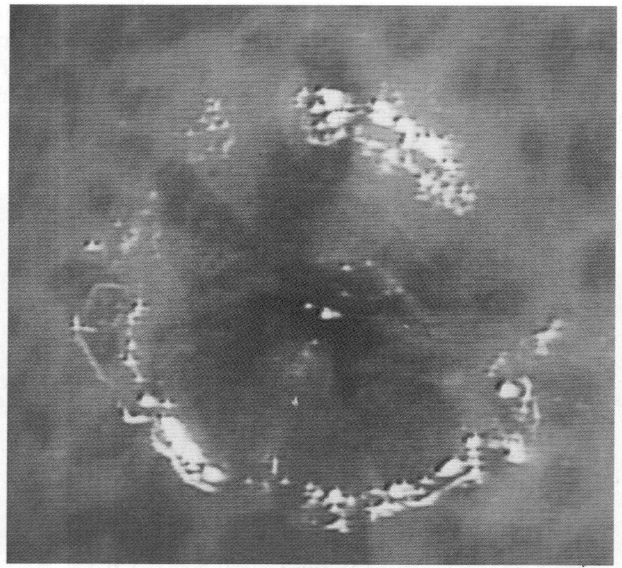

Figure 4

(A) Avoid sun overexposure
(B) Avoid alcohol
(C) Avoid milk products
(D) Avoid taking on an empty stomach

11 A 26-year-old, G0, woman presents to your clinic. One of her recent sexual partners has been treated for a sexually transmitted disease but she cannot remember what the specific infection was called. Review of systems is negative for rash or malaise. She also denies painless or painful vulvar lesions. Recently, she has noticed an increase in odorless discharge and some pelvic cramping. Examination reveals no lymphadenopathy or vulvar lesions. Speculum examination reveals a slightly friable cervix with scant yellow discharge and minimal discomfort on examination. Gram stain and wet prep of her cervical mucus show many WBCs, but no clue cells, moving organisms, or gram-negative diplococci. Which of the medications would be the best treatment for this patient?

(A) Penicillin G 2.4 million units IM once
(B) Acyclovir 400 mg orally three times a day for 1 week
(C) Ceftriaxone 250 mg IM once
(D) Doxycycline 100 mg two times a day for 1 week
(E) Metronidazole 500 mg orally twice a day for 2 weeks

---

12 You start your night shift in labor and delivery and are asked to assess a 19-year-old G2P0101 at 39 weeks who arrived in active labor with subsequent spontaneous rupture of membranes but has been 5/100/−1 for the last 3 hours. You arrive to find a category 1 strip and contractions every 3 to 4 minutes. Her cervix is unchanged. What is your recommendation?

(A) Start an amnioinfusion
(B) Place an intrauterine pressure catheter (IUPC) to measure Montevideo units
(C) Start a fluid bolus to ensure adequate hydration
(D) Perform a Cesarean section due to arrest of dilation

---

13 You are making morning rounds with the gyn residents when the nurse calls you about a patient who is post-op day 1 from an abdominal hysterectomy you assisted with yesterday. The patient complained of dizziness when she got her up this morning and her vital signs are T 97.8, BP 100/65 mmHg, pulse (P) 100 beats/min, and R 16 breaths/min. What further information do you want to know?

(A) "What are her medication allergies?"
(B) "What is her post-op hemoglobin and hematocrit?"
(C) "What is her intravenous (IV) rate?"
(D) "What are her O_2 sats?"

---

14 A 43-year-old patient who is 7 days post-op from a laparoscopic hysterectomy for heavy menstrual bleeding and anemia presents to the clinic with fever. Her past medical history is complicated by diabetes that is moderately well controlled. She has a temperature of 100.8; pulse 90 beats/min; and BP 140/88 mmHg. She has normal bowel movements, urinary function, and decreased appetite. She denies any other

complaints. Her abdomen is examined and the infraumbilical incision is erythematous and tender to palpation. What is the next step in the management of this patient?

(A) Order computed tomography (CT) abdomen/pelvis
(B) Wound debridement
(C) Initiate antibiotics
(D) Plan surgical repair for umbilical hernia
(E) Reassure the patient

15 You are making post-op rounds with the gyn team and see a 42-year-old who is post-op day 3 from a total abdominal hysterectomy for fibroids and was to be dis charged but was noted to have a temperature of 100.3 at 0400 hours. She denies nausea, vomiting, diarrhea, constipation, chest pain, or shortness of breath. The patient has no allergies and has no other medical conditions. What is the next step in the management of this patient?

(A) Reassure the patient and send her home
(B) Begin antibiotics and send her home
(C) Order a urinalysis (UA)
(D) Order a CT angiogram
(E) Order a chest X-ray

16 A 38-year-old woman, G3P2002 at 38 weeks, presents to labor and delivery in the first stage of labor. She has had an uncomplicated pregnancy so far but at 5 cm she undergoes artificial rupture of membranes and thick meconium is noted. Later, at 8 cm, she is noted to have severe variable decelerations from her baseline of 130s to the 60s lasting 30 to 45 seconds. Variability remains moderate throughout. Luckily she undergoes a spontaneous vaginal delivery within an hour but the 1- and 5-minute Apgar scores are 6 and 9, respectively. Which of the following is an appropriate use of the Apgar score?

(A) To define the degree of birth asphyxia
(B) To assess the future risk of cerebral palsy
(C) To grade the overall health of the neonate
(D) To evaluate the need for neonatal resuscitation

17 You are assisting a senior resident on a Cesarean section. The patient is a 30-year-old G4P2103 at 39 weeks admitted for her fourth Cesarean. Once the uterus is visualized the resident points out an area of marked vascularity. "That's not a good sign," she says. After delivery of the baby, the patient undergoes Cesarean hysterectomy for uncontrollable bleeding. What does the uterine pathology report reveal?

(A) Placental tissue with large areas of calcification
(B) Placental tissue with large underlying clot
(C) Placental tissue penetrating into the myometrium
(D) Placental tissue penetrating through the full thickness of the myometrium

---

18 A 16-year-old G0 presents to the emergency room (ER) complaining of lower abdominal pain, nausea, and vomiting. Her last period was 1 week ago and she admits to being sexually active on no contraception. On examination she was noted to have the following: T 101, P 100 beats/min, and BP 128/84 mmHg. Her abdomen is slightly tender with no rebound. Her pelvic examination is remarkable for a thick yellow mucopurulent discharge. Left untreated, what is this patient at risk for?

(A) Chronic pelvic pain
(B) Ovarian cancer
(C) Cervical cancer
(D) Ovarian torsion

---

19 A 70-year-old woman presents with complaints of leaking of urine with a cough or sneeze, or while walking daily. It is significantly impacting her life. Medical history is complicated by hypertension controlled on hydrochlorothiazide. Vital signs are BP 149/90 mmHg and P 87 beats/min. Physical examination is remarkable for loss of her mid-urethral angle and minimal cystocele. There is no uterine prolapse or rectocele. The patient undergoes urodynamic testing confirming your suspected diagnosis of her urinary incontinence. What is the next best step in therapy for this patient?

(A) Oxybutynin
(B) Midurethral sling
(C) Trimethoprim–sulfamethoxazole
(D) Tolterodine

---

20 You are seeing an infertility patient in clinic. She is a 26-year-old G0 who has been trying to get pregnant for over a year. Her husband had a normal semen analysis. Her periods are regular and predictable but they last 6 to 7 days and are very painful. She has never had a sexually transmitted infection. She had been on oral contraceptive pills (OCPs) since her teens and did not have much pain until she stopped them to try to get pregnant. To make matters worse she is now having increasing pain with intercourse. What would be the most probable findings of a diagnostic laparoscopy?

(A) Filmy adhesions from the liver to the diaphragm
(B) Black pinpoint lesions on the appendix
(C) Red, white, or blue lesions on the ovaries
(D) Abscess adjacent to the uterosacral ligaments
(E) Erythema in the posterior cul-de-sac

---

21 A 37-year-old woman, G3P3003, status post three Cesarean sections and a tubal ligation presents to your office complaining of gradually worsening dysmenorrhea and heavy menstrual bleeding, though her cycles remain regular. Bimanual examination reveals a nontender, 12-week-sized globular uterus. Abdominal ultrasound reveals a uniformly enlarged uterus without evidence of discrete masses (see *Figure 5*). What is the most likely diagnosis?

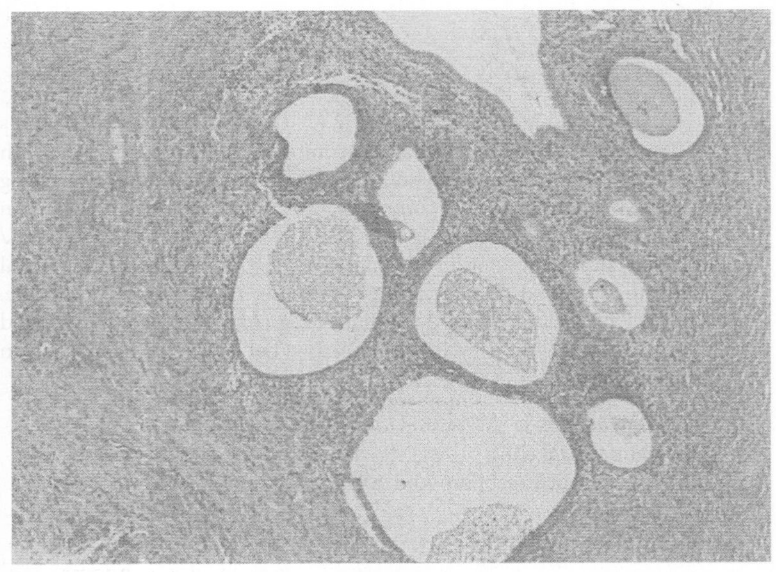

Figure 5

(A) Endometrial hyperplasia
(B) Adenomyosis
(C) Endometriosis
(D) Leiomyomata
(E) Leiomyosarcomata

22 A 25-year-old woman, G2P0101, presents to the hospital in active labor. She has received no prenatal care. Fundal height is 33 cm. Vital signs are T 98.2, BP 130/78 mmHg, and P 88 beats/min. She is 5 cm dilated and states she had a gush of fluid more than 24 hours prior to her presentation to the hospital. Ultrasound is consistent with a term pregnancy. Her labor is progressing normally and the fetal HR tracing is category 1. What should she be treated with?

(A) Azithromycin
(B) Penicillin
(C) Magnesium sulfate
(D) Betamethasone
(E) Acyclovir

23 A 26-year-old G2P1 presents for her routine prenatal care visit at 36 weeks 2 days by sure last menstrual period (LMP) and consistent with a second-trimester ultrasound. She denies loss of fluid, bleeding, or contractions. She admits to frequent fetal movement. She is a gestational diabetic requiring insulin. She has no other complications with her pregnancy. She plans to use the intrauterine device (IUD) for postpartum birth control. What test is indicated at this visit?

(A) Hemoglobin A1c
(B) Quad screen
(C) Transvaginal ultrasound for cervical length
(D) Rectovaginal culture for group B strep

24 A 34-year-old G2P2002 presents to clinic with intermittent bilateral milky discharge for the past 6 months. The discharge is non-bloody and is not associated with increased breast tenderness. The discharge occurs spontaneously without manual stimulation and she denies any recent changes in bra size. Until recently, the patient has had regular periods but they have become irregular over the last 6 to 9 months. Her last period was 6 weeks ago. She uses condoms. The patient is currently not taking any medications. In the office, BP is 120/75, HR 82, T 98.5, H 5′5″, and W 179 which is 20 lb heavier than when you saw her last year. On physical examination the breasts are symmetric and no breast lesions or masses are appreciated. A thin white discharge can be manually expressed bilaterally. Microscopy reveals fat globules. What is the most likely mechanism leading to these findings?

weight gain?

(A) Hyperprolactinemia from microadenoma of the pituitary gland
(B) Underlying intraductal papilloma
(C) Decreased clearance of prolactin due to renal failure
(D) Hyperprolactinemia from increased thyrotropin-releasing hormone due to hypothyroidism
(E) Cushing disease leading to increased growth hormone causing hyperprolactinemia

---

25 A 32-year-old G0 last period 1 week ago on oral contraceptives presents for her annual examination. The patient is concerned about hair loss, weight gain, and unusually light periods for the past 4 months. The patient attributes most of these symptoms to stress and wonders if there is anything you can do to help. The patient's only current medication is an oral contraceptive pill (OCP). The patient is currently not sexually active. The pelvic and breast examinations are normal. What is the next best step in the care of this patient?

(A) Refer the patient to a psychiatrist
(B) Prescribe alprazolam 0.25 mg PO TID with follow-up in 1 month
(C) Perform a pregnancy test
(D) Tell the patient to keep a daily basal body temperature log and return in 1 month
(E) Obtain a thyroid-stimulating hormone (TSH) test

---

26 A 22-year-old graduate student comes to see you for her annual examination. She is a G0, last period 3 weeks ago on oral contraceptives. Her gyn history is unremarkable but her medical history reveals a seizure disorder that is well controlled on medication. She is also being treated for anxiety and depression. You notice that aside from her seizure medication and antidepressant she is presently on a course of antibiotics for strep throat. Which of the following medications will decrease the effectiveness of her combined oral contraceptives?

(A) Carbamazepine
(B) Fluoxetine
(C) Ampicillin

---

27 A 16-year-old G1P0 at 10 weeks by last period presents to the clinic with 5 days of intractable nausea and light vaginal bleeding. Pelvic examination is significant for a 14-week-sized uterus. Quantitative hCG level is 150,000 and ultrasound imaging reveals a "snowstorm" appearance (see *Figure 6*). There are no fetal parts seen. The patient undergoes an uncomplicated dilation and evacuation in the operating room and the tissue is sent for genetic testing. What is the most likely genetic constitution of the specimen?

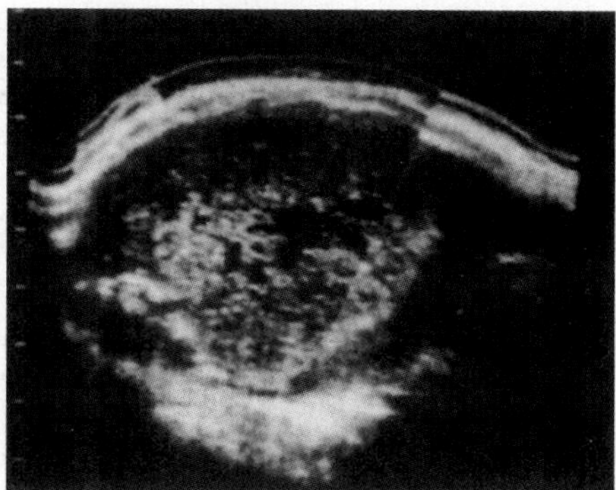

Figure 6

(A) 69, XXX
(B) 69, XXY
(C) 46, XX
(D) 46, XY

---

28 A 36-year-old G2P1 decides to undergo first-trimester genetic screening. At 11 weeks her blood is drawn and an ultrasound performed. The results are positive for a risk of trisomy 21 above her age-related risk. She is offered chorionic villus sampling as a diagnostic test. Which of the following findings was most likely seen on her first-trimester screening?

(A) Decreased level of hCG
(B) Decreased level of pregnancy-associated plasma protein A
(C) Decrease in size of the nuchal translucency
(D) Decreased level of α-fetoprotein

---

29 A 38-year-old G0 is being seen for preconception counseling. She is concerned about advanced maternal age and is inquiring about early detection of Down syndrome. What are the advantages of the quadruple screen over the triple screen?

(A) Adding hCG to the triple screen improves the detection rate of trisomy 18 to approximately 80%
(B) Adding hCG to the triple screen improves the detection rate of trisomy 21 to approximately 80%
(C) Adding inhibin to the triple screen improves the detection rate of trisomy 18 to approximately 80%
(D) Adding inhibin to the triple screen improves the detection rate of trisomy 21 to approximately 80%

30 A 33-year-old G1 had normal first-trimester genetic screening at 12 weeks. Her pregnancy has been uncomplicated and she presents for a routine obstetric visit at 16 weeks. What is the next step to further screen her pregnancy for aneuploidy?

- **(A)** Independent second-trimester serum screening with the quadruple screen
- **(B)** Ultrasound screening once at 26-week gestation
- **(C)** Integrated or sequential screening
- **(D)** 18-Week ultrasound with amniocentesis

31 A 23-year-old G0 is about to undergo diagnostic laparoscopy for severe pelvic pain consistent with endometriosis. During the consent process, the risks, benefits, and alternatives are explained to the patient and she is given the opportunity to ask questions. What is the primary purpose of the consent process?

- **(A)** To protect the physician from lawsuits
- **(B)** To protect patient autonomy
- **(C)** To disclose information relevant to the surgery
- **(D)** To establish a satisfactory physician–patient relationship

32 You are seeing a 16-year-old girl who is brought in by her mother because she has not started her period yet. Her medical history is unremarkable. She is a sophomore in high school and does well academically and in sports. When interviewed without her mother's presence, she admits to attempting intercourse once but her boyfriend "could not get in and it was very painful." She asks you not to tell her mother. A urinary pregnancy test is negative. She denies nausea, vomiting, abdominal pain, or cramping. On examination, she is 5′7″ tall and weighs 138 lb (body mass index [BMI] 21.6). She has Tanner stage V breast development with minimal pubic or axillary hair. Her mother prohibits a pelvic examination so an ultrasound is ordered. What would an ultrasound show?

- **(A)** Hematocolpos—a vagina filled with menstrual blood due to imperforate hymen
- **(B)** Hematometra—a uterus filled with blood due to transverse vaginal septum
- **(C)** Absent uterus and ovaries
- **(D)** Absent ovaries and rudimentary uterus
- **(E)** Normal female anatomy

33 A 26-year-old G0P0 presents to the resident clinic complaining of amenorrhea for 3 months. Menarche occurred at age 14 and although never regular, she has never gone this long without a period. She has been married for 4 years and used condoms until 2 years ago when they started trying to get pregnant. A urinary pregnancy test in the office is negative. She has no history of sexually transmitted infections. She is 5′6″ and weighs 193 lb (BMI 31.1). What physical examination finding would assist you in diagnosing the patient?

(A) Ambiguous genitalia
(B) Moderate acne
(C) Alopecia
(D) Cervical motion tenderness

34 A 32-year-old G3P2012 presents to her primary care physician complaining of several months of insomnia, heat intolerance, and decreased libido. She has not had a period in 2 years since getting her levonorgestrel intrauterine system placed. She denies recent changes in weight, diet, or activity. Her obstetric history includes two uncomplicated, full-term vaginal deliveries and one first-trimester spontaneous abortion. On examination, she is thin and tired-appearing, without thyromegaly. Vital signs are T 36.8°C, respiratory rate (RR) 14, P 82, and BP 132/78. Her weight is unchanged since last year. Her breasts are nontender, without masses or nipple discharge. Pelvic examination reveals moderately well-estrogenized vaginal mucosa and a small, nontender uterus with regular contours and no palpable adnexal masses. A urinary pregnancy test is negative. What test would best help you to assess the cause of the patient's symptoms?

(A) Follicle-stimulating hormone (FSH)
(B) Thyroid-stimulating hormone (TSH)
(C) Endometrial biopsy
(D) 24-Hour cortisol

35 A 17-year-old G2P1001 at 32-week gestation, comes to see you for a routine prenatal appointment. She complains of being tired all the time and short of breath. She is not taking her prenatal vitamins because her friends told her they make you gain more weight. BP is 100/60 and HR is 90. Heart and lung examinations are unremarkable. Fundal height is 31.5 and fetal heart tones (FHTs) are in the 150s. Labs show a hemoglobin of 9 g/dL. What is the most likely cause of the patient's fatigue?

(A) Iron deficiency
(B) Folate deficiency
(C) Hypothyroidism
(D) Physiologic changes
(E) Glucose-6-phosphate dehydrogenase deficiency

---

36 A 23-year-old G1 comes to see you for her first prenatal visit at 12 weeks. At the appointment, the patient informs you that she has a history of epileptic seizures but she stopped her medication when she found out she was pregnant because of fear of birth defects. The patient denies any complications since stopping the medication on her own. She has been seizure free for 5 years or so. What do you inform the patient?

(A) She stopped the medication just in time as intrauterine exposure to antiepileptic drugs is the main cause of birth defects in epileptic patients
(B) There is an increased risk of fetal anomalies associated with epilepsy itself
(C) She will be treated with magnesium sulfate in labor to prevent seizures
(D) She should restart the antiepileptic drugs immediately

---

37 A 37-year-old G2P2 comes to see you because she has recently noticed spotting between her periods that is progressively getting worse. Furthermore, her periods have gotten very heavy since her tubal ligation at age 33. She started her periods at age 13 and they have always been regular lasting about 5 days. Now they are lasting 7 to 8 days and are very heavy. She is also bleeding for a few days about a week after her period stops. She used pills for contraception until after her last pregnancy when she was diagnosed with gestational diabetes and had her tubes tied. Subsequently she was diagnosed with "real diabetes" and is now on oral medications with "OK" control. Her HgbA1c is 8. She is 5′4″ and weighs 188 lb. Vital signs are stable. Her examination is remarkable only for a 10-week smooth, nontender uterus. What is your immediate assessment and plan?

(A) The patient's abnormal uterine bleeding necessitates an endometrial biopsy to rule out endometrial hyperplasia and cancer
(B) The patient's abnormal uterine bleeding is likely due to premature ovarian failure and chromosomal analysis is indicated to rule out a genetic cause
(C) The patient's abnormal uterine bleeding should be treated with endometrial ablation since further childbearing is not desired
(D) The patient's abnormal uterine bleeding is likely due to anovulation necessitating workup for hypothalamic–pituitary–gonadal axis dysfunction

38 A 22-year-old G0 last period 6 weeks ago comes to see you for her annual examination. She has never been sexually active. Her past medical and surgical histories are unremarkable. The patient has seen her family medicine doctor for evaluation of inability to lose weight despite dieting and aerobic exercise. The doctor performed a thyroid test that was negative. On examination, the patient's BP is 112/82, P 68, height 5′3″, and weight 155. The thyroid, cardiac, pulmonary, breast, and pelvic examinations are all normal, but she is noted to have excessive hair on her chest and pubic region along with darkly pigmented axillae. What is the most likely cause of this patient's symptoms?

- **(A)** Pregnancy
- **(B)** Idiopathic hirsutism
- **(C)** Stein-Leventhal syndrome
- **(D)** 21-α-Hydroxylase deficiency
- **(E)** Pseudohermaphrodite

39 A 38-year-old G0 and her 40-year-old husband present for evaluation of infertility. His semen analysis is normal. She has monthly cycles with minimal cramping and positive ovulation indicator for the entire 6 months they have been trying. Their past medical histories are negative as are their family histories. They are nonsmokers and deny history of sexually transmitted infections. They have been married for 4 years and used a levonorgestrel-releasing intrauterine device (IUD) until 1 year ago. Today the patient appears in good health with HR 70 beats/min, BP 110/72 mmHg, RR 18 breaths/min, T 98.6, H 63, and W 125. What is the next best step in the management of this couple's infertility?

- **(A)** Counsel the couple on good conception practices and if still unsuccessful at 12 months inform the couple to return for infertility assessment
- **(B)** Perform a hysterosalpingogram to evaluate possible tubal infertility secondary to scaring from the patient's levonorgestrel-releasing IUD
- **(C)** Inform the patient that it is likely due to advanced maternal age and immediately begin an infertility workup with an follicle-stimulating hormone (FSH level) for ovarian reserve
- **(D)** Due to advanced maternal age, schedule an appointment in 1 month to harvest eggs and plan for in vitro fertilization at 12 months if couple has not conceived naturally

40 A 20-year-old G0 presents to the emergency room (ER) with nausea, vomiting, headaches, and dizziness for several days. She uses condoms

for contraception but noted her last period was 6 weeks ago. She claims they have been regular since menarche at age 12. Her past medical history is unremarkable. Vital signs are T 36.8, P 100 beats/min, BP 160/100 mmHg, and RR 16 breaths/min. On examination you note a nervous young woman with slight hand tremor. Her pelvic examination is remarkable for bright red bleeding from a 10-week-sized uterus. What is the most likely diagnosis?

(A) Missed abortion
(B) Incomplete abortion
(C) Gestational hypertension
(D) Molar pregnancy
(E) Ectopic pregnancy

---

41 A 14-year-old G0 presents with her mother complaining of painful periods. Menarche was at age 12 and her periods are monthly and predictable, lasting 5 days. She has always had painful periods but her menstrual cramping now is so severe for the first 3 days of her period that she misses school and had to drop out of the basketball team. She has tried heating pads to no avail. She is not sexually active and has no significant medical history. Her physical examination is unremarkable. What would you recommend for this 14-year-old patient.

(A) Acetaminophen
(B) Nonsteroidal anti-inflammatory drugs
(C) Diagnostic laparoscopy
(D) Oral contraceptive pills (OCPs)
(E) Gonadotropin antagonists

---

42 A 19-year-old G0 presents for an annual well-woman examination. She is sexually active with multiple male partners, receives depot medroxyprogesterone injections every 3 months for contraception, and says that she "almost always" uses condoms. During the initial interview she breaks down crying and tells you she really made the appointment because of a bump on her vagina. On examination, you notice a single 1-cm round ulcer with a clean-cut margin on the inner surface of the patient's left labia majora. The patient reports that she had noticed this lesion about a week ago, but that it is not painful. Which of the following pathogens is the likely cause of this patient's lesion?

(A) Herpes simplex
(B) *Haemophilus ducreyi*
(C) *Treponema pallidum*
(D) *Chlamydia trachomatis*
(E) Varicella zoster

43 A 32-year-old G2P1 presents to triage at 38 weeks and 5 days with ruptured membranes and meconium. She is having no contractions. The patient's first baby was delivered by Cesarean at term for footling breech presentation. She had discussed the possibility of a trial of labor after Cesarean section (TOLAC) during her prenatal visits and desires to proceed with this. What is this patient's greatest risk if she undergoes induction?

(A) Placental abruption
(B) Uterine rupture
(C) Cord prolapse
(D) Meconium aspiration
(E) Pulmonary embolism

44 A 35-year-old G2P2 is calling back for the results of a loop electrical excision procedure performed for possible severe dysplasia. She became sexually active at 15 and has had 15 or more lifetime male partners. She has a Mirena intrauterine device (IUD) and therefore does not use condoms regularly. She had chlamydia twice in her teens along with trichomoniasis. Her recent HIV test was negative. She drinks four to six beers per weekend and admits to smoking three to four cigarettes a day and more on weekends. Which of the following is the most significant risk factor for cervical squamous cell carcinoma in this patient?

(A) History of cigarette smoking
(B) Age of first intercourse
(C) Use of an IUD
(D) Number of sexual partners in her lifetime
(E) History of sexually transmitted infections

45 A 58-year-old P0 obese woman with a 40 pack-year history presents to her gynecologist for vaginal bleeding. The bleeding started as intermittent spotting about a month ago and now is daily and requires a panty liner. There is no pain or cramping. She reports menarche at age 11 and menopause at age 52. She has had no abnormal Pap smears. She was on combination hormone replacement therapy for the first year after menopause. Which of the following is thought to be protective against endometrial cancer?

(A) Negative Pap/human papilloma virus (HPV) history
(B) Obesity
(C) Nulliparity
(D) Late menopause
(E) Smoking

46 An 18-year-old primigravida underwent a spontaneous vaginal delivery under no epidural. Following delivery of the head she screamed uncontrollably resulting in rapid delivery of the shoulders and a second-degree midline laceration along with bilateral sidewall tears. During inspection prior to repair, a non-enlarging hematoma, 3 cm in diameter, is noted adjacent to the right sidewall tear. After repairing the lacerations, what is the next step in the management of this patient?

(A) Manage expectantly with frequent evaluation
(B) Surgically open the area of clotted blood at its most dependent portion and drain
(C) Apply drains and vaginal packs to the area of clotted blood
(D) Apply heat packs to the affected area

47 A 16-year-old primigravida undergoes a spontaneous vaginal delivery of a 3,400 g male after a long induction for preeclampsia at 39 weeks including 3 hours of pushing. She is stable on magnesium sulfate and an epidural. After spontaneous delivery of an intact placenta, the uterus is noted to be boggy despite administration of oxytocin intravenously. What is the next step in the management of this patient?

(A) Cesarean hysterectomy
(B) Manual uterine massage
(C) Wait 10 minutes and reassess
(D) Blood type and screen the patient
(E) Apply uterine compression sutures

48 A 46-year-old woman presents with abnormal menses. She usually has regular periods every month lasting 5 to 6 days but over the last 9 months they have been very irregular, ranging from every 15 to 45 days. They also last up to 7 days. Additionally she is experiencing some difficulty sleeping and is often awakened by hot flashes. She denies weight gain, hair loss, or temperature intolerance. She also denies nipple discharge or visual changes. What is the most likely cause of this patient's abnormal uterine bleeding?

(A) Hypothyroidism
(B) Menopause
(C) Pituitary prolactinoma
(D) Polycystic ovarian syndrome (PCOS)
(E) Anovulatory bleeding

49 A 24-year-old G1 at 39 weeks presents at 4/50/−2 with complaint of regular contractions every 3 minutes and spontaneous rupture of membranes 3 hours ago. Reevaluation 4 hours after arrival confirms no change in her cervical examination despite contractions every 3 to 4 minutes. The patient is concerned because a friend of hers underwent a Cesarean section when she "got stuck" at 4 cm for 3 hours. What advice can you give this patient?

(A) A prolonged latent phase is considered a risk factor for Cesarean section
(B) Modern labor patterns confirm the findings of Friedman in the 1950s
(C) Multiparous women begin active labor at lesser dilation than primiparous women
(D) Ninety percent of women will be in active labor at 5-cm dilation
(E) Perceived pain level has been demonstrated to be reliable at differentiating latent from active phase of labor

---

50 A 24-year-old G1 at term is taken to the operating room for a stat Cesarean for fetal distress with fetal heart tones (FHTs) in the 60s for over 10 minutes despite repositioning and other efforts. The newborn has an HR of less than 100, a slow RR, flaccid muscle tone, a grimace, and blue coloring. What is the appropriate Apgar score?

(A) 1
(B) 2
(C) 3
(D) 4
(E) 5

---

51 A 17-year-old G1 at 10 weeks presents for her prenatal visit to discuss her initial labwork. A urine culture performed at her first prenatal visit was positive for *Escherichia coli.* She denies history of urinary tract infection and also denies dysuria, frequency, or urgency. She has no drug allergies. What is the appropriate management?

(A) Repeat the culture
(B) Prescribe cephalexin
(C) Prescribe ciprofloxacin
(D) Order a renal ultrasound
(E) No treatment

---

52 A 20-year-old G2P1 at 12 weeks presents for a follow-up to her new obstetric visit. As you review her routine prenatal labs you note a positive urine culture for *Staphylococcus saprophyticus.* Review of systems is negative for urinary frequency, urgency, or other symptoms. A urinalysis (UA) today reveals negative nitrites. What is your rationale for antibiotic treatment?

(A) Decrease the risk of chorioamnionitis
(B) Prevent preterm premature rupture of membranes
(C) Prevent kidney stones
(D) Prevent preterm labor
(E) Prevent the development of antibiotic resistance

---

53 A 23-year-old G0P0 of Ashkenazi descent, presents with a 3-week history of a painful right breast lump that is about the "size of a jelly bean." Her last menstrual period (LMP) was 2 weeks ago on oral contraceptive pills (OCPs). She has no medical problems. Family history is positive for premenopausal breast cancer in her mother and a maternal aunt who were diagnosed at 39 and 42, respectively. Her maternal grandmother died from ovarian cancer at age 62. Physical examination confirms a mobile, tender mass on the right at 10 o'clock about 2 cm from the nipple edge. There are no associated skin changes or axillary nodes. What is your next step?

(A) Diagnostic mammogram
(B) Helical CT scan
(C) Magnetic resonance imaging
(D) Screening mammogram
(E) Ultrasound

---

54 A 25-year-old G0P0 last menstrual period (LMP) was 3+ weeks ago using condoms presents for evaluation of a breast mass she found yesterday. Her maternal aunt was diagnosed with breast cancer recently. This news, along with cyclic breast pain, made her do a breast examination and she noted a lump in her right breast. There is no other family history of cancer.

Breast examination reveals moderate nodularity bilaterally with a single, 1-cm, mobile, tender mass in the upper outer quadrant of her right breast. No lymphadenopathy or nipple discharge is noted. The remainder of her history, review of systems, and physical examination are unremarkable. What is the next step?

(A) Ultrasound
(B) Biopsy
(C) Mammogram
(D) Re-examine after the next menses
(E) Routine follow-up in 1 year

---

55 A 45-year-old G4P4003 presents for an annual gynecologic examination. She had a tubal ligation and is having regular periods. She complains of fullness in her vagina after being active a few hours and has had difficulty inserting tampons. She is sexually active and notes no

difficulty with intercourse. She denies leakage of urine or any difficulty having a bowel movement. She had four vaginal deliveries, each one greater than 4,000 g. Her last delivery was 18 years ago. She had a third-degree laceration that was repaired without incident.

Physical examination is remarkable for prolapse of the anterior vaginal wall. What is the diagnosis?

(A) Cystocele
(B) Enterocele
(C) Rectocele
(D) Urethrocele

---

56 A 58-year-old woman presents with severe pain when attempting intercourse for the first time in several years. She was recently widowed after taking care of her ailing husband and had not had intercourse in over 5 years. She had been on estrogen therapy for about 2 to 3 years after a hysterectomy for fibroids in her late 40s. On examination you note thinned tissue around the urethra and at the introitus. No discharge is noted externally. There is no discoloration. On speculum examination, pale, thin vaginal epithelium with scant thin clear vaginal secretion is noted. Measurement of pH is 6.0. Whiff test is negative. KOH prep is negative. What will you find on her wet mount?

(A) Columnar cells
(B) Parabasal cells
(C) Ciliated cells
(D) Clue cells
(E) Pseudohyphae

---

57 A 44-year-old woman, G2P2, presents for a routine annual examination. Until 4 months ago, her menses were normal. Over the past 3 months she has not had a period and has noticed symptoms associated with "the change of life." These include moodiness, vaginal dryness, difficulty sleeping throughout the night, occasional hot flashes, and excessive fatigue during the day. As a result, she has stopped exercising which she feels contributed to her recent 7-lb weight gain.

Past medical history reveals hypothyroidism followed by her primary care physician. She is otherwise healthy and reports no other remarkable history. Her general physical examination is unremarkable, as are her vital signs. On pelvic examination, you note an irregular, mildly enlarged uterus. Which of the following tests is the most appropriate?

(A) Follicle-stimulating hormone (FSH)
(B) Luteinizing hormone (LH)
(C) Pregnancy test
(D) Sonogram
(E) Thyroid-stimulating hormone (TSH)

---

58 A 26-year-old G1 with no prenatal care presents to labor and delivery because of bright red, painless vaginal bleeding that occurred after intercourse. Her gestational age of 29 weeks by last period is confirmed by fundal height and ultrasound that also reveals a complete placenta previa. There are no contractions and fetal heart tones (FHTs) are reactive. The bleeding has subsided. Hemoglobin is 12.6 and platelets are 199K. Management of this patient includes which of the following?

(A) Blood transfusion
(B) Double setup examination
(C) Hospitalization
(D) Immediate Cesarean section
(E) Immediate Pitocin induction of labor

---

59 A 30-year-old G2P2 presents to the clinic for preconception counseling. Her last pregnancy was remarkable for severe postpartum depression requiring medication. Looking back, the symptoms started during the pregnancy and were present but milder during her first pregnancy. She is currently taking selective serotonin reuptake inhibitor (SSRI) and wants advice about pursuing another pregnancy. Which of the following would you have her switch for another SSRI?

(A) Citalopram
(B) Fluoxetine
(C) Fluvoxamine
(D) Paroxetine
(E) Sertraline

---

60 A 37-year-old G1P0 Chinese exchange student presents 9 weeks after her last normal menstrual period to the emergency room (ER). Her BP on arrival was 205/115 mmHg and she is in a postictal state. A pregnancy test is positive with a qualitative β-hCG of 1,500,000 mIU. What would you expect to find on ultrasound?

(A) Twin gestation
(B) Anembryonic pregnancy
(C) Snowstorm pattern
(D) Ectopic pregnancy

---

61 You are making obstetric rounds and see a 24-year-old G1P1 who is status post Cesarean 4 days ago for arrest of descent. She has been on gentamicin and clindamycin for 2 days for temperature 39°C associated with a tender uterus. She has continued to spike daily. Her white blood count is 18K and her examination remains unchanged with clear lungs and tender uterus. What is the next step?

(A) Add ampicillin
(B) Add cephazolin
(C) Order ultrasound
(D) Order chest X-ray

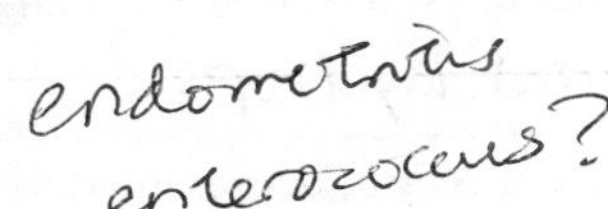

62 A 29-year-old, G1P0010, woman with regular menses (every 28 days lasting 5 days) is currently trying to conceive. She has not used contraception for 6 months. Her ovulation predictor kit revealed an luteinizing hormone (LH) surge 7 days ago. She presents with acute left lower quadrant pain. The ultrasound reveals fluid in her cul-de-sac. A pregnancy test is negative. What is the most likely diagnosis?

(A) Cystic teratoma
(B) Ectopic pregnancy
(C) Follicular cyst
(D) Hemorrhagic corpus luteum cyst
(E) Serous cystadenoma

63 A 23-year-old G2P1 who recently moved to the United States from Vietnam presents at 32-week gestation by last period with no prenatal care. Her previous birth was a normal spontaneous vaginal delivery at home in the countryside attended by a lay midwife. Examination is remarkable for fundal height of 36 cm. Ultrasound examination revealed fetal skin edema (7 mm), fetal ascites, polyhydramnios, and a thickened placenta (see *Figure 7*). What prenatal lab will assist in the diagnosis and treatment of this patient?

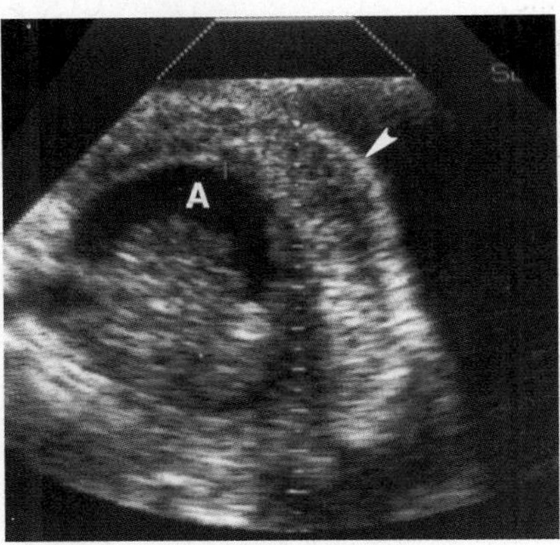

Figure 7

(A) Complete blood count (CBC)
(B) Rubella titer
(C) Test for syphilis
(D) Blood type and Rh
(E) HBsAg

---

64 A G2P1 at 33 weeks presented to Triage with ruptured membranes and fully dilated. She subsequently underwent a precipitous vaginal delivery before being moved to a delivery room. The neonate cried spontaneously and received an Apgar score of 7 at 1 minute. Although the neonatal team had been called, they did not arrive until 4 minutes after the delivery. The Triage room was not equipped with a baby warmer. What is the most effective method to keep this neonate warm after initially drying it until the neonatal team arrives?

(A) Move to the warmer immediately
(B) Cover the neonate's head with a stocking net
(C) Swaddle the neonate
(D) Place in a plastic bag
(E) Place the baby skin-to-skin with the mother

---

65 A 31-year-old G1P0 at 40 weeks presents with premature rupture of membrane. Her cervix is cl/th/high. She progressed to 4 cm after a single dose of misoprostol, but over the past 3 hours she has not changed her cervix. An intrauterine pressure catheter (IUPC) is placed and the Montevideo unit per 10 minutes equals 40. What is the next step?

(A) Give subcutaneous terbutaline
(B) Administer oxytocin
(C) Prepare for Cesarean
(D) Start amnioinfusion
(E) Re-examine in 2 hours

---

66 A 24-year-old G2P1011 just delivered a 29-week neonate via primary low vertical Cesarean section for breech and severe preeclampsia. Estimated blood loss was over 1,200 cc. Which of the medications is most likely responsible for the postpartum hemorrhage (PPH)?

(A) Cephazolin
(B) Betamethasone
(C) Oxytocin
(D) Magnesium sulfate

67 A 23-year-old G1P1 just delivered a 3,120 g neonate via spontaneous vaginal delivery after a long induction for postdates and pushing for over 2 hours. Estimated blood loss was 800 cc. Her medical history is significant for seasonal allergies and asthma. Her pregnancy was complicated by gestational diabetes. Which of the following should be avoided when in this patient?

(A) Methylergonovine
(B) Misoprostol
(C) Oxytocin
(D) Prostaglandin E1
(E) Carboprost tromethamine

68 A 33-year-old G3P3003 presents to the emergency room (ER) 10 days postpartum with fever and right flank pain. She had one isolated spike in her temperature postpartum day 1 and was not started on antibiotics. On arrival to the ER, vital signs are T 39.2, P 120 beats/min, and R 16 breaths/min. A complete blood count (CBC) reveals WBC of 15.2K, hemoglobin 11.6/hematocrit 33. A voided midstream urinalysis (UA) is leukocyte esterase positive and nitrite negative. There are 15 WBCs/high power field with WBC casts present. Homan sign is negative. Breast examination is normal, non-engorged. Costovertebral angle tenderness (CVAT) is positive on the right. Her uterus is nontender. What is the most likely organism?

(A) Enterococci
(B) *E. coli*
(C) *Klebsiella* spp.
(D) *Pseudomonas aeruginosa*
(E) *S. saprophyticus*

69 You see a 17-year-old G1 at 37 week's who was admitted for mild preeclampsia. A sonogram that was performed today reveals a singleton gestation with estimated fetal weight of 2,800 g consistent with last menstrual period (LMP), vertex presentation, anterior grade 2 placenta, amniotic fluid index (AFI) 2.6. A cervical examination today is cl/th/−3. The plan is induction if symptoms worsen. The mother expresses concern because she had a postpartum hemorrhage (PPH) after delivering her daughter, receiving 3 units of blood and subsequently developing

hepatitis C. She wants to know if there are ways to prevent PPH and thus avoid blood products during her daughter's delivery. You tell them that the daughter's risk factors include:

(A) Preeclampsia
(B) A possible induction of labor
(C) Oligohydramnios
(D) A family history of PPH

---

70 A 25-year-old G3P2002 at 10 weeks presents to the emergency room (ER) with severe cramping and bleeding. She says she has passed large clots but is unsure of passing tissue. On examination T 98, BP 100/60 mmHg, P 100 beats/min, and R 16 breaths/min. She appears to be in pain, but cooperative. Her abdomen is tender in the midline. Pelvic reveals an open cervical os with tissue protruding. An ultrasound reveals large amounts of tissue and clot in the uterus. Her Hgb is 7.8. What is the most appropriate plan for this patient?

(A) Admit for serial quantitative hCGs
(B) Admit for immediate transfusion
(C) Admit for immediate dilatation and curettage
(D) Discharge with prescription for misoprostol
(E) Discharge with prescription for methylergonovine

---

71 A 23-year-old G2P0100 at 25 weeks presents with regular contractions and cervical dilation to 2/75/−2. Luckily the contractions respond to hydration and slow down. Her first pregnancy was delivered at 26 weeks and the baby died of pulmonary complications. She has been offered weekly progesterone injections but could not afford them. During your conversation, her membranes rupture copious, clear fluid. What is your next step?

(A) Discuss cerclage
(B) Discuss antenatal corticosteroids
(C) Discuss emergency Cesarean
(D) Discuss tocolysis

---

72 A 20-year-old G1P1 presents to the clinic with fever and chills 2 weeks postpartum. Vital signs are P 110 beats/min, R 16 breaths/min, and T 39°C. She appears to be in mild distress. Breast examination: bilateral engorgement with the right side being much larger with cracked nipple and surrounding erythema. Her pelvic and abdominal examinations are completely benign. You advise her to start dicloxacillin immediately. What is the next step?

(A) Continue to breastfeed on both sides
(B) Bind breasts with cabbage leaves and ace wraps and stop breastfeeding
(C) Breastfeed on the left, pump the milk on the right side, and dump it
(D) Pump on both sides and dump it

---

73 A 30-year-old G2P2 last period 3 weeks ago status post tubal ligation presents to the emergency room (ER) for the fourth time in 3 months. She complains of intermittent left lower quadrant pain associated with severe vomiting. The pain is 7/10 now but she says it comes and goes at lesser intensities. It is triggered by exercise and relieved by lying down and turning onto her stomach. Her bowel movements are normal and she has no bladder symptoms. The previous ER visits of her pain resolved spontaneously while awaiting an ultrasound so she left. This time the pain has lasted longer and is stronger than usual. What is your next step?

(A) Order a CT scan
(B) Order an ultrasound with color-flow Doppler
(C) Order serial quantitative hCGs
(D) Set her up for emergency laparoscopy
(E) Set her up for a hysteroscopy

---

74 While working in the emergency department, a 15-year-old female patient is brought in by her parents who are concerned she may have appendicitis. They state she started having abdominal pain last night and developed a fever to 100.8 along with chills. She has been nauseated and did not go to school today for the pain. The patient is in the fetal position and appears to be in pain. She flinches when you accidently bump the bed. When her parents leave the room for her examination, the patient tells you her period started a week ago and she is sexually active on no contraception. Her temperature is 101.2, P 100 beats/min, BP 134/80 mmHg, and R 18 breaths/min. Her abdomen is tense with decreased bowel sounds and tenderness to palpation in all four quadrants. On pelvic examination you note a light yellow discharge with no odor and marked cervical motion tenderness. Aside from appendicitis, what is the most likely diagnosis?

(A) Ovarian torsion
(B) Endometriosis
(C) Pelvic inflammatory disease
(D) Ectopic pregnancy
(E) Ruptured ovarian cyst

75 Refer to the patient in Question 74 to answer the question. What is the most appropriate next step in patient management?

(A) Prescribe methotrexate and ask her to follow up as an outpatient
(B) Admit the patient to the hospital and treat with cefotetan
(C) Perform a Pap smear with high-risk human papilloma virus (HPV) testing and ask her to follow up as an outpatient
(D) Rush the patient to the operating room for emergent laparoscopic evaluation
(E) Prescribe metronidazole and ask her to follow up as an outpatient

76 A 30-year-old G3P2002 at 28 weeks presents to the emergency room (ER) with right-sided flank pain, dysuria, and fever of 101. Examination revealed right Costovertebral angle tenderness (CVAT) and urinalysis (UA) confirmed the diagnosis of pyelonephritis. After 3 days in hospital on intravenous (IV) antibiotics the patient is ready to go home on a 14-day course of antibiotics. What will you advise after her follow-up visit?

(A) We will order an outpatient renal ultrasound
(B) We should start a 24-hour urine collection for total protein
(C) We will start her on prophylactic antibiotics in labor
(D) We will start prophylactic daily antibiotics for the rest of her pregnancy

77 A 25-year-old G3P2002 presents for her 36-week prenatal visit and states that she is not feeling the baby move as often. This pregnancy has been uncomplicated as were her previous two. The patient's BP is 100/68 mmHg with a pulse of 80 beats/min. Fetal HR is in the 140s by Doppler. Fundal height is measured to be 35 cm. What is the next step in the management of this patient?

(A) Reassure the patient that babies slow down near term
(B) Send the patient for an immediate nonstress test (NST)
(C) Send the patient for an immediate contraction stress test
(D) Order an ultrasound
(E) Admit her for 24-hour observation

78 A 22-year-old G2P1001 at 32 weeks presents to the obstetric clinic complaining of leaking fluid for the past 18 hours. The patient denies fever, abdominal cramping, vaginal bleeding, or dysuria. She is afebrile and the uterus is nontender. Fetal heart tones (FHTs) are reactive and there are no contractions noted on the monitor. Vaginal examination shows a copious amount of clear fluid in the vaginal vault. Microscopy reveals ferning. What is the next step in the management of this patient?

(A) Perform an urgent Cesarean section.
(B) Start Pitocin induction after confirming vertex presentation
(C) Admit to the hospital to begin latency antibiotic therapy
(D) Perform ultrasound to determine the amniotic fluid index (AFI)

---

79 A 22-year-old G2P0101 at 30 4/7 weeks presents to her prenatal appointment. A 20-week growth scan confirmed her dates but the patient has had poor weight gain and her fundal height has been consistently 2 cm behind her gestational age for the last 3 visits. Today she again fails to gain weight and her fundal height is only 26 cm. Fetal heart tones (FHTs) are 140s. She denies leaking of fluid or fever and confirms fetal movement. What is the next step in the management of this patient?

(A) Schedule an appointment with the dietician
(B) Schedule a growth ultrasound
(C) Schedule biweekly nonstress tests (NSTs)
(D) Admit to hospital for fetal monitoring
(E) Schedule a biophysical profile (BPP)

---

80 You are examining a placenta from a recently delivered neonate. The mother was a 40-year-old G5P0222 who was delivered at 32 weeks by stat Cesarean for ominous fetal tracing. The Apgar scores were 2 at 1 minute/4 at 5 minutes/6 at 10 minutes. The placenta is small for dates, calcified, and has adherent clot covering 25% of the surface area. What do you think the fetal tracing shown in *Figure 8*?

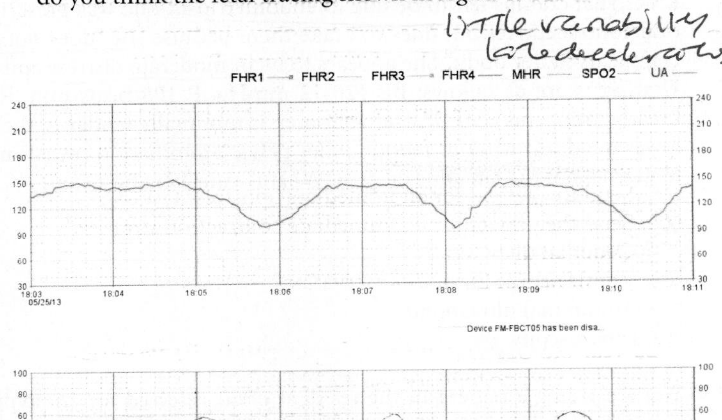

Figure 8

(A) Late decelerations with moderate variability
(B) Late decelerations with absent variability
(C) Variable decelerations to the 80s
(D) Variable decelerations to the 50s

---

81 A 24-year-old G0 presents to the clinic as a referral from a local family practitioner with an atypical squamous cells of undetermined significance (ASCUS) Pap. She had a Pap about 2 to 3 years ago and it was normal. She became sexually active at age 17 and has had five lifetime partners. She and her male partner have been together for over a year. She started having periods at age 13 and has regular cycles on her own. Her last period was 1 week ago on oral contraceptives. She has a history of Herpes simplex virus (HSV) well controlled with daily acyclovir. Her physical examination is normal. What is the next step?

(A) Repeat the Pap
(B) Get high-risk human papilloma virus (HPV) typing
(C) Get low-risk HPV typing
(D) Perform colposcopy
(E) Perform a conization

---

82 You are in the emergency room (ER) seeing a 19-year-old college student, last menstrual period (LMP) 6 weeks ago, with moderate left lower quadrant pain and minimal spotting. She did not know she was pregnant until today when she took a urine pregnancy test at the request of her roommate who brought her in. She has a history of severe menstrual cramps felt to be due to endometriosis. She was prescribed oral contraceptives but does not take them because she "does not like chemicals in her body." She appears to be in moderate distress and her vital signs are as follows: BP 120/72 mmHg, P 108 beats/min, R 18 breaths/min, and BMI 27. Her abdomen is minimally tender in the left lower quadrant without rebound; her pelvic examination reveals mild tenderness in the left adnexal area. What is your next best step?

(A) Qualitative hCG
(B) Quantitative hCG
(C) Vaginal ultrasound
(D) Abdominal ultrasound
(E) Laparoscopy

---

83 You are seeing a patient in the resident clinic referred for an atypical squamous cells of undetermined significance (ASCUS) Pap. The patient is a 22-year-old college student, G0 last period 2 weeks ago on oral contraceptives. She became sexually active at 16 and has three life partners. She has never had a sexually transmitted infection and has not had Gardasil. What is the next step?

(A) Offer colposcopy
(B) Offer cryotherapy
(C) Offer repeat Pap in 6 months
(D) Offer high-risk human papilloma virus (HPV) typing
(E) Offer low-risk HPV typing

---

84 You are in the resident clinic seeing a 19-year-old white woman requesting an annual examination. What information would best guide you in contraceptive counseling?

(A) Her obstetric history
(B) Her sexual history
(C) Her family history
(D) Her past medical history
(E) Her smoking history

---

85 A 54-year-old white woman, G2P2002, presents to your clinic who is 3 years postmenopause with history of vaginal bleeding for 3 to 4 days last month. She has hypothyroidism and hypertension well controlled by her family medicine doctor. She had a normal mammogram less than a year ago and a Pap 2 years ago. Menopause was unremarkable with the patient using hormones for less than a year. Her history is otherwise unremarkable. On examination she is in no apparent distress. She is afebrile with BP 138/82 mmHg, P 88 beats/min, and BMI 35. Her pelvic examination is remarkable for marked vaginal atrophy, making her bimanual somewhat uncomfortable. Her cervix is noted to be small and stenotic. She is not bleeding and her uterus is of 6-week size. Her ovaries are not palpable. What is your next step?

(A) Perform in-office endometrial biopsy
(B) Start vaginal estrogen cream and return for endometrial biopsy in 6 weeks
(C) Perform vaginal ultrasound
(D) Schedule dilatation and curettage in hospital
(E) Schedule office hysteroscopy

---

86 You are in the emergency room (ER) seeing a 20-year-old G0 last menstrual period (LMP) 2 weeks ago on oral contraceptive pills (OCPs) who complains of painful bumps near her vagina. She is currently sexually active with a new male partner of 3 to 4 months and rarely uses condoms. She became sexually active at age 16 and has had six lifetime partners. She denies any history of sexually transmitted infections. Her past medical history and surgical history are unremarkable. On physical examination she is anxious but in no distress. Her vital signs are stable and she is afebrile. Her examination is remarkable for

HSV

left inguinal lymphadenopathy and a cluster of tender vesicles on her left labia majora. What is the next step?

(A) GC/chlamydia DNA, Herpes simplex virus (HSV) I and II IgM and IgG; Pap
(B) GC/chlamydia DNA, HSV I and II IgA and IgG
(C) GC/chlamydia DNA, HSV I and II IgM and IgG, lipid profile
(D) Call in acyclovir after discussing the diagnosis

---

87 A 27-year-old G2P1011 presents to your clinic for preconception counseling. Two years ago she had a second-trimester miscarriage, and postmortem examination of the fetus detected spina bifida. She desires another child and wants to know how to prevent a recurrence. Which of the following recommendations can decrease the risk of another fetus being affected with spina bifida?

(A) 1,000 mg/day omega 3
(B) 2,000 mg/day omega 3
(C) 400 μg/day folic acid
(D) 2 mg/day folic acid
(E) 4 mg/day folic acid

---

88 A 26-year-old G2P2 presents for her annual gynecologic examination. Her mother is 46 and recently diagnosed with ovarian cancer. She would like to discuss her risk of ovarian cancer. Menarche occurred at age 10. She used oral contraceptive pills (OCPs) for 3 years prior to the birth of her first child when she was 23. She had her second child at age 25. She breastfed both of her children for 1 year. She had a maternal aunt who passed away in her 80s from breast cancer. She does not smoke or consume excessive alcohol. She admits to a high-fat diet though and has had little time to exercise since the birth of her children. What is this woman's greatest potential risk factor for developing ovarian cancer?

(A) BRCA mutation
(B) Poor diet and limited exercise
(C) Family history
(D) Early menarche
(E) Late childbearing

---

89 A 27-year-old G2P1001 at 37 week's presents to your clinic for a routine prenatal care visit. She complains of mild discomfort while urinating so you decide to perform a urinalysis (UA). The UA shows large leukocytes, positive nitrites, negative protein, and trace blood. What is the most appropriate next step in managing this patient?

(A) Treat with a 7- to 10-day course of ciprofloxacin
(B) Treat with a 7- to 10-day course of amoxicillin
(C) Treat with a 7- to 10-day course of cephalexin
(D) Treat with nitrofurantoin daily for the remainder of the pregnancy
(E) Perform a urine culture prior to initiating any form of treatment

---

90 A 21-year-old G0 presents to the emergency room (ER) with temperature of 101 at home and severe left lower quadrant pain. Her last menstrual period (LMP) was 2 weeks ago. She denies any medical problems and has not had any surgical procedures. She has several sexual partners and reports inconsistent condom use. Review of systems is positive for nausea and vaginal discharge. Physical examination findings include T 101.2, P 105 beats/min, and BP 110/60 mmHg. She is noted to have involuntary guarding along with left lower quadrant tenderness to palpation and rebound. There is yellow discharge at the cervical os (which is tender) and a palpable left adnexal mass. WBC count is 19,000. β-hCG is negative. What is the most appropriate next step?

(A) Admit to hospital for serial quantitative β-HCGs
(B) Admit to hospital for intravenous (IV) antibiotics
(C) Admit to hospital for surgical intervention
(D) Discharge home with oral antibiotics
(E) Obtain a CT scan

---

91 A 33-year-old G0 patient comes to the clinic for preconception counseling. She has had regular periods since age 13 and was on oral contraceptives until a year ago when she developed hypertension so now she uses condoms. She was tried on several high BP medications before settling on enalapril. She may not really need it though since her hypertension may have been due to anxiety now well controlled with sertraline. She has a family history of hypertension and diabetes. In fact both of her sisters got gestational diabetes. Her vitals today are BP 120/76 mmHg, HR 72 beats/min, RR 18 breaths/min, and T 98.0. She has a BMI of 34. What is the most urgent advice you give her?

(A) Start prenatal vitamins as soon as possible
(B) Lose weight before you attempt pregnancy
(C) Switch enalapril to another antihypertensive
(D) Discontinue Zoloft immediately

---

92 A 37-year-old G3P0020 at 37 week's gestation comes to clinic for her weekly nonstress test (NST) due to chronic hypertension. The NST has one acceleration in 40 minutes. What is the next step?

(A) Obtain a biophysical profile (BPP)
(B) Obtain an ultrasound for estimated gestational weight
(C) Admit for induction
(D) Admit for Cesarean
(E) Repeat the Newborn Screening Ontario in 24 hours

93 A full biophysical profile (BPP) is ordered. In a 30-minute period you observe diaphragmatic movement for 1 minute, an amniotic fluid index (AFI) of 4 with the largest pocket being 1.5 cm, five discrete periods of fetal movement, as well as flexion and extension of the extremities. Based on this information what would your clinical evaluation and management be?

(A) Her BPP is 8, recommend to repeat BPP in 1 week
(B) Her BPP is 4, you should plan for delivery today
(C) Her BPP is 6, recommend delivery due to gestational age of 37
(D) Her BPP is 5, recommend delivery due to oligohydramnios
(E) Her BPP is 2, she needs to be sent by ambulance for stat Cesarean section

94 A 49-year-old woman comes into your office due to concerns of changes in her menses for the past year and a half. Although unpredictable, her cycles have been farther apart and lighter. She had no period for the last 7 months but bled for 3 days last month. Her last Pap smear was 9 months ago and was normal. She has no history of abnormal Pap smears or sexually transmitted infection. Her mother had breast cancer at the age of 65. The patient reports taking levothyroxine and hydrochlorothiazide. When should the patient receive an endometrial biopsy?

(A) In the office today
(B) After 12 months of irregular bleeding
(C) She should never have an endometrial biopsy
(D) If she bleeds after 12 months of amenorrhea

95 You are in labor and delivery when a 26-year-old multiparous woman arrives who appears to be in active labor. She has had no prenatal care and is 38 weeks by last period. Fetal heart tones (FHTs) are noted high in the abdomen and are 140s. Fundal height is 34 cm and you suspect breech presentation by Leopold maneuvers. Pelvic examination confirms footling breech presentation (see *Figure 9*). Which of the following counseling statements is most accurate?

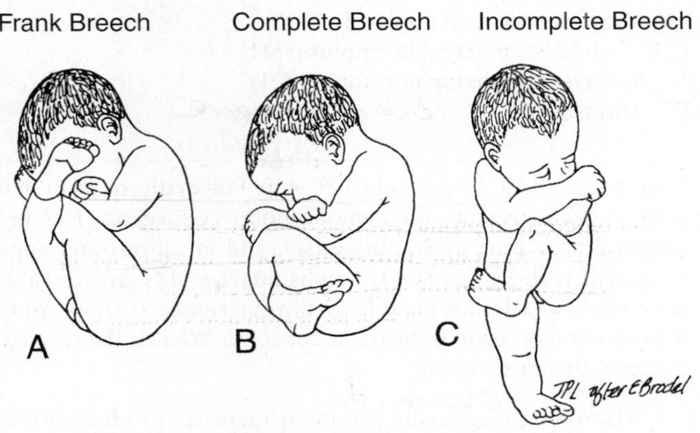

Figure 9

(A) A footling or incomplete breech should be delivered vaginally depending on the skill of the physician
(B) A complete breech is a contraindication to vaginal delivery
(C) A frank breech can be delivered vaginally depending on the skill of the physician
(D) No breech should ever be delivered vaginally

---

96 A 24-year-old female law student presents to the office with the inability to conceive after 12 months of unprotected intercourse. She had menarche at age 13 and has regular, monthly periods. She used condoms until she married at age 22 but did have chlamydia at age 17. Her husband has one child from a previous relationship. Medical history is positive only for migraines. Surgical history is positive for appendectomy at age 15. What is the most likely cause of her infertility?

(A) Male factor
(B) Premature ovarian failure
(C) Tubal factor
(D) Polycystic ovarian syndrome (PCOS)

---

97 A 42-year-old G2P2 presents with her new husband and is interested in trying to conceive. She is in good health, has no history of sexually transmitted infections, and does not smoke. Her husband has fathered a child in the past and she did not have any difficulty getting pregnant in the past. Her periods are regular, monthly, and last 5 to 6 days. Her pelvic examination is normal. What single test will assess her chances of getting pregnant?

(A) Progesterone level on day 21
(B) Thyroid-stimulating hormone (TSH)
(C) Follicle-stimulating hormone (FSH)
(D) Ultrasound

98 Your patient is a 28-year-old G0 with Polycystic ovarian syndrome (PCOS) who presents for preconception counseling. Her history is significant for long cycles, hirsutism, and an ultrasound appearance consistent with PCOS. She is a nonsmoker and is already taking prenatal vitamins. Her husband has a normal semen analysis. You discuss the use of medication to help her conceive. What is the mechanism of action of this medication?

(A) It is an antiestrogen which results in increased production of Follicle-stimulating hormone (FSH) and luteinizing hormone (LH)
(B) It decreases the conversion of androgens into estrogens which reduces the negative feedback loop on the hypothalamus which increases FSH
(C) It inhibits gluconeogenesis and therefore allows the ovary to respond to normal gonadotropin signals
(D) It interferes with the pulsatile release of FSH and LH from the anterior pituitary

99 A 29-year-old G1P0010 presents to your clinic desiring pregnancy. She had one ectopic pregnancy in the past treated with methotrexate. She has not been able to become pregnant despite 2 years of unprotected intercourse. Her husband has a normal semen analysis. She is otherwise healthy and has normal menstrual cycles. What is the next step in her workup?

(A) Intrauterine insemination
(B) Diagnostic laparoscopy
(C) Hysterosalpingogram
(D) In vitro fertilization

100 A 28-year-old G0 and her husband present to your office for preconception counseling. She has not attempted pregnancy to date because based on her family history, she is concerned about her future pregnancies and wants to know about preimplantation genetic diagnosis. From her statement you ask her about her other medical and family history. Which of the following diagnoses is she likely to have?

(A) Seizure disorder
(B) Tay-Sachs disease
(C) Poorly controlled diabetes
(D) Family history of neural tube defect

Answer Key

1)	E
2)	D
3)	E
4)	B
5)	D
6)	B
7)	A
8)	D
9)	D
10)	B
11)	D
12)	B
13)	B
14)	C
15)	C
16)	D
17)	D
18)	A
19)	B
20)	C
21)	B
22)	B
23)	D
24)	D
25)	E
26)	A
27)	C
28)	B
29)	D
30)	C
31)	B
32)	C
33)	B
34)	A
35)	A
36)	B
37)	A
38)	C
39)	C
40)	D
41)	B
42)	C
43)	B

44) D
45) E
46) A
47) B
48) A
49) D
50) D
51) B
52) D
53) E
54) D
55) A
56) B
57) C
58) C
59) D
60) C
61) A
62) D
63) D
64) E
65) B
66) D
67) E
68) E
69) B
70) C
71) B
72) A
73) B
74) C
75) B
76) D
77) B
78) C
79) B
80) B
81) B
82) B
83) D
84) B
85) C
86) D
87) E

88) A
89) C
90) B
91) C
92) A
93) C
94) E
95) C
96) C
97) C
98) A
99) C
100) B

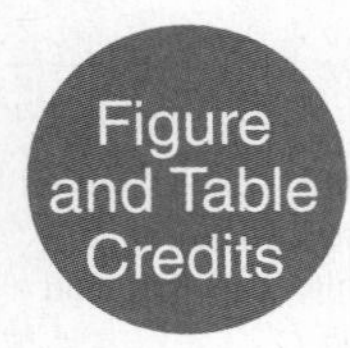

Figure and Table Credits

Figure 3-1 From Topol EJ, Califf RM, Prystowsky EN, et al. *Textbook of Cardiovascular Medicine*. 3rd ed. Philadelphia, PA: Lippincott Williams & Wilkins; 2006.

Figure 3-2 From LifeART image copyright © 2013 Lippincott Williams & Wilkins. All rights reserved.

Figure 3-3 From Sadler T, PhD. *Langman's Medical Embryology, Ninth Edition Image Bank*. Baltimore, MD: Lippincott Williams & Wilkins; 2003.

Figure 3-4 Courtesy of Dr. Kathleen Rao, Department of Pediatrics, University of North Carolina.

Figure 3-5 LifeART image copyright © 2013 Lippincott Williams & Wilkins. All rights reserved.

Figure 4-1 From Pillitteri A. *Maternal and Child Health Nursing: Care of the Childbearing and Childrearing Family*. 6th ed. Philadelphia, PA: Lippincott Williams & Wilkins; 2009.

Figure 4-2 From Beckmann CRB, Ling FW, Laube DW, et al. *Obstetrics and Gynecology*. 4th ed. Baltimore, MD: Lippincott Williams & Wilkins; 2002.

Figure 4-3 LifeART image copyright © 2013 Lippincott Williams & Wilkins. All rights reserved.

Table 5-1 From Anbazhagan A. Obstetric ultrasound and biophysical scoring, Obs Gynae & Midwifery News. Harrogate, North Yorkshire: Barker Brooks Communications Ltd.; 2012.

Table 5-2 From Anbazhagan A. Obstetric ultrasound and biophysical scoring, Obs Gynae & Midwifery News. Harrogate, North Yorkshire: Barker Brooks Communications Ltd.; 2012.

Figure 5-7 Beckmann CRB, Ling FW, Smith RP, et al. *Obstetrics and Gynecology*. 5th ed. Philadelphia, PA: Lippincott Williams & Wilkins; 2006.

Figure 6-1 Courtesy of Ellen Deutsch, MD.

Figure 6-2 From Scott JR, Gibbs RS, Karlan BY, et al. *Danforth's Obstetrics and Gynecology*. 9th ed. Philadelphia, PA: Lippincott Williams & Wilkins; 2003.

Figure 6-3 From Scott JR, Gibbs RS, Karlan BY, et al. *Danforth's Obstetrics and Gynecology*. 9th ed. Philadelphia, PA: Lippincott Williams & Wilkins; 2003.

Figure 6-4 From Eisenberg RL. *An Atlas of Differential Diagnosis*. 4th ed. Philadelphia, PA: Lippincott Williams & Wilkins; 2003.

Figure 9-1 Data from Munro MG, Critchley HO, Broder MS, et al. FIGO classification system (PALM-COEIN) for causes of abnormal uterine bleeding in nongravid women of reproductive age. FIGO Working Group on Menstrual Disorders. *Int J Gynaecol Obstet.* 2011;113:3-13.

Figure 9-2 From Mills SE. *Histology for Pathologists*. 3rd ed. Philadelphia, PA: Lippincott Williams & Wilkins; 2007.

Figure 9-3 Baggish MS, Valle RF, Guedj H. *Hysteroscopy: Visual Perspectives of Uterine Anatomy, Physiology and Pathology*. Philadelphia, PA: Lippincott Williams & Wilkins; 2007.

Figure 9-4 From Zuber TJ, Mayeaux EF. *Atlas of Primary Care Procedures.*

Philadelphia, PA: Lippincott Williams & Wilkins; 2003.

Figure 9-5 From Zuber TJ, Mayeaux EF. *Atlas of Primary Care Procedures*. Philadelphia, PA: Lippincott Williams & Wilkins; 2003.

Figure 9-6 From Zuber TJ, Mayeaux EF. *Atlas of Primary Care Procedures*. Philadelphia, PA: Lippincott Williams & Wilkins; 2003.

Figure 9-7 From Baggish MS, Valle RF, Guedj H. *Hysteroscopy: Visual Perspectives of Uterine Anatomy, Physiology and Pathology*. Philadelphia, PA: Lippincott Williams & Wilkins; 2007.

Figure 10-1 From Baggish MS, Valle RF, Guedj H. *Hysteroscopy: Visual Perspectives of Uterine Anatomy, Physiology and Pathology*. Philadelphia, PA: Lippincott Williams & Wilkins; 2007.

Figure 10-2 Courtesy of Keith H. Charlton, Robert D. Maxwell (Chiro), Brisbane, Australia.

Figure 10-3 From Pillitteri A. *Maternal and Child Nursing*. 4th ed. Philadelphia, PA: Lippincott, Williams & Wilkins; 2003.

Figure 12-1 From Sweet RL, Gibbs RS. *Atlas of Infectious Diseases of the Female Genital Tract*. Philadelphia, PA: Lippincott Williams & Wilkins; 2005.

Figure 12-2 From Beckmann CRB, Ling FW, Smith RP, et al. *Obstetrics and Gynecology*. 5th ed. Philadelphia, PA: Lippincott Williams & Wilkins; 2006.

Figure 12-3 From Sweet RL, Gibbs RS. *Atlas of Infectious Diseases of the Female Genital Tract*. Philadelphia, PA: Lippincott Williams & Wilkins; 2005.

Figure 12-4 From Willis MC. *Medical Terminology: A Programmed Learning Approach to the Language of Health Care*. Baltimore, MD: Lippincott Williams & Wilkins; 2002.

Figure 12-5 From Sweet RL, Gibbs RS. *Atlas of Infectious Diseases of the Female Genital Tract*. Philadelphia, PA: Lippincott Williams & Wilkins; 2005

Figure 12-6 From Rubin E, Farber JL. *Pathology*. 3rd ed. Philadelphia, PA: Lippincott Williams & Wilkins; 1999.

Figure 12-7 From Sweet RL, Gibbs RS. *Atlas of Infectious Diseases of the Female Genital Tract*. Philadelphia, PA: Lippincott Williams & Wilkins; 2005.

Figure 12-8 From Sweet RL, Gibbs RS. *Atlas of Infectious Diseases of the Female Genital Tract*. Philadelphia, PA: Lippincott Williams & Wilkins; 2005.

Figure 12-9 From Sweet RL, Gibbs RS. *Atlas of Infectious Diseases of the Female Genital Tract*. Philadelphia, PA: Lippincott Williams & Wilkins; 2005.

Figure 12-10 From Sweet RL, Gibbs RS. *Atlas of Infectious Diseases of the Female Genital Tract*. Philadelphia, PA: Lippincott Williams & Wilkins; 2005.

Figure 12-11 From McConnell TH. *The Nature of Disease Pathology for the Health Professions*. Philadelphia, PA: Lippincott Williams & Wilkins; 2007.

Figure 13-1 From Beckmann CRB, Ling FW, Smith RP, et al. *Obstetrics and Gynecology*. 5th ed. Philadelphia, PA: Lippincott Williams & Wilkins; 2006.

Figure 13-2 Modified from Berek JS, Hacker NF. *Practical Gynecologic Oncology*. 4th ed. Philadelphia, PA: Lippincott Williams & Wilkins; 2005.

Figure 1 From Sweet RL, Gibbs RS. *Atlas of Infectious Diseases of the Female Genital Tract*. Philadelphia, PA: Lippincott Williams & Wilkins; 2005.

Figure 2 From Beckmann CRB, Ling FW, Smith RP, et al. *Obstetrics and Gynecology*. 5th ed. Philadelphia, PA: Lippincott Williams & Wilkins; 2006

Figure 3 From Willis MC. *Medical Terminology: A Programmed Learning Approach to the Language of Health Care*. Baltimore, MD: Lippincott Williams & Wilkins; 2002.

Figure 4 From Sweet RL, Gibbs RS. *Atlas of Infectious Diseases of the Female Genital Tract*. Philadelphia, PA: Lippincott Williams & Wilkins; 2005.

Figure 5 From Sweet RL, Gibbs RS. *Atlas of Infectious Diseases of the Female Genital Tract*. Philadelphia, PA: Lippincott Williams & Wilkins; 2005.

Figure 6 From Beckmann CRB, Ling FW, Smith RP, et al. *Obstetrics and Gynecology*. 5th ed. Philadelphia, PA: Lippincott Williams & Wilkins; 2006.

Figure 7 From Eisenberg RL. *An Atlas of Differential Diagnosis*. 4th ed. Philadelphia, PA: Lippincott Williams & Wilkins; 2003.

Figure 9 From McConnell TH. *The Nature of Disease Pathology for the Health Professions*. Philadelphia, PA: Lippincott Williams & Wilkins; 2007.

Figure 10 From Beckmann CRB, Ling FW, Laube DW, et al. *Obstetrics and Gynecology*. 4th ed. Baltimore, MD: Lippincott Williams & Wilkins; 2002.

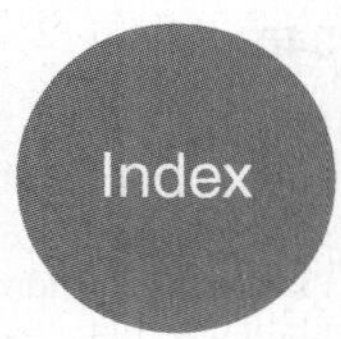

Index

Note: Page numbers followed by *f* indicate figures; those followed by *t* indicate tables.

A

B

K

L

M

Q

R

S

V

W

X

Y